NEUROANATOMY RESEARCH AT THE LEADING EDGE

FOCUSED NEUROANATOMY FOR MEDICAL STUDENTS

NEUROANATOMY RESEARCH AT THE LEADING EDGE

Additional books in this series can be found on Nova's website under the Series tab.

Additional e-books in this series can be found on Nova's website under the e-book tab.

NEUROANATOMY RESEARCH AT THE LEADING EDGE

FOCUSED NEUROANATOMY FOR MEDICAL STUDENTS

OR COHEN-INBAR, M.D., PHD

NOVA BIOMEDICAL

New York

Library of Congress Cataloging-in-Publication Data

ISBN: 978-1-63482-298-5
Library of Congress Control Number: 2015932938

Published by Nova Science Publishers, Inc. † New York

To my mother Malka Cohen-Inbar, who encouraged me to dream
To my wife Tal Cohen-Inbar, dreaming with me
and to my children, Ofek Bar-Sheli and Gaya Cohen-Inbar,
for changing what dreaming is all about.

To all the Neuroanatomy teachers, especially the great ones.

Contents

Preface

The "Focused Neuroanatomy for Medical Students" textbook fulfills a unique role by combining the necessity of rote learning the names of the different neuroanatomical structures, with their connections, and their physiological and neurological function. The problems that students face in learning about the nervous system is that it has so many parts, each one separately named and each one has its own intricate connections web. Moreover, each of these parts is housed in a complex structure of considerable importance. To learn by rote all those parts, their connections and structure in which they are contained is difficult and once learned, easily forgotten. This very innovative and well written textbook answers this problem by placing the brain within the context of its embryology, its chemistry and physiology. As the title implies each neuroanatomical region receives a separate focus that includes gross and microscopic anatomy, function and clinical correlations. The spinal cord, peripheral nervous system, brainstem and cranial nerves are considered separately.

The idea of a focused view was conceived by the author, Dr. Or Cohen-Inbar MD, PhD thruough his teaching of neuroanatomy, his own basic science work and in his clinical work as an active neurosurgeon, "Focused Neuroanatomy for Medical Students" is an exceptionally successful attempt to solve a perpetual pedagogic problem.

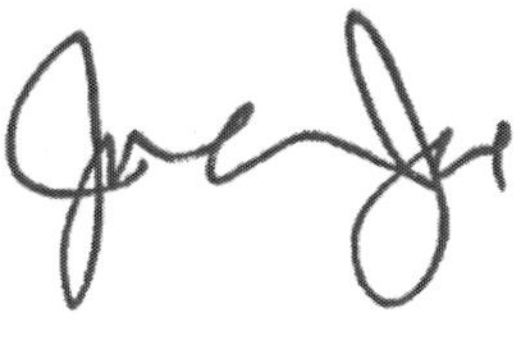

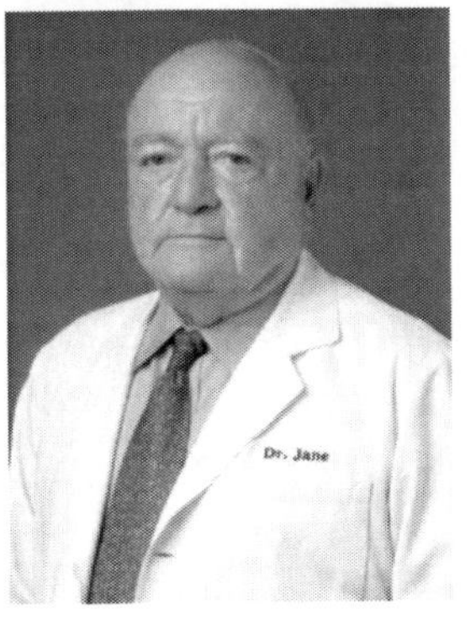

John A. Jane, Sr., MD, PhD, FRCS(C)
Professor of Neurosurgery
Editor Emeritus, Journal of Neurosurgery Publishing Group

Author Degree and Affiliations

Or Cohen-Inbar, MD, PhD

Attending Neurosurgeon at the department of Neurosurgery,
Rambam Health Care Campus, Haifa Israel

Clinical Instructor of Surgical Neuro-Oncology and Radiosurgery,
University of Virginia Health Care System and Gamma Knife Center.

A Lecturer at the Ruth and Bruce Rappaport Faculty of Medicine,
Technion Israel institute of Technology.

Laboratory of Molecular Immunology & Antibody Engineering
Technion Israel institute of Technology.

Correspondence: orcoheni@tx.technion.ac.il; oc2f@virginia.edu.

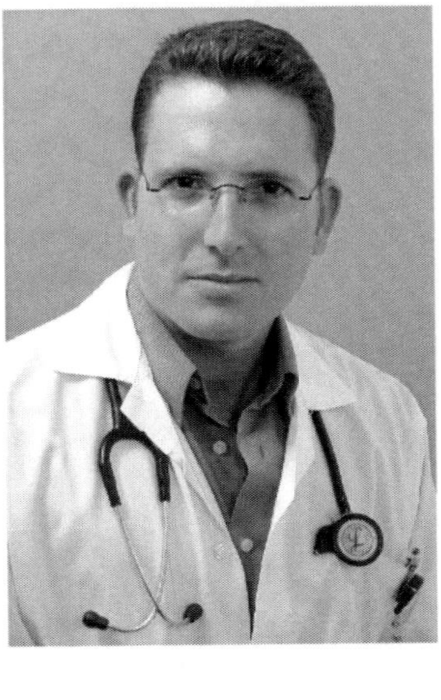

Book Description

The grasp of neuroanatomy, maybe more than in other organ systems, is closely related to function, neurophysiology and neuro-biochemistry. Its understanding requires a working knowledge of the pivotal neuro-embryological events as well as a working knowledge of general anatomy. For these reasons, it remains one of the greatest challenges encountered during medical studies, both for the aspiring student and for the dedicated mentor. The span of books used as references in teaching neuroanatomy is either too detailed or too simplistic in their attempt to balance the time constraints against the key points for each subject. In addition, since the neurosciences are at the forefront of research, many of the textbooks are written by researchers rather than clinicians, and as a result they tend to suffer a lack of clinical focus. This book, written by a tutor of neuroanatomy and a practicing neurosurgeon, attempts to offer a better balance and a more useful formula. This book is composed for the medical student, relying on comments from past medical students.

The book begins with an introduction chapter which discusses the organization of the nervous system, anatomical planes, introduction to neuro-embryology, as well as relevant scalp and skull anatomy. The next succeeding six chapters discuss the central nervous system regionally. Each chapter begins with the key embryological processes that shape the anatomy and function of that region. The gross anatomical description is followed by a short discussion of microscopic anatomy, gray and white matter anatomical features, major connections and key clinical correlations. First, The spinal cord and the organization of the somatomotor and somatosensory systems are presented, accompanied with a short overview of the peripheral nervous system. The brainstem is examined next with a special subchapter presenting a synopsis of cranial nerves. The diencephalon and the third ventricle are then presented together, followed by a focused review of the basal ganglia and the cerebellum, each presented in separate chapters. A discussion about the cerebrum and the cerebral cortex follows, including a short review of the laminar and columnar cortical organization concepts, the limbic system and higher order cerebral functions, including a discussion about memory and memory disorders, as well as dominant hemisphere clinical syndromes.

The next three chapters tackle specific problematic topics separately. The meninges, the cerebrospinal fluid and the lateral ventricles are discussed first, followed by an overview of the cerebral blood supply. A unique chapter focusing on specific skull base complex structures, such as the cavernous sinus region, the sphenoid sinus, and the jugular foramen is subsequently presented. The book ends with two chapters presenting the special sensory senses, vision and audition. These chapters are organized in a system rather than in regional anatomy forms, with an in-depth discussion of related anatomical features.

Acknowledgment

I thank Prof. Rhoton (the Rhoton collection), Dr. Maxim Shapiro (www.neuroangio.org), Dr. Francesco Gaillard (www.radiopaedia.org), and Dr. Rubin Smithuis (www.radiology assistant.nl) for their support and valuable contributions to this book. We encourage curious readers to visit these authors' masterpieces and websites. We thank Prof. John A. Jane Sr. M.D., Ph.D., FRCS for his guidance and mentoring as well as his time honored contribution to the field of modern neurosurgery. He is truly one of this profession's founding fathers, leaving a legacy in the form of today's neurosurgical leaders trained by him.

Chapter 1

Introduction to Neuroanatomy and the Skull

1.1. Abstract

This is the opening chapter of the book, designed to ease the introduction of Neuroanatomy and related knowledge sets to the aspiring medical student. First we discuss the concept of reflex arcs (in both the motor and sensory systems as well as in higher brain functions) and the organization of the central and peripheral nervous systems. Taxonomy of the nervous system is presented shortly. Next, a short description of the concept of anatomical and neuroanatomical planes is presented. An introduction to neuro-embryology follows, with presentation of the initial steps in the development of the nervous system. This part presents only the general initial steps in neuro-embryology, since each of the following chapters dealing with different segments of the CNS presents the specific developmental key points for that segment. Next, a short description of the focused anatomy of the scalp and skull is detailed. Skull development, skull base fossae and the cranial foramina are presented. These details will prove crucial for the understanding of future chapters.

1.2. Reflex Arcs and the Organization of the Nervous System

The role of the nervous system can be grouped into three main functions:

1) Sensing - The ability to recognize stimuli of various significance.
These can be Internal or external to the body and hence sensed by “sensors” (receptor) located at different locations. The world and reality as we know it, is only that part of reality for which we have receptors, and within these receptor’s range. Thus, the appearance of the world is very different for organism with a different spectrum visual auditory or a proprioceptive system spectrum.

2) Integration - This is the actual “Neural processing”. This phase may be a simple unisynaptic connection (as is the case of the spinal unisynaptic patellar reflex) or a multisynaptic conditioning type of a reflex arch (emotions, learning etc).
3) Response - The output of the nervous system, which manifests as a muscle Contraction, glandular secretion etc.

As insulting as it may seem, most of human actions and behavior patterns can be described in terms of reflex arcs. A reflex arc is the term given to the anatomical points of decision along the path of a certain action. A reflex arc can be simple or complex and may be independent or conditioned. The five key components of the reflex arc include:

1) Receptor type - describing the sensing part of the arc and the threshold needed to evoke an action potential form of information transmission.
2) Afferent pathway - the anatomical nerve conducting the information into the central nervous system.
3) The integrating center - this may be the spinal cord solely, brainstem solely or multiple interconnected centers all through the central nervous system.
4) Efferent pathway - the anatomical nerve conducting the output information from the central nervous system.
5) The effector organ / tissue - Manifesting the output response of the nervous system.

1.3. Organization of the Nervous System

Before diving into the detailed description of the different parts and components of the central nervous system, a short overview of organizational hierarchy is in place.

Both the central and the peripheral nervous systems have sensory and motor functions. The central nervous system (CNS, detailed in figures 1.1, 1.2) is a single organ tissue, separated artificially for our ease of grasping into its evolutionally based segments. The most ancient part, the spinal cord, is located within the spinal canal formed by the vertebral laminae. The brainstem, immediately continuous with the spinal cord, occupies the anterior (ventral) aspects of the posterior fossa (explained later), and to which the cerebellum is directly connected. The brainstem is subdivided to three evolutionary progressive segments, starting from the medulla oblongata (directly continuous with the spinal cord), the pons (the word means “bridge”, for its role in bridging and connecting to the cerebellum) and the midbrain. The diencephalic structures (ventral thalamus and related structures) are directly continuous with the midbrain (the upper segment of the brainstem). The dual cerebral hemispheres are connected to the diencephalon. For a detailed description of each segment refer to the relevant chapters. Refer to table 1.1 for an overview of the nervous system organization. We will discuss the peripheral nervous system (PNS) only briefly, not being a part of the scope of this book. A fluid filled cavities system (i.e., the ventricles), span the center of the different segments of the CNS. The two lateral ventricles (formerly called first and second ventricles) are located in the depth of the cerebral hemispheres. Both lateral ventricles drain into the third ventricle, the diencephalic cavity. This in turn drains into the fourth ventricle, the brainstem and cerebellar cavity, through a narrow passage within the midbrain, termed as the aqueduct (of Sylvius). The central canal is the narrow continuation of this cavities system, located within the spinal cord. For a detailed description of the ventricular system, refer to the relevant chapter.

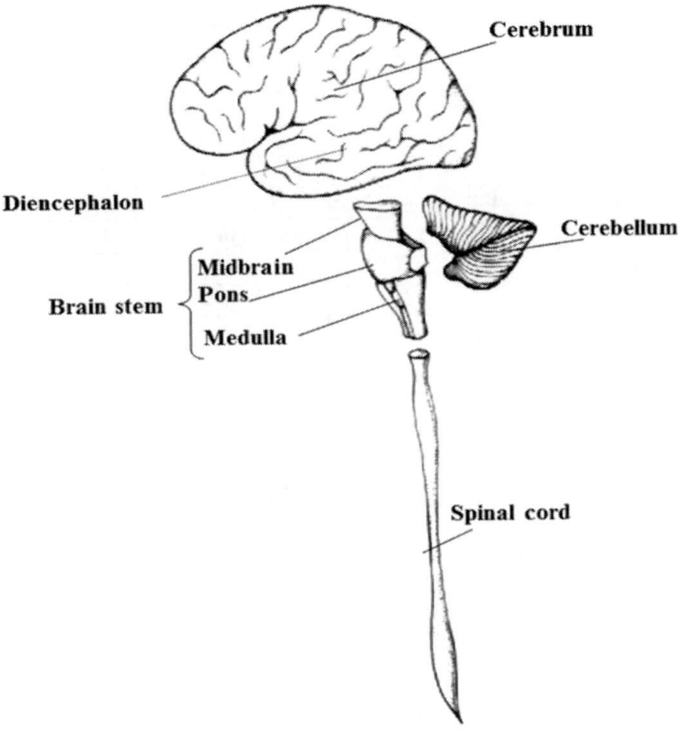

Figure 1.1. Organization of the CNS (Central Nervous System).

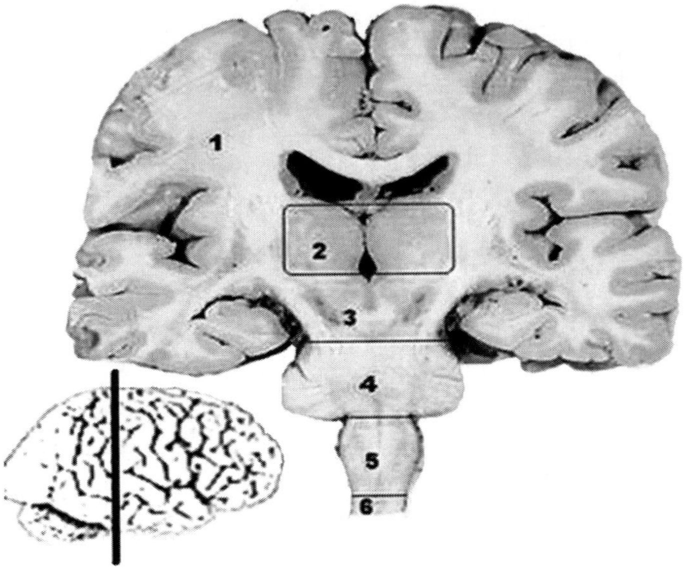

Figure 1.2. Brain dissection. The divisions of the brain are seen in a coronal slice of the brain. 1. Cerebrum 2. Thalamus 3. Midbrain 4. Pons 5. Medulla oblongata 6. Spinal cord. Taken with permission from www.Radiopaedia.org.

Table 1.1. The organization of the Nervous System

CNS*	Spinal cord			
	Brainstem	Medulla Oblongata		
		Pons		
		Midbrain		
	Cerebellum			
	Diencephalon	Thalamus		
		Hypothalamus	Hypothalamus	
			Pituitary gland (Hypophysis)	
		Ventral Thalamus (Subthalamic nucleus)		
		Epithalamus	Pineal gland	
			Habenular nuclei,	
			Stria Medullaris Thalami	
	Basal Ganglia	Corpus striatum	Neostriatum	Caudate nucleus
				Putamen
			Paleostriatum	Globus Pallidum
			Lentiform nucleus	Globus Pallidum and Putamen
		Ventral striatum (Nucleus Accumbens)		
		Substancia Innominate (Ventral Pallidum)		
	Cerebral cortex	Lobes	Frontal, Parietal, Occipital, Temporal, Insula	
		White matter tracts		
PNS+	SNS (Somatic Nervous System)	Sensory Component		
		Motor Component		
	ANS (Autonomic Nervous System)	Sensory Component		
		Motor component	Sympathetic (sometimes confusingly abbreviated as SNS)	
			Parasympathetic (sometimes confusingly abbreviated as PNS)	
	ENS (Enteric Nervous System)	Sensory Component		
		Motor component		

*Central Nervous System, +Peripheral Nervous System.

1.4. Anatomical Planes

In the description of different neuro-anatomical structures and their relative positions in space, a uniform language and terminology should be utilized. As shown in figure 1.3, the conventional 3-axis system is widely utilized. The coronal plane, divides the tissue into an anterior and posterior portions. The sagittal plane, divides the tissue into a left-sided and a Right-sided portions, whereas the horizontal plane (also termed as the axial plane) divides the tissue into a superior and inferior portions. In each of these planes, a section can be performed in the midline (creating a midsagittal section for example) or through any other point of reference (for example, a coronal view at the level of the anterior commissure etc).

Still, in the description of Neuroanatomical structures, the 3-axis system may prove at times insufficient. Thus, a second system, relying on the embryological development of the primary brain vesicles (discussed later as well as in chapter 7) is superimposed. With development, the prosencephalic cells (discussed later) proliferate faster than those of the other segments, and hence the prosencephalon bends anteriorly. The posterior surface of the initial prosencephalon is oriented in the developed brain at a superior-posterior position, now termed as the dorsal surface. The anterior portion of the initial prosencephalon is oriented in the developed brain at an anterior inferior position, now termed the ventral surface.

Dorsal thus refers to the back aspect of the neuroaxis, which in 3-dimentional space is actually positioned posterior-superior. The ventral surface refers to the front aspect of the neuroaxis, which in 3-dimentional space is actually positioned anterior-inferior. Refer to figure 1.4.

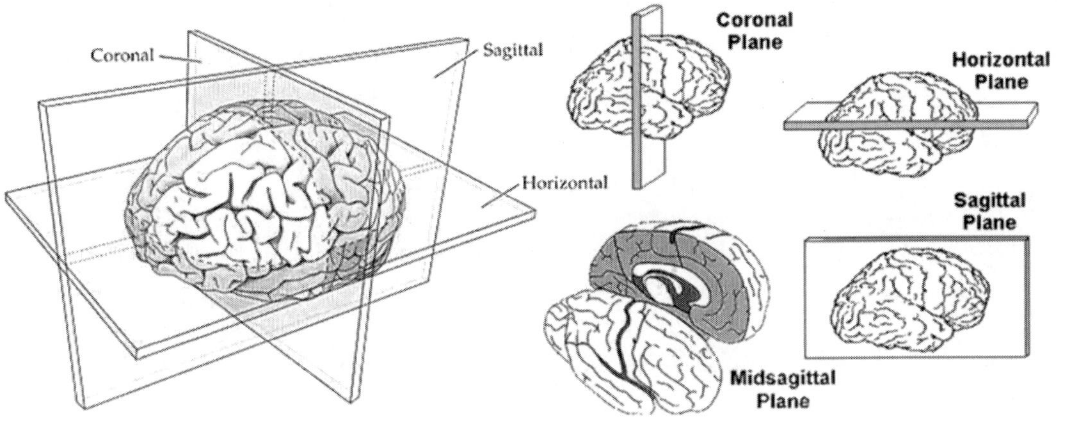

Figure 1.3. Anatomical Planes. The three Axis system.

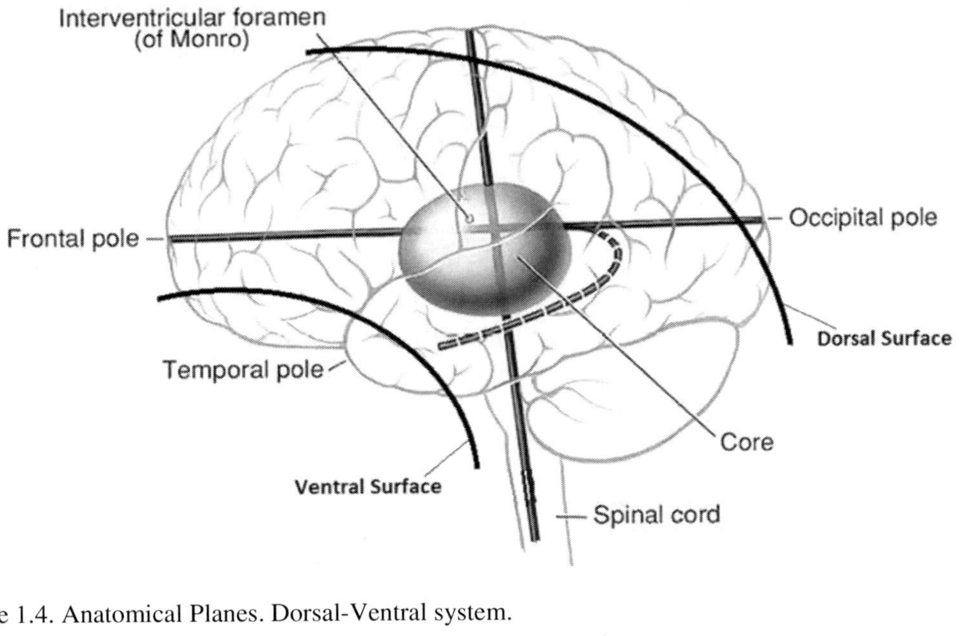

Figure 1.4. Anatomical Planes. Dorsal-Ventral system.

1.5. An Introduction to Neuro-Embryology

The CNS Appears at the beginning of the third week (Gastrulation) after fertilization, Gastrulation refers to the process in which the cranial-caudal and left-right axes are defined. Neurolation is the process where the overlying ectoderm thickens into the neural plate (slipper shaped plate of thickened ectoderm).

Edges of the neural plate form the neural fold. At the dorsal edge of each fold, a group of cells pinches off to form the neural crest. The neural folds later approach each other in the midline, fusing to form the neural tube. Fusion begins in the cervical region, than proceeds in cephalic and caudal directions, but it is delayed there, and the cranial and caudal neuropores form temporarily (connecting the neural tube lumen and the amniotic cavity). Final closure occurs at 18~20 somite stage (25th day and 27th day for caudal neuropore). Refer to figure 1.5 for a short illustration of the process.

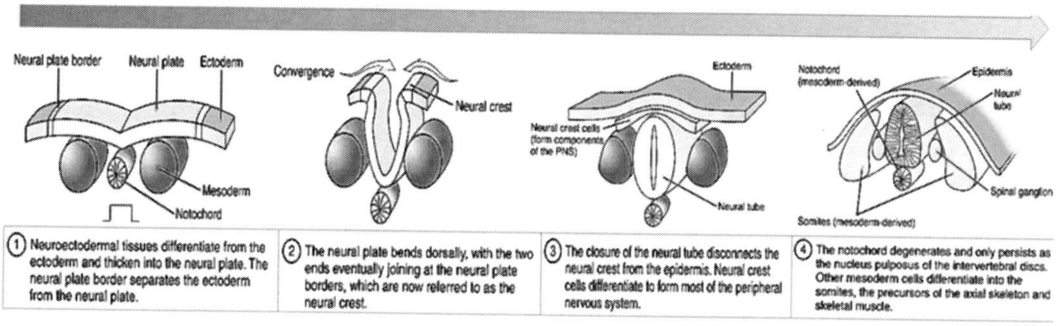

Figure 1.5. Neuro-embryology. The Process of Neurolation begins by the end of the third week after fertilization, progressing in successive steps.

The primary brain vesicles are three dilations in the cephalic end of the neural tube. The Prosencephalon (later becomes the forebrain), Mesencephalon (later becomes the midbrain) and the rhombencephalon (later becomes the hindbrain). Simultaneously, two flexures form, the cervical flexure (at hindbrain-spinal cord junction) and the cephalic flexure (in midbrain region). By the fifth week of fertilization, each of the primary vesicles further differentiates. Refer to figures 1.6-1.7 for an illustration of this process. Parallel to the development and proliferation of the walls of the brain vesicles, the lumen (i.e., the future ventricular lumen) shapes as well.

The telencephalic cavity will form the lateral ventricles, the diencephalic cavity will form the third ventricle, and the rhombencephalic cavity will form the fourth ventricle. The latter two are connected through the lumen of the mesencephalon, that with wall cell proliferation narrows substantially and is designated as the Aqueduct of Sylvius. The fourth ventricle is continuous with the central canal (i.e., the lumen of the spinal cord).

The cranial nerves (discussed in chapter 3) have their origin from the different segments of the primary brain vesicles, as summarized in table 1.2. The relevant focused embryological development of each segment of the CNS is discussed in the relevant chapters.

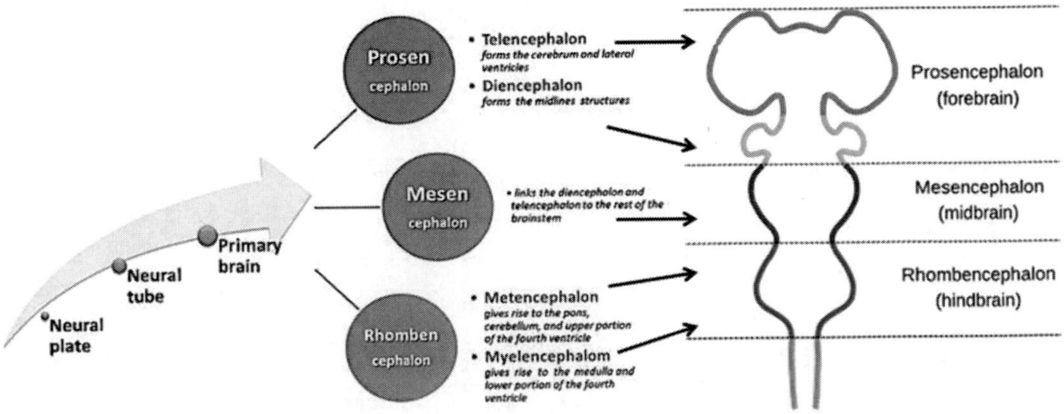

Figure 1.6. The development of the neural tube. Taken with permission from www.Radiopaedia.org.

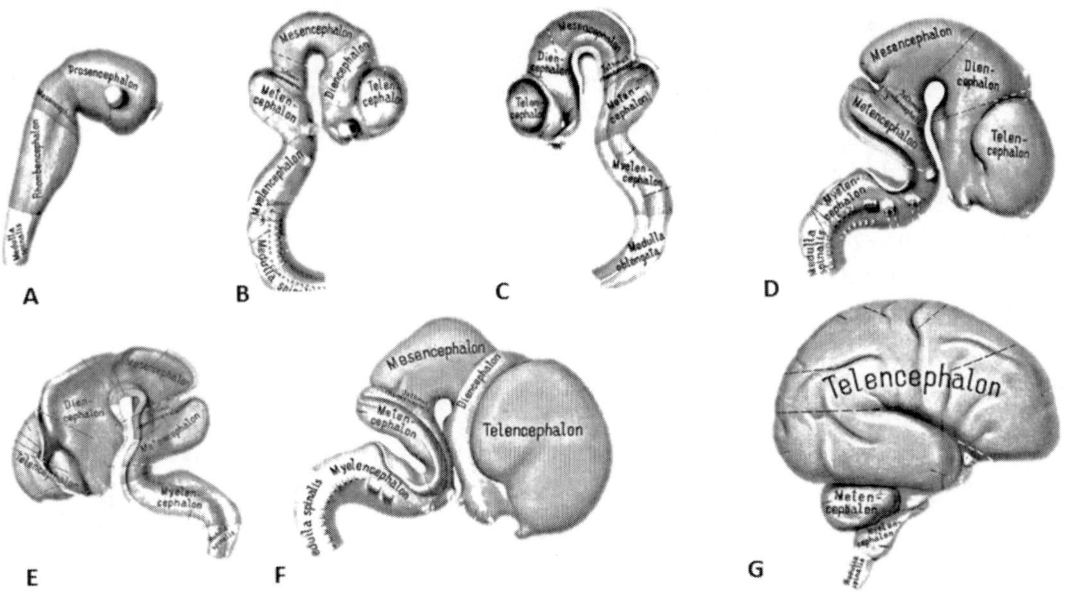

Figure 1.7. Stepwise illustration of the development of the neural tube. A-G, starting from 8-9 weeks age in 2 weeks differences between the figures. Taken from Gray's anatomy, now out of copyright and in the public domain.

Table 1.2. The Origin of the Cranial Nerves

Brain Vesicle	Cranial Nerve	Composition	Ganglia	Comments
Telencephalon	Olfactory	Sensory		
Diencephalon	Optic	Sensory		
Mesencephalon	Oculomotor	Motor and Parasympathetic	Ciliary	

Table 1.2. (Continued)

Brain Vesicle	Cranial Nerve	Composition	Ganglia	Comments
Metencephalon	Trochlear	Motor		final location is mesencephalone
	Trigeminal	Sensory and Motor	Trigeminal	sensory ganglia arise in Metencephalon & Myelencephalon
	Abducens	Motor		
	Facial	Sensory, Motor, Parasym.	Superior, Inferior, Sphenopalatine, Submandibular.	
	Vestibulocochlear	Sensory	Acoustic, vestibular	
Myelencephalon	Glossopharyngeal	Sensory, Motor, Parasym.	Superior, Inferior, Otic	
	Vagus	Sensory, Motor, Parasympathetic	Superior, Inferior, Parasympathetic.	
	Spinal Accessory	Motor		
	Hypoglossal	Motor		

1.6. Focused Anatomy of Scalp

The scalp is composed of five layers (See figure 1.8), with the outer three layers—skin, subcutaneous tissue and galea fixed together as a unit that glides easily over the pericranium (Figure 1.9). The scalp skin (epidermis and dermis) is the thickest skin in the body. Due to its apneurosis, dissecting the subcutaneous fat, compartmentalizing this space and related traveling blood vessels and nerves, manual compression with immediate suturing is a more effective means of controlling bleeding in the scalp than any other mean. Scalp vessels travel within the subcutaneous layer superficial to the galea. The galea is the aponeurotic layer connecting the frontalis muscle to the occipitalis muscle. The superficial temporal fascia is a thin, highly vascular layer that is contiguous with the galea and lies deep to the subcutaneous tissue of the lateral aspect of the scalp. The superficial temporal artery and vein are housed within the fascia, thus rendering this layer vital to the viability of temporoparietal skin flaps designed in surgery. In the temporal region, the galea becomes adherent to the underlying subgaleal fascia, but the subgaleal fascia can easily be detached from it or the layer covering the temporalis muscle. The deep temporal fascia is a thick white fascial layer on the external surface of the temporalis muscle.

The anterior aspect of the face is supplied by musculo-cutaneous perforators, whereas the scalp is supplied by fascio-cutaneous perforators. These perforators pierce the deep fascia at fixed skin margins (the supraorbital rim, tragus, mastoid process, masseter, parotid, and superior nuchal line). Within these areas of mobile skin, the vessels become superficial and connect to the subdermal plexus. Clinical studies have demonstrated that an adjacent vascular territory can be included when raising a flap on one to two perforators, but problems arise when attempts are made to include more than two successive angiosome territories (see figure 1.8).

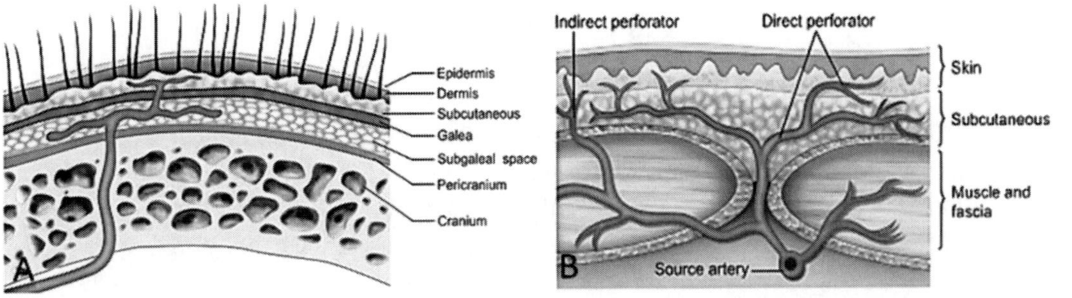

Figure 1.8. The Scalp. A, General anatomy B, Angiosome. A regional artery, termed a source artery, provides blood supply to the skin either directly through fascial and septocutaneous arteries or indirectly through musculocutaneous perforators.

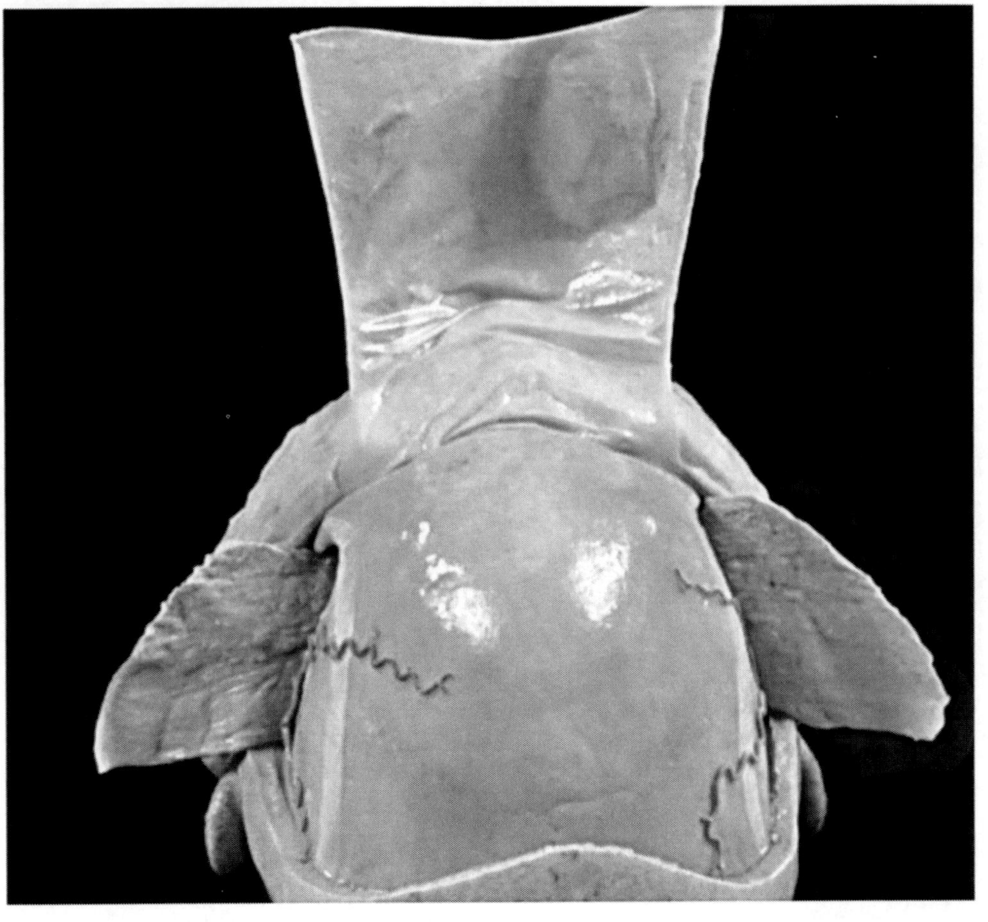

Figure 1.9. Dissection of the Pericranium. The pericranium is seen retracted superiorly. The two temporalis muscles are retracted laterally. Adapted with permission from the Rhoton Collection.

1.7. The Skull

The skull, a flat bone, is formed by the union of different bones formed via an intramembranous ossification process. Eight different bones form the cranial vault (Frontal, Parietal X2, Temporal X2, Occipital, Sphenoid, and Ethmoid). Fourteen bones form the face (Nasal, Maxilla X2, Zygomatic X2, Lacrimal X2, Palatine, X2, Inferior nasal conchea X2, Vomer, and Mandible). A suture is formed whenever two bone meet, forming a non-moving joint. A fontanelle is formed whenever more than two bones meet. Refer to figures 1.10-1.13 for the normal adult skull anatomy.

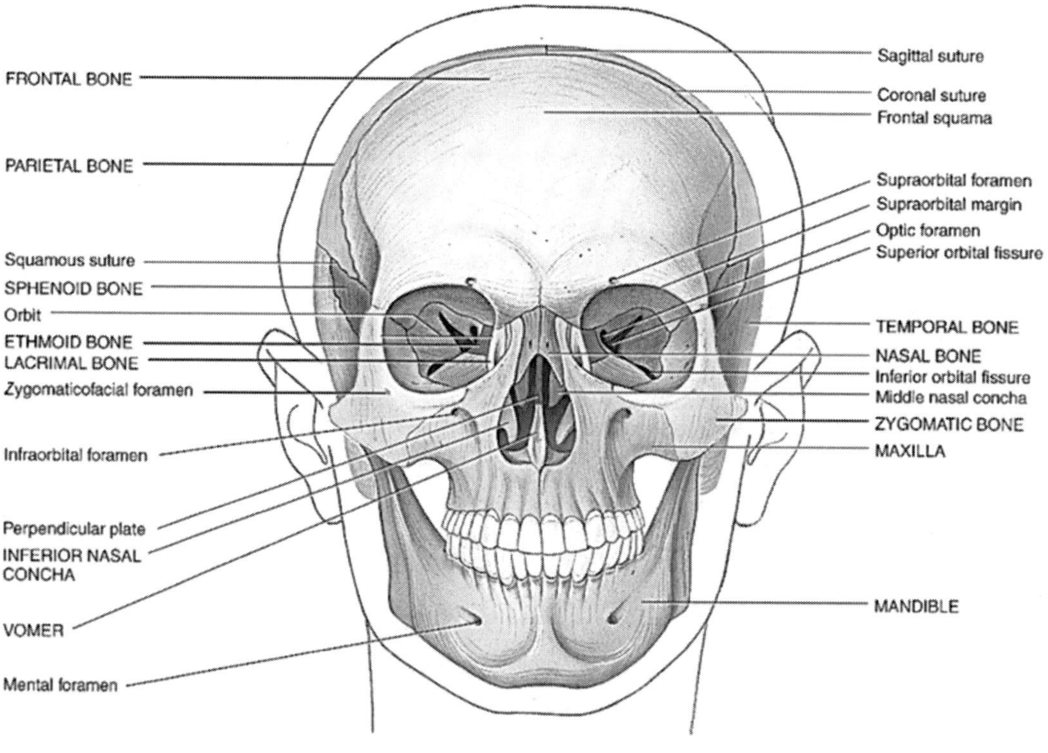

Figure 1.10. The Skull, Anterior view.

The anterior part of the cranial base is separated from the middle fossa by the sphenoid ridge and the chiasmatic sulcus. The middle cranial base is separated from the posterior cranial base by the dorsum sellae and the petrous ridges. The upper surface of the anterior cranial base is formed by the frontal bone, which roofs the orbit; the ethmoid bone, which is interposed between the frontal bones and is the site of the cribriform plate; and the lesser wing and anterior part of the body of the sphenoid, which forms the posterior part of the floor of the anterior fossa. The upper surface of the middle cranial base floor is formed by the greater sphenoid wing and posterior two-thirds of the sphenoid body anteriorly and the upper surface of the temporal bone posteriorly. The posterior part of the cranial base is formed by the temporal and occipital bones. The cribriform plate, sella, and clivus are located in the medial part of the cranial base. The lateral part of the cranial base is located above the orbits, pterygopalatine and infratemporal fossae, and the subtemporal and lateral part of the suboccipital areas (figure 1.12a).

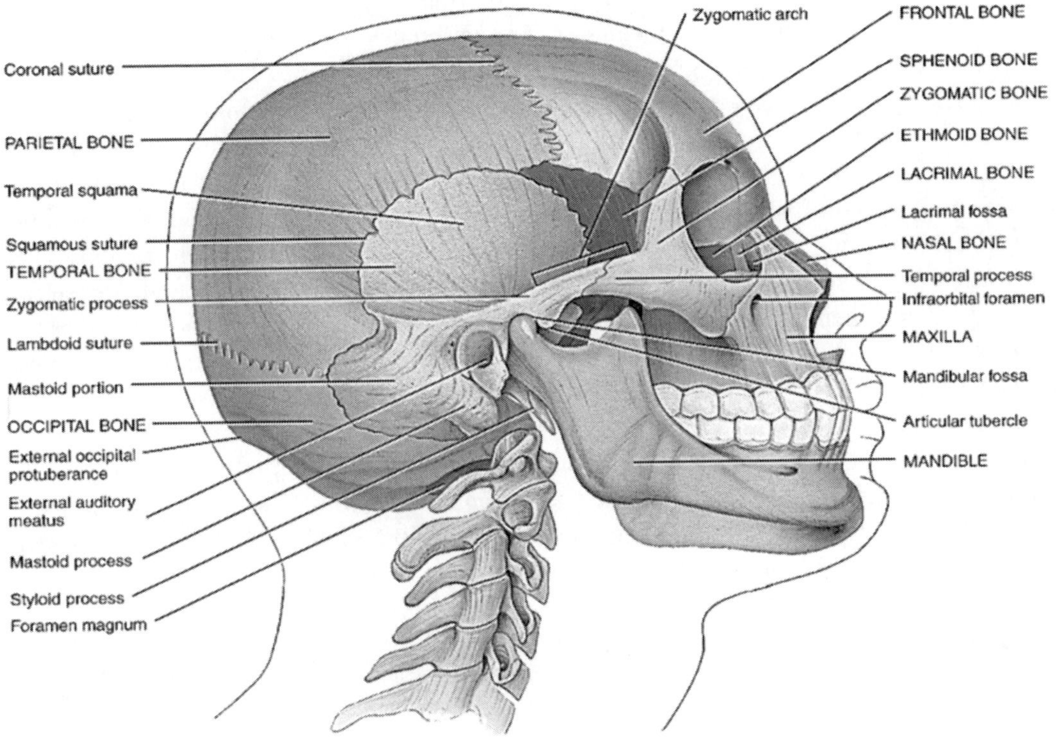

Figure 1.11. The Skull, Lateral view.

The exocranial surface of the cranial base, is formed by the maxilla, the zygomatic, palatine, sphenoid, temporal, and occipital bones, and the vomer. The maxilla, orbits, and nasal cavity are located below the anterior fossa. The mandibular fossa on the lower surface of the temporal squama is located below the posterior part of the middle fossa. The vomer attaches to the lower part of the body of the sphenoid and forms the posterior part of the nasal septum (figure 1.12b).

The orbital rim is formed by the frontal bone, zygoma, and maxilla. The roof of the orbit is formed by the frontal and sphenoid bones; the lateral wall by the greater sphenoid wing and the zygomatic bone; the floor by the maxilla, except for a small part of the posterior floor formed by the palatine bone; and the medial wall of the orbit by the maxilla and lacrimal and ethmoid bones. The nasal cavity is located between the ethmoid bones above and the maxillae, palatine bones, and sphenoid pterygoid process below. It is roofed by the frontal and ethmoid bones and the floor is formed by the maxillae and palatal bones. The osseous nasal septum is formed by the perpendicular ethmoid plate and the vomer. The inferior concha is a separate bone, and the middle and superior conchae are appendages of the ethmoid bone. The orbit opens through the superior orbital fissure into the middle fossa and through the inferior orbital fissure into the pterygopalatine and infratemporal fossae (figure 1.12c). The anterior part of the hard palate (figure 1.12d) is formed by the maxillae and the posterior part is formed by the horizontal plate of the palatine bone. The vomer forms the posterior part of the nasal septum and divides the posterior nasal aperture in the midline.

The walls of the orbit are formed by seven bones (figure 1.13a). They are the frontal, zygomatic, sphenoid, lacrimal, ethmoid, and palatine bones, and the maxilla. The lateral border of the orbital opening is formed by the frontal process of the zygoma, except the upper part, which is formed by the zygomatic process of the frontal bone. The lower margin of the orbital opening is formed laterally by the zygoma and medially by the maxilla. The upper part of the medial border is formed by the frontal bone and the lower part is formed by the frontal process of the maxilla. The medial part of the upper border contains the frontal sinus. The superior orbital fissure is bounded above by the lesser wing of the sphenoid bone, below by the greater wing, and medially by the sphenoid body. The frontal bone forms the narrow lateral apex of the superior orbital fissure. The inferior orbital fissure is bounded posteriorly by the greater sphenoid wing and anteriorly by the maxilla. The supraorbital margin is notched or is the site of one or several small foramina that transmit the supraorbital nerves and vessels. The inferior concha is a separate bone, which protrudes into the nasal cavity from the maxilla (figure 1.13b). The middle and superior concha are appendages of the ethmoid bone. The maxillary ostium is located between the perpendicular plate of the palatine bone behind, the ethmoid superiorly, and the medial maxillary wall below. The maxillary and frontal sinus and the anterior ethmoid air cells drain into the middle meatus, and the posterior ethmoid air cells drain into the superior meatus.

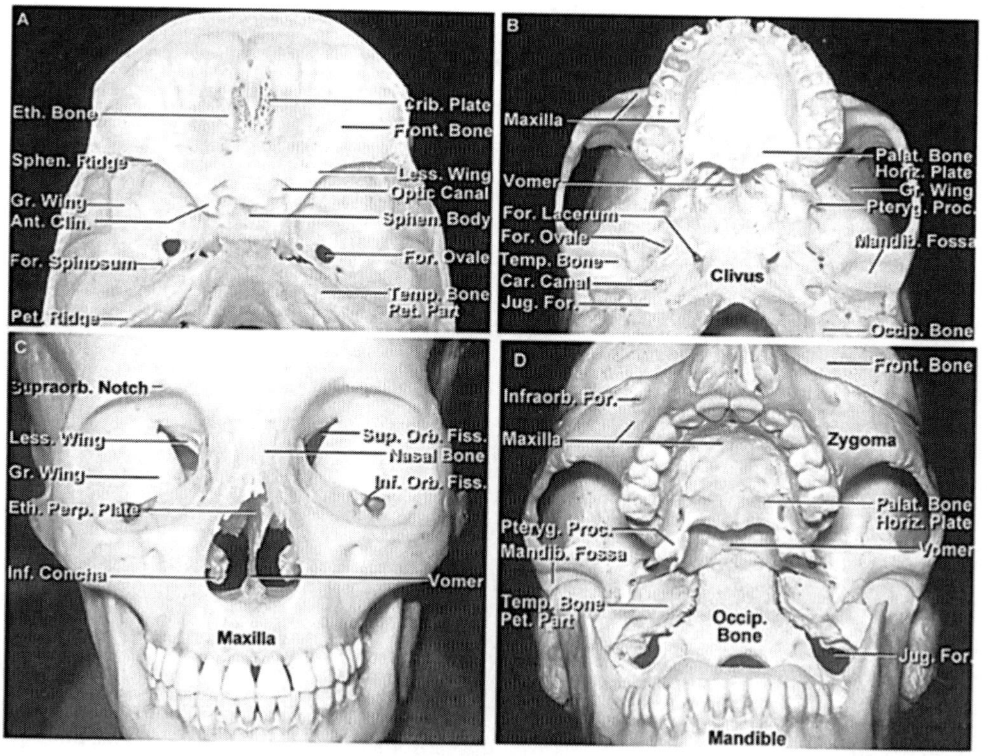

Figure 1.12. Osseous relationships of the anterior and middle cranial base. A, the skull fossae. B, exocranial surface of the cranial base. C, anterior view. D, an anteroinferior view of the cranial base. Adapted with permission from the Rhoton Collection.

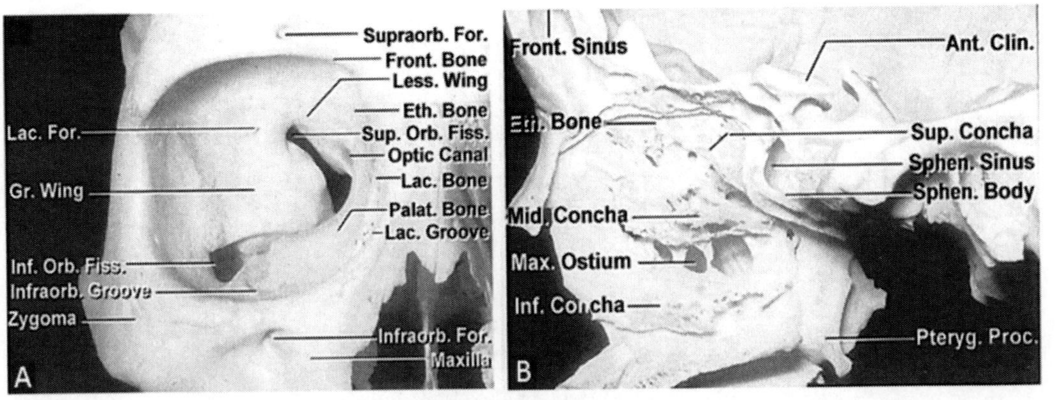

Figure 1.13. A. Anterior view of the right orbit. B, Sagittal view, the nasal septum has been removed. Adapted with permission from the Rhoton Collection.

1.7.1. Craniometric Points

1) Pterion - The junction of temporal, frontal, parietal, sphenoid bone. 2 fingers above the zygomatic arc, 1 finger posterior to frontal process of zygomatic bone.
2) Asterion – The junction of occipitomastoid, parietomastoid and lambdoid sutures. The junction of the sigmoid and transverse venous sinuses.
3) Vertex - The topmost point of the skull.
4) Lambda - The junction of lambdoid and sagittal sutures.
5) Bregma - The junction of coronal and sagittal sutures.
6) Stephanion - The junction of coronal suture and superior temporal line.
7) Opisthion - The posterior margins of foramen magnum in the midline.

1.7.2. Skull Development, Sutures and Fontanelles

The fontanelles serve a crucial role in the extra-uterine normal brain and skull development occurring in early childhood. Together with the sutures, they allow for some mobility and deformity during delivery and accommodate for cerebral development. These are membranous covering, serving also as important clinical clues (in infectious meningitis, intracerebral hemorrhage or other causes of increased intracranial pressure in a infant, a bulging anterior fontanelle serves as the first hint).

The anterior fontanelles is the most prominent one (at the junction of the coronal and sagittal sutures, forming in the adult the Bregma), usually closes (ossifies) by 20-22 months of age.

The posterior fontanelle (at the junction of the sagittal and the lambdoid sutures, forming in the adult the Lambda) normally ossifies by 9 months of age. Any delay or premature closure of the fontanelles requires an immediate neurosurgical consult. Refer to Figure 1.14 for an illustration of an infant's skull.

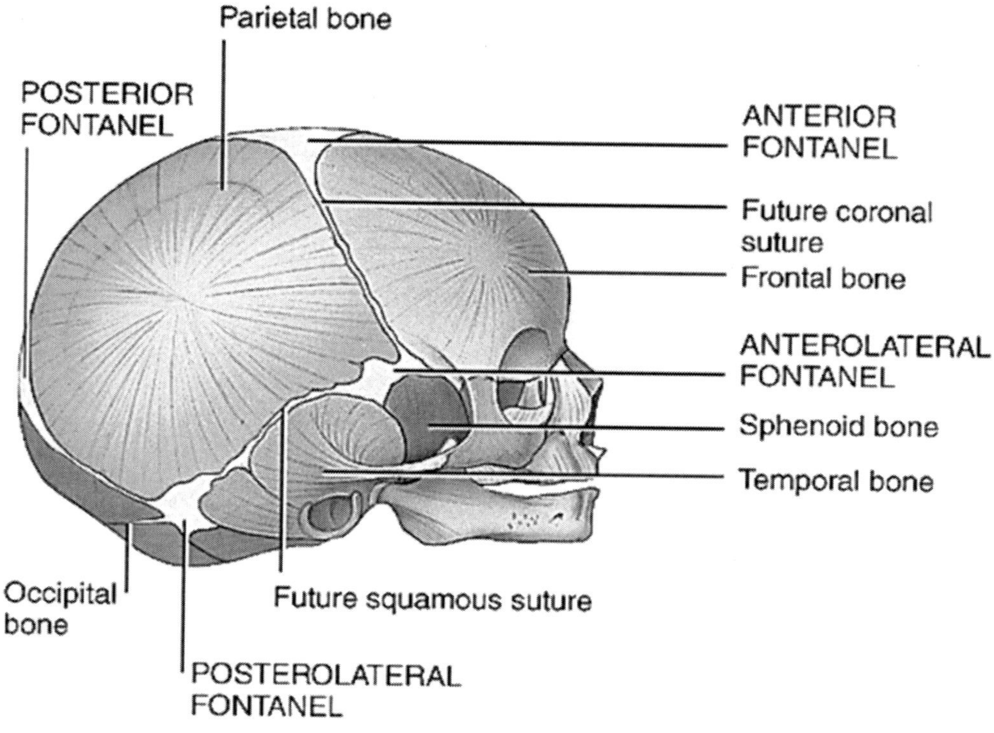

Figure 1.14. Infant's Skull showing sutures and fontanelles. These close (ossify) at different time points post-partum. The anterior fonatelle normally closes by 20-22 months of age.

1.7.3. Skull Base Fossae and the Cranial Foramina

The skull floor, with the vault and brain removed, reveal a compartmentalized type of surface, classically described as composed of three unique cranial fossae. Each fossa is discussed in details in the chapters to come, yet an introductory overview is appropriate.

Figures 1.15, 1.16 present an illustration and image of the skull floor, Table 1.3 summaries the important skull base foramina its related content.

The anterior cranial fossa, as viewed in Figure 1.15, is formed mostly by the frontal bone. The frontal bone forms the majority of the floor of the anterior fossa (the orbital roof), as well as the anterior and lateral walls. The posterior margin of the anterior fossa is formed by the lesser wings of the sphenoid bone, with their posteriorly projecting anterior clinoid processes. In the center of the anterior fossa floor, the cribriform plate, housing the passage of the olfactory fibers of the first cranial nerve, reaching the olfactory bulb and tract from the nasal cavity can be seen. In its center, the Crista galli, a sharp bridge can be seen. The nasal slits, on the lateral edges of the cribriform plate, house the anterior Ethmoidal nerve artery and veins.

The middle cranial fossa, by far the most elaborate of the cranial fossae is composed of the lesser wings of the sphenoid bone forming its anterior aspects, the greater wings of the sphenoid bone forming the majority of its floor and central portion and the temporal bone forming its lateral floor and wall, as well as its posterior border at the petrous (a bony ridge which houses among other structures the vestibular and cochlear organs). The crescent of four foramina, spanning the sides of its central mass is composed from posterior to anterior of foramen Spinosum, foramen Ovale, foramen Rotundum and the Superior orbital fissure. Refer to figure 1.16 for details. Other structures and passages in this fossa are the inferior orbital fissure opening to the Sphenopalatine fossa and foramen Lacerum. Refer to table 1.3 for details. The central bony mass of the middle cranial fossa, formed by the sphenoid sinus, has a Turkish saddle shape (hence termed as the Sella Turcica), whose floor is the sphenoid sinus, and houses the pituitary gland. A layer of dural covering roofs this sella (the diaphragma sellae), as well as carpeting it, resulting in the pituitary gland being both intradural and subdural. On both sides of the sella turcica, an elaborate neurovascular structure exists. This is the cavernous sinus (a venous blood containing sinus discussed in length later), housing the fourth segment of the internal carotid artery in its Medial wall and several cranial nerves in its medial and lateral walls. The details of these structures are referred to in the chapters to come.

The posterior cranial fossa is bordered anteriorly by the petrous portion of the temporal bone, and the occipital bone forming its inferior, posterior and central anterior walls (the clivus). The floor of the posterior fossa is housed by the foramen magnum, through which the spinal cord is continuous with the medulla oblongata portion of the brainstem. The foramen magnum allows also passage for the vertebral and related arteries as well as entry of the spinal accessory nerve (cranial nerve 11, not a true cranial nerve). The Occipito-petrous junction houses the jugular foramen, and the posterior petrous aspect houses the internal acoustic meatus (all discussed in table 1.3 and in great details in the brainstem and other chapters). On the outer inferior rim of foramen magnum, the occipital condyles are present, articulating with the first cervical vertebrae (the Atlas). The fissue between the condules and the rim of foramen magnum houses the entrance to the hypoglossal canal, through which the so named cranial nerve leaves the skull.

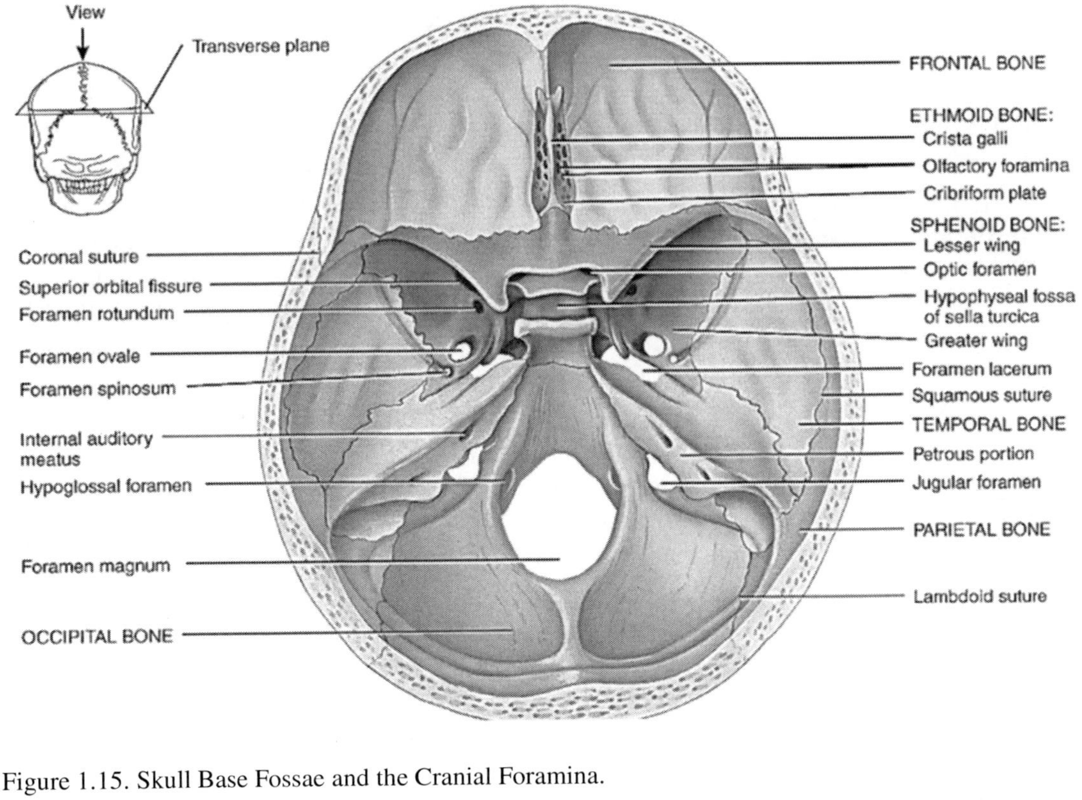

Figure 1.15. Skull Base Fossae and the Cranial Foramina.

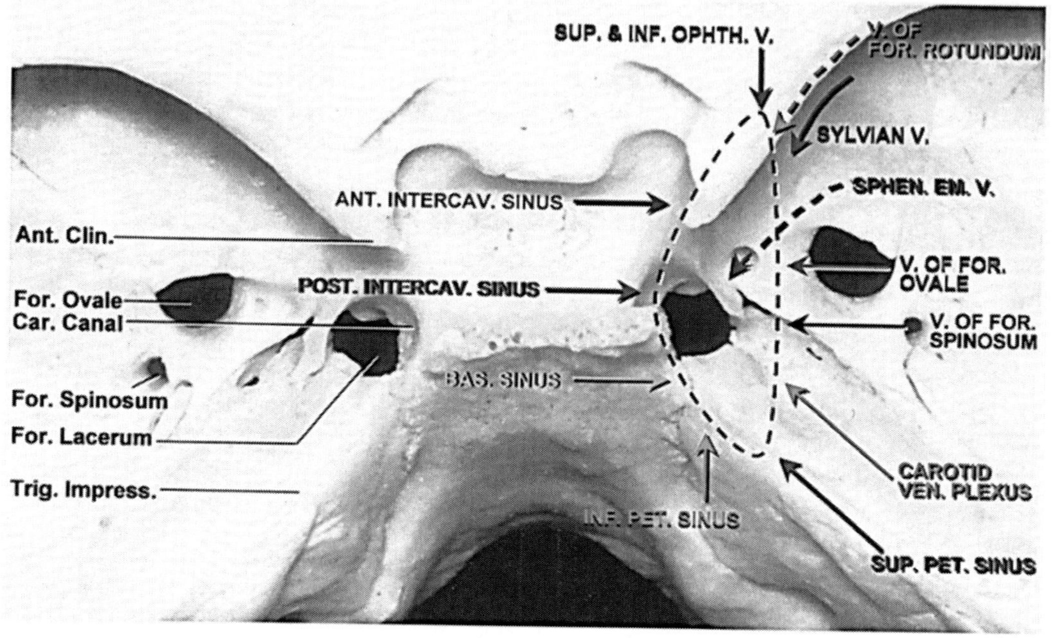

Figure 1.16. Superior view of the cranial base in the region of the cavernous sinus. The left side demonstrates the foraminal anatomy. The cavernous sinus anatomy and venous connections is presented on the right. Adapted with permission from the Rhoton Collection.

1.7.4. External Scalp and Bone Landmarks

Approximating the site of the sylvian fissure and central sulcus on the scalp begins by noting the position of the nasion, inion, and the fronto-zygomatic point. The nasion is located in the midline at the junction of the nasal and frontal bones. The inion is the site of a bony prominence that overlies the torcula herophili (the bony protrusion indication and intersection of the superior sagittal, occipital and the straight sinus, draining into the transverse sinus). The frontozygomatic point is located on the orbital rim 2.5 cm above the level where the upper edge of the zygomatic arch joins the orbital rim and just below the junction of the lateral and superior margins of the orbital rim. The next steps are to construct a line along the sagittal suture and, using a flexible measuring tape, to determine the distance along this line from the nasion to inion and mark the midpoint and three-quarter points (50% and 75% points).

The sylvian fissure is located along a line that extends backward from the frontozygomatic point across the lateral surface of the head to the three-quarter point. The pterion, the site on the temple approximating the lateral end of the sphenoid ridge, is located 3 cm behind the frontozygomatic point on the sylvian fissure line. The central sulcus is located by identifying the upper and lower rolandic points.

The upper rolandic point is located 2 cm behind the midpoint (50% plus 2 cm point) on the nasion-to-inion midsagittal line. The lower rolandic point is located where a line extending from the midpoint of the upper margin of the zygomatic arch to the upper rolandic point crosses the line defining the sylvian fissure. A line connecting the upper and lower rolandic points approximates the central sulcus. The lower rolandic point is located approximately 2.5 cm behind the pterion on the sylvian fissure line. Refer to figure 1.17 for an illustration of these markings.

Table 1.3. Cranial foramina

Anterior Fossa	Cribriform plate	Olfactory nerve	
	Incisive foramen	Nasopalatine nerve.	
	Greater palatine foramen	Greater palatine nerve, artery, vein.	
	Lesser palatine foramen	Lesser palatine nerve.	
	Nasal slits	Anterior Ethmoidal nerve, artery, vein.	
Middle Fossa	Superior Orbital Fissure	CN-III (Oculomotor), CN-IV (Trochlear), CN-VI (Abducens)	
		$CN-V_1$ (Ophthalmic)	All $CN-V_1$ branches (Nasociliary, frontal, lacrimal).
		Superior ophthalmic vein.	
		Recurrent meningeal artery.	
		Orbital branch of middle meningeal artery.	
	Inferior Orbital fissure	$CN-V_2$ (Maxillary).	
		Zygomatic nerve.	
		Infra-orbital artery and vein.	
	Foramen lacerum	Nothing, Internal carotid traverses its upper portion.	
	Carotid canal	Internal carotid artery (ICA).	
		Postganglionic Sympathetic nerve fibers on ICA wall.	
	Optic canal	CN-II (optic nerve).	
		Ophthalmic artery.	
	Foramen Rotundum	$CN-V_2$ (Maxillary).	
		Artery of foramen Rotundum.	
	Foramen Ovale	$CN-V_3$ (Mandibular).	
	Foramen Spinosum	Middle Meningeal artery and vein	
Posterior Fossa	Internal acoustic meatus	CN-VII (Facial nerve).	
		CN-VIII (Vestibulocochlear).	
	Hypoglossal canal	CN-XII (hypoglossal)	
		Meningeal branch of ascending pharyngeal artery	
	Foramen magnum	Medulla oblongata	
		CN-XI (spinal accessory)	
		Vertebral artery	
		Anterior and posterior spinal arteries (corona arteria).	
	Jugular foramen	CN-IX (Glossopharyngeal).	
		CN-X (Vagus).	
		CN-XI (Spinal Accessory).	
		Internal jugular vein (IJV).	
	Stylomastoid foramen	CN-VII (facial).	
		Stylomastoid artery.	
	Condyloid foramen	Veins from the transverse sinus.	
	Mastoid foramen	Veins to mastoid sinus.	
		Branch of the occipital artery	

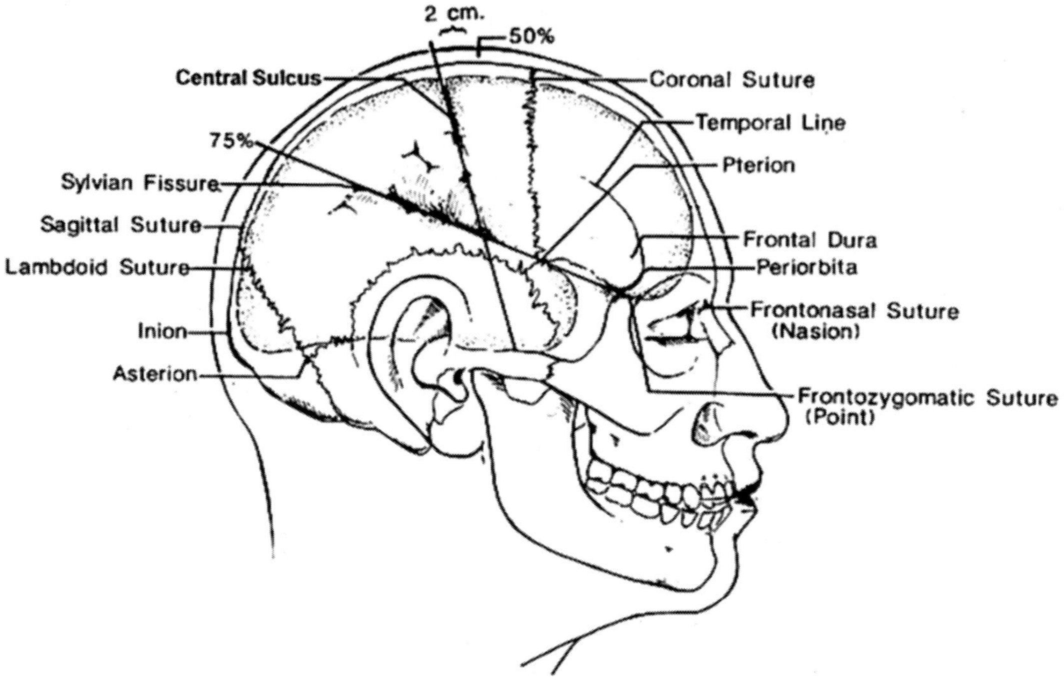

Figure 1.17. External Scalp and Bone Landmarks. Adapted with permission from the Rhoton Collection.

Chapter 2

The Spinal Cord and the Organization of the Somatosensory and Somatomotor System

2.1. Abstract

This chapter reviews the anatomy of the spinal cord, Somatomotor and somatosensory systems. The chapter begins with a short overview followed by a few key points regarding the anatomy of the occipito-atlanto-axial complex. Next, a focused discussion on the peripheral nervous system is presented, aimed at bringing the reader up to speed, and helping in forming a concise dataset. Clinically important anatomical details are stated together with clinical examples (entrapment syndromes etc.). Next, a short overview of spinal cord development is given. Spinal cord arterial supply and venous drainage are discussed next. Gross anatomy of the spinal cord follows, describing the surface features as well as gross anatomy of white and gray matter and regional characteristics of the spinal cord. The discussion then turns to a didactic overview of the important ascending and descending tracts, organized according to function and anatomy. Neuroanatomy of micturition is discussed next, and the chapter closes with a focused clinical correlation summary, offering the reader a focused look at key clinical definitions, physical neurological examination points and important syndromes.

2.2. Overview

The spinal cord is the major conduit through which motor and sensory information travels between the brain and the body. The spinal cord contains longitudinally oriented spinal tracts (a tract by definition is part of the white matter) surrounding central areas (gray matter) where most spinal neuronal cell bodies are located. The gray matter is organized into segments and regions comprising sensory and motor neurons. Axons from spinal sensory neurons (whose soma is located in the dorsal root ganglia) enter the spinal cord whereas axons from motor neurons leave the spinal cord via segmental spinal nerves or roots. The spinal roots are numbered and named according to the foramina through which they enter/exit the vertebral column. For example, the two C6 spinal nerve roots (left and right) pass through foramina situated between the C5 and C6 vertebrae. This holds true for the cervical region only, where a spinal nerve is located above the so named vertebrae. Upon transition to the thoracic spinal cord and column, this changes. Since there are eight cervical spinal nerves, but only seven cervical vertebrae, the C8 spinal nerve root passes below the C7 vertebrae. From this point on, the spinal nerves pass below the so named vertebrae. This holds true for the thoracic, lumbar and sacral segments of the spinal cord.

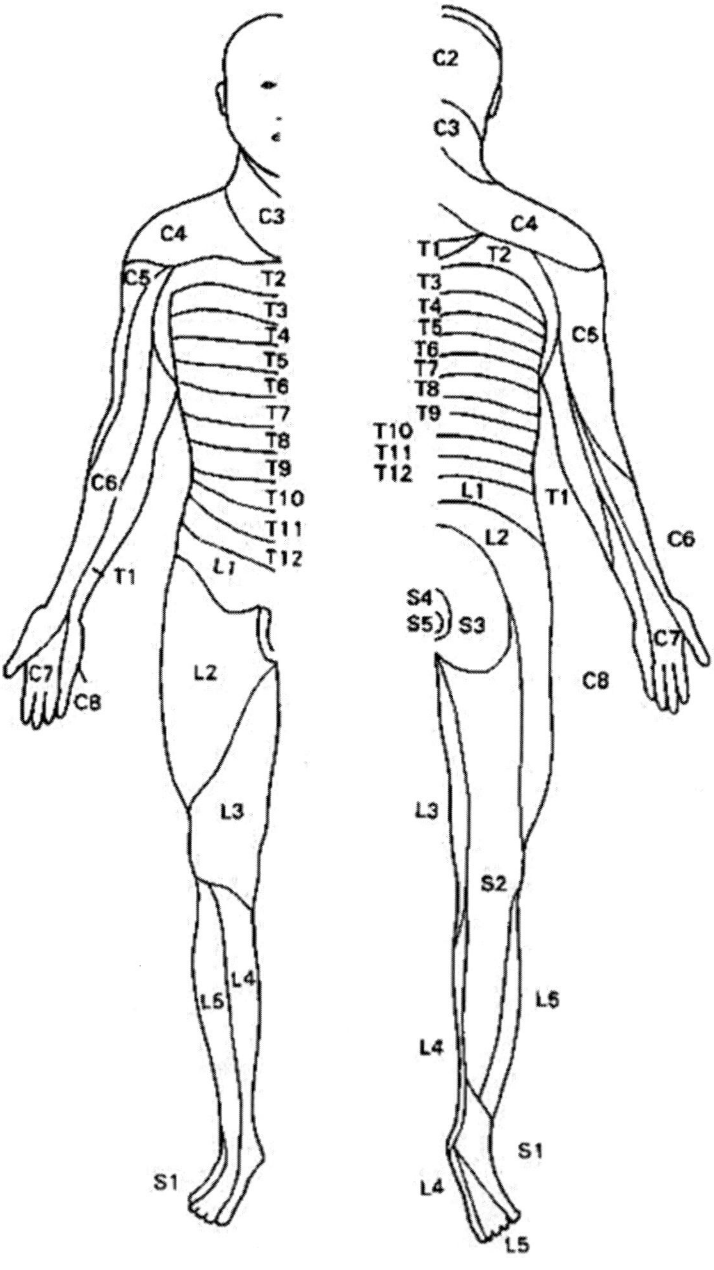

Figure 2.1. The dermatomes in front and back views.

Each spinal nerve root receives sensory information from a skin area. The skin area corresponding to a single spinal nerve root is called a dermatome. Similarly, each spinal nerve root innervates a group of muscles. A group of muscles innervated by a single nerve root is called a myotome. While a dermatome usually represents a discrete and contiguous skin area, unique for a specific spinal nerve root, most spinal nerve roots innervate more than one muscle, and most muscles are innervated by more than one spinal nerve root. Refer to figure 2.1 for an illustration of the spinal nerve root dermatomes.

The detailed knowledge of these territories forms a basic part of a neurological assessment. Checking for different sensory modalities in the different dermatomes, comparing both sides, is a very available, effective and worthwhile step in formulating a differential diagnosis. Spinal cord injury (SCI, described later) affects conduction of sensory and motor signals across the site(s) of lesion(s). By systematically examining the dermatomes and myotomes, as described in this chapter, one can determine the cord segments affected by spinal cord injury. From such an examination, several measures of neurological damage are generated, e.g., neurological level, sensory level and motor level (on right and left sides).

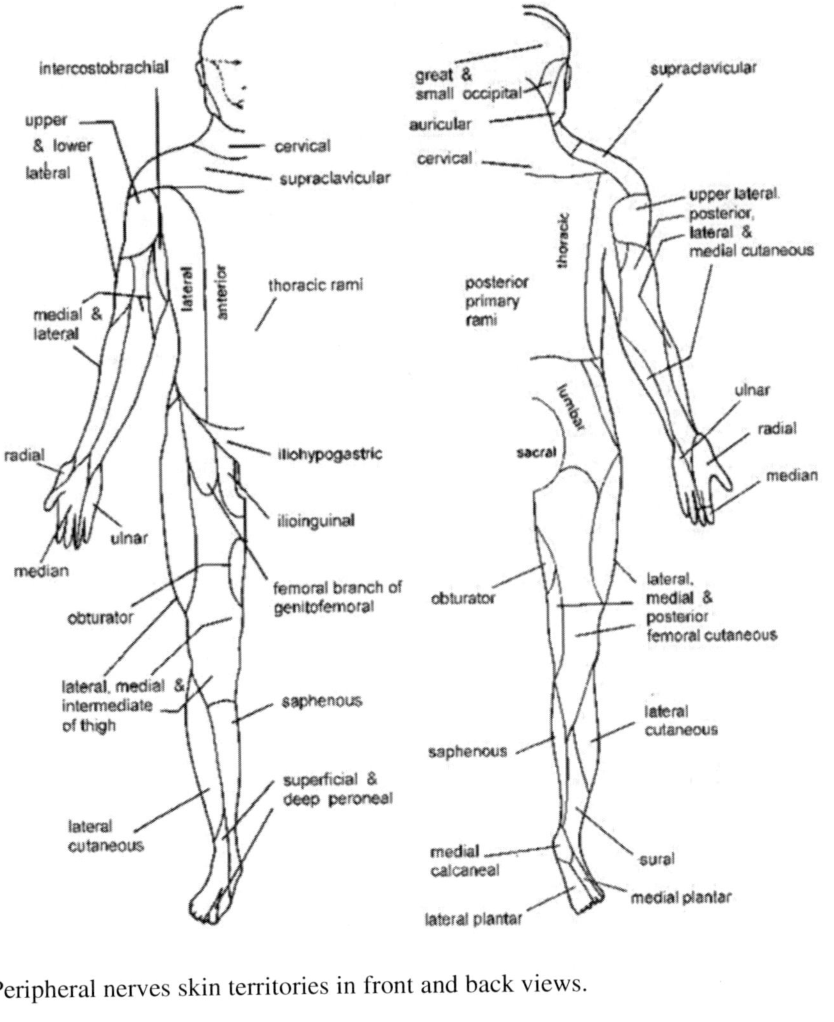

Figure 2.2. Peripheral nerves skin territories in front and back views.

Yet, another territorial division is superimposed on the dermatomal and myotomal system. Since most spinal nerve roots (specifically the ventral rami of the spinal nerve roots) undergo rearrangement outside of the spinal cord and canal, in structures termed as plexuses (The cervical, brachial, and lumbosacral plexuses described later). In these networks, the axons from different ventral spinal nerve roots are arranged in peripheral nerves innervating specific muscles and receiving sensory information from specific territories. A single peripheral nerve may be composed from axons originating from different spinal nerve roots. As such, a separate map, delineating the skin regions innervated by a single peripheral nerve and the muscles innervated by a single peripheral nerve may be composed. Refer to figure 2.2 for such an illustration. A detailed knowledge of peripheral nervous system anatomy is crucial for patient neurologic evaluation and formulating a differential diagnosis and location for a certain pathology. This is detailed in the next section.

2.3. Focused Review of the Occipito-Atlanto-Axial Complex

Although not in the frame of this book, the detailed knowledge of bony vertebral, ligamentous and muscular anatomy is important for any clinician in general, particularly so for the inspiring neurologist or neurosurgeon. This should be addressed in the frame of general anatomy. Still, the bony and ligamentous complex defining the relation between the occipital bone and its condules at foramen magnum and the first two cervical vertebrae carries unique points which merit mentioning. The first cervical vertebrae (the Atlas) and the second cervical vertebrae (the axis) relate to each other and to the occiput (both) in a unique joint structure allowing for a multiaxial and multiplaner movement. Refer to figure 2.3 for details. The stability of this joint complex is primarily due to ligaments, with very little contribution from bony articulations and joint capsules. The most important structures in maintaining the atlanto-occipital stability are the tectorial membrane and the alar ligaments. Without these, the cruciate ligament and apical dentate ligament are insufficient.

Ligaments that connect atlas to occiput:

A. Anterior atlanto-occipital membrane – A cephalad extension of the anterior longitudinal ligament arising from the anterior margin of foramen magnum (FM) to the anterior arch of the atlas (C1 vertebrae).

B. Posterior Atlanto-occipital membrane connects the posterior margins of FM to the posterior arch of the atlas (C1 vertebrae).

C. The ascending band of the cruciate ligament

Ligaments that connect the axis to the occiput:

A. The tectorial membrane – composed of two components:

i. Superficial part – A cephalad continuation of the posterior longitudinal ligament (PLL). This is a strong band connecting the dorsal surface of the dens (C2 vertebrae process) to the ventral surface of the FM above, and dorsal surface of C2 & C3 vertebral bodies below.

ii. Accessory (deep) - Located laterally, connects the axis (C2 vertebrae) to the occipital condyles

B. Alar ("check") Ligament – has three components:

i. Occipito-alar portion – connects the side of the dens (of C2) to the occipital condyle.

ii. Atlanto-alar portion – connects the side of the dens (of C2) to the lateral mass of the atlas (C1).

iii. Apical odontoid ligament – connects the tip of the dens (C2) to the FM. It has very little mechanical strength.

Ligaments that connect the axis to the atlas:

A. Transverse (Atlanto-axial) ligament - It is the horizontal component of cruciate ligament. It holds the dens (C2) to the anterior atlas (C1) via a strap-like mechanism. It is the strongest ligament of the spine.

B. Atlanto-alar portion of the alar ligament.

C. The descending band of the cruciate ligament

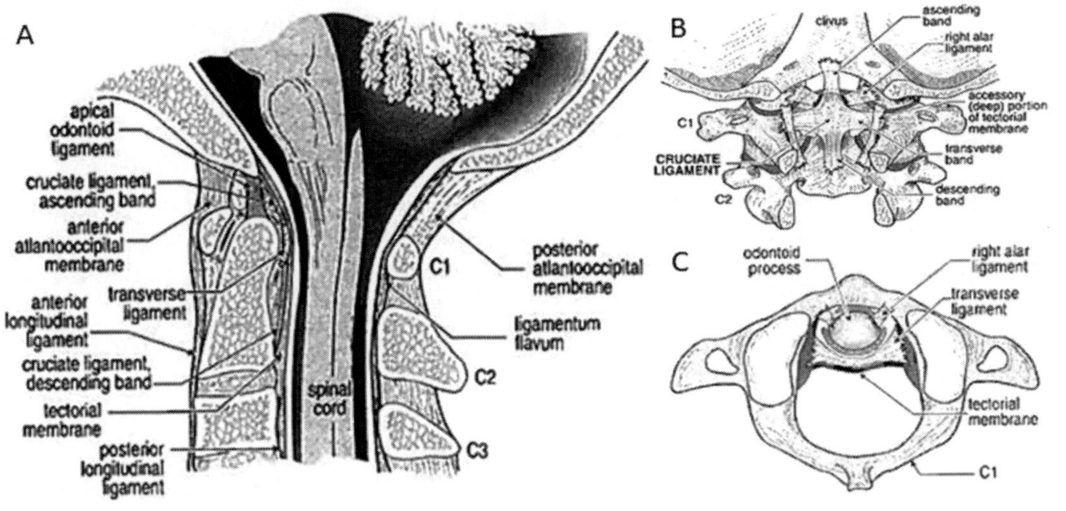

Figure 2.3. The Occipito-atlanto-axial complex anatomy. A, Sagittal view. B, Dorsal view of the cruciate and alar ligaments with tectorial membrane removed. C, C1 vertebrae (atlas) viewed from above, showing the transverse and alar ligaments. Modified from "In vitro cervical spine biomechanical testing" BNI quarterly, no.4 1993.

2.4. Focused Review of the Peripheral Nervous System

The peripheral nervous system (PNS) consists of many structures. These include the cranial nerves III-XII (excluding the olfactory and optic nerves considered part of the central nervous system (CNS)), spinal nerves, nerves of the extremities and the cervical, brachial and lumbosacral plexuses. Thus, all neural structures that connect the CNS with motor and sensory, somatic as well as visceral end (effector) organs. A detailed description of the PNS is not in the scope of this book. Therefore, for the sake of relevancy and practicability, we choose to present the spinal nerve fiber types, the brachial plexus and key muscular innervations in table format (tables 2.1, 2.2). Next we discuss common (mainly in examinations) related clinical syndromes.

2.4.1. The Spinal Nerves

The spinal nerves are formed by the union of the dorsal and ventral roots. Thus, thirty-one pairs (corresponding to number of spinal cord levels). Each spinal nerve contains Affarent fibers, conveying sensory input from the periphery to the spinal cord, and Efferent fibers, arising from the spinal motor neurons at the ventral horn (discussed later). These sensory and motor components, together with local interneuronal circuits in spinal gray matter, are the anatomical basis for spinal reflexes. The Spinal nerves contain up to four fiber types (two sensory types of neurons having their cell-body in the dorsal root ganglion, and two motor types of neurons, having their cell body in the spinal cord gray matter). Sensory input may originate from the body surface (previously termed somatosensory), from deep structures (like muscles, tendons, joints etc) or from internal organs (previously termed viscerosensory).

Sensory fibers are classified as general somatic afferent (GSA) or general visceral afferents (GVA). The GSA fibers (previously termed somatosensory) are further classified to exteroreceptive, receptors sensitive to discriminative touch or vibratory stimulus and proprioceptors. The exteroreceptors are mechanoreceptors, thermoreceptors or chemoreceptors. These are slowly conducting unmyelinated A-δ, C fibers, entering the cord via the lateral division of the dorsal root, and ascend or descend in the dorsolateral fasciculus (discussed later) before entering the dorsal horn to terminate at Rexed laminae I-IV (discussed later). The receptors sensitive to discriminative touch or vibratory stimuli are fast conducting, myelinated, A-β fibers. These enter the cord through the medial division of dorsal root and after entering the dorsal funiculus, may give rise to ascending or descending collaterals. Proprioceptors originate from receptors in muscles, tendons or joints. These are sensitive to stretch or pressure, much less to vibratory stimuli. These are myelinated A-β fibers, entering the cord via the medial division of the dorsal root as well. Their central process (as well as that of exteroreceptors), may directly enter, and ascend in the dorsal columns, or may branch into the spinal gray to synapse in relay nuclei (like Clarke's, discussed later), or in the ventral horn to participate in reflexes.

GVA neurons, previously termed as viscerosensory (VS), carry sensory information from the viscera. It is an interoceptive input, originating from receptors that are sensitive to nociceptive stimuli. These fibers travel (for example) via the splanchnic nerve, traversing the Sympathetic chain and white rami to enter the spinal nerve. Their central process enters the lateral division of the dorsal root and terminates at Rexed lamina I, V-VII (discussed later). These are slow conducting, lightly myelinated, A-δ fibers.

Motor fibers are classified as general somatic efferent (GSE previously termed as somatomotor) or general visceral efferent (GVE previously termed as visceromotor). GSE fibers directly innervate skeletal muscle, originate in the ventral spinal gray mater horn. GSE fibers also supply motor innervation to the specialized intrafusal muscle fibers of the muscle spindles (sensory structures in the muscles that detect muscle length and various aspects of contraction dynamics). These large nerve fibers are organized in two general, overlapping patterns. Nerve fibers directed to proximal muscles are situated more medially and those directed to more distal muscles are progressively organized more laterally. This arrangement explains why the ventral horn is smaller and narrower at the thoracic than at the cervical and lumbar segments of the spinal cord. Within the ventral horn at the cervical (C4-T1) and lumbar (L1-S2) regions, motor nerves to extensor muscles are ventrally located, while those to flexors are more dorsally located.

GVE fibers are autonomic fibers (part of the autonomic nervous system, preganglionic sympathetic and parasympathetic fibers) that synapse on secondary neurons in peripheral ganglia. These secondary neurons (postganglionic fiber) than reaches its target tissue, namely smooth muscle, cardiac muscle or glandular epithelium. GVE cell bodies are located at Rexed lamina VII of the spinal cord at the T1-L2 levels for the sympathetic preganglionic fibers. Lamina VII at this region belongs to the intermediolateral cell column (discussed later). GVE cell bodies are also located at the Rexed lamina VII of the spinal cord S2-S4 segments, forming the preganglionic parasympathetic sacral VM nucleus. Both GSE (SM) and GVE (VM) nerve fibers exit the spinal cord at the ventral root into the spinal nerve. GVE (VM) fibers than leave the spinal nerve to join the Sympathetic trunk via the white communicating ramus, and rejoin the spinal nerve via the gray communicating ramus.

2.4.2. The Brachial Plexus

For an illustration of the brachial plexus and innervation of the shoulder and upper extremity refer to table 2.1 and figures 2.4-2.6. The brachial plexus originates from the ventral rami of spinal nerves C5 to T1. It emerges between the anterior and middle scalene muscles, courses through the posterior triangle of neck posterior to the clavicle before becoming closely associated with the axillary artery in the axilla before giving up its terminal branches. A shown in figure 2.4-2.5, major branches include the median nerve, ulnar nerve, radial nerve, axillary nerve, and the musculocutaneous nerve. Motor supply includes the upper limb and pectoral girdle. Sensory supply includes the upper limb and part of the upper thorax. The brachial plexus consists of roots, trunks, divisions, cords and terminal branches as it travels from proximal to distal upper limb. Roots are formed behind scalenus anterior by the anterior rami of C5-C8 and T1. Three branches arise from the roots; these are the dorsal scapular nerve, the subclavian nerve and the long thoracic nerve.

Trunks form from the roots as they pass between scalenus anterior and medius muscles, then go on to traverse the posterior triangle. C5 and C6 roots combine to form the upper trunk, C7 root makes up the middle trunk, C8 and T1 roots combine to form the lower trunk. One branch arises from the trunks, i.e., the suprascapular nerve. Each trunk divides to form an anterior and posterior division behind the clavicle. The divisions then combine to form cords, which are named for their relation to the second part of the axillary artery. The lateral cord is formed by the union of the upper two anterior divisions at the lateral border of the first rib. The medial cord is a continuation of the lower anterior division. The posterior cord consists of the united three posterior divisions the prevertebral fascia of the neck extends down to ensheath the axillary artery and cords. It is into this axillary sheath that local anesthetic is injected when performing a brachial plexus block. Various peripheral nerves then branch from these cords.

Branches from the lateral cord:	Lateral pectoral nerve Musculocutaneous nerve Lateral root of the median nerve
Branches from the medial cord:	Medial pectoral nerve Medial root of the median nerve Medial cutaneous nerve of the arm Medial cutaneous nerve of the forearm Ulnar nerve
Branches from the posterior cord:	Upper subscapular nerve Thoracodorsal nerve Lower subscapular nerve Radial nerve Axillary nerve

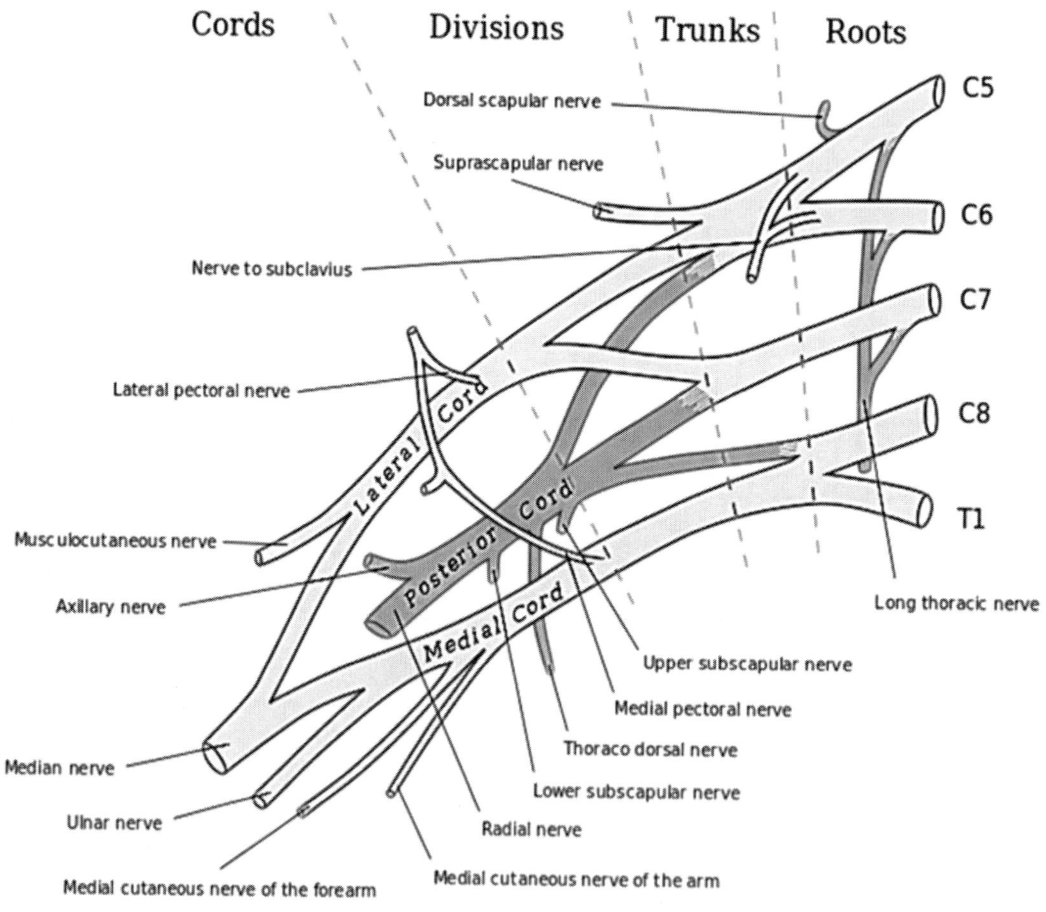

Figure 2.4. The brachial plexus scheme. Images from Gray's anatomy (out of copyright).

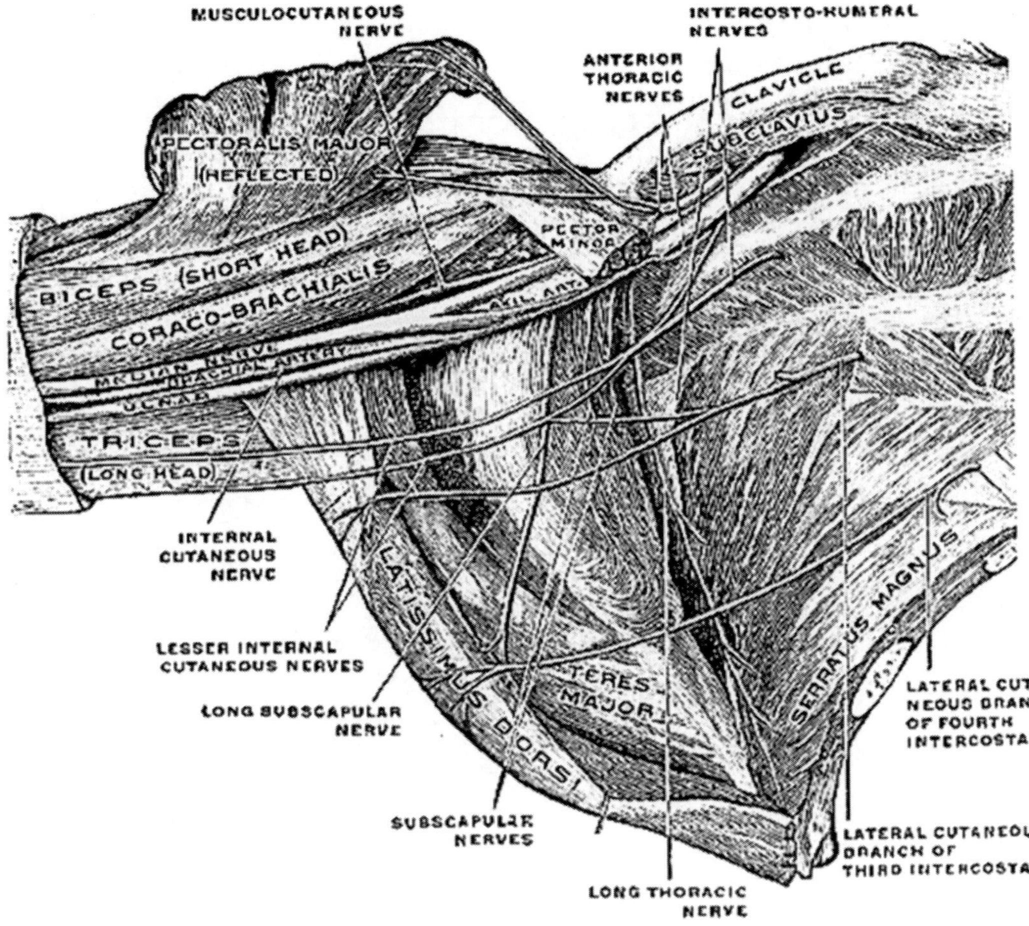

Figure 2.5. The brachial plexus in situ. Images from Gray's anatomy (out of copyright).

Table 2.1. Muscle Innervation of the Shoulder and Upper extremity

Nerve	Muscles	
Radial (C5-C8)	1	Triceps (all 3 heads)
	2	Brachioradialis
	3	Extensor carpi radialis longus & brevis.
	4	Supinator (originates near the terminal branch)
	5	Continues into forearm as posterior interosseous nerve (C7,C8)
	6	Extensor carpi ulnaris
	7	Extensor digitorum
	8	Extensor digiti minimi
	9	Extensor pollicis brevis & longus
	10	Abductor pollicis longus
	11	Extensor indicis
Axillary (C5, C6)	1	Teres minor
	2	Deltoid

Table 2.1. (Continued)

Nerve	Muscles			
Median (C5-T1)	Nothing in arm			
	1	All forearm pronators and flexors except The two supplied by ulnar nerve	Pronator teres	
	2		Flexor carpi Radialis	
	3		Palmaris longus	
	4		Flexor digitorum superficialis	
	5	In the hand the "LOAF muscles"	Lumbricals I & 2	
	6		Opponens pollicis	
	7		Abductor pollicis brevis	
	8		Flexor pollicis brevis	
	9	Anterior interosseous nerve	Flexor digitorum profundus I & II	
	10		Flexor pollicis longus	
	11		Pronator Quadrates	
Ulnar (C8, T1)	Nothing in arm			
	1	In the forearm	Flexor carpi ulnaris	
	2		Flexor digitorum profundus III & IV	
	3	In the hand all muscles excluding "LOAF"	Adductor pollicis	
	4		Flexor pollicis brevis	
	5		All dorsal& palmar interossei	
	6		Lumbricals 3 & 4	
	7		Hypothenar muscles	Abductor
	8			Opponens
	9			Flexor digiti minimi
Musculocutaneous (C5, C6)	1	Coracobrachialis		
	2	Biceps		
	3	Brachialis		
	4	Lateral cutaneous nerve of the forearm		
Dorsal scapular (C4, C5)	1	Rhomboids (major & minor)		
	2	Levator scapulae		
Suprascapular (C5, C6)	1	Supraspinatus		
	2	Infraspinatus		
Subscapular (C5-7)	1	Teres major		
	2	Subscapularis		
Thoracodorsal (C6-C8)	1	Latissimus dorsi		
Long thoracic (C5-7)	1	Serratus anterior		

Innervation of the thumb occurs via three nerves. Abduction / flexion / opposition is innervated by the median nerve, adduction is innervated by the ulnar nerve and extension is innervated by the radial nerve.

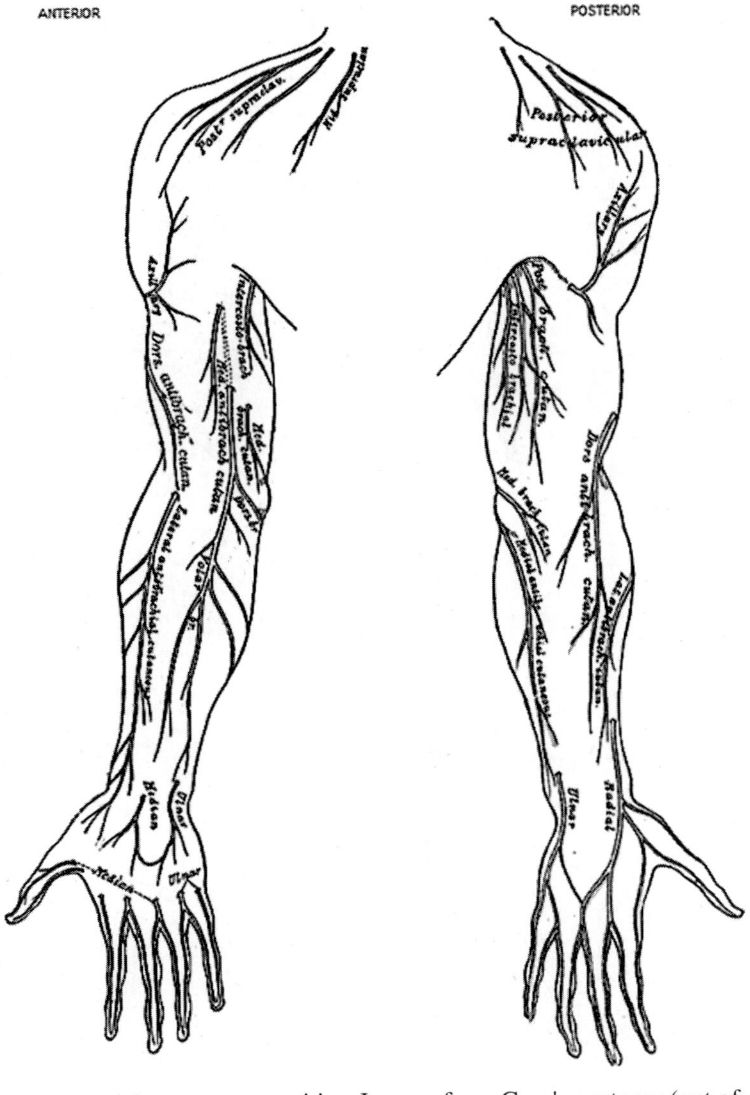

Figure 2.6. Innervation of the upper extremities. Images from Gray's anatomy (out of copyright).

2.4.3. The Lumbosacral Plexus

For an illustration of the lumbosacral plexus and innervation of the hip and lower extremity refer to table 2.2 and figures 2.7-2.8. A handy mnemonic to recall the branches of the lumbar plexus is “Indecent Ian Gets Laid On Fridays Luckily”. These are the iliohypogastric nerve (I), ilioinguinal nerve (I), genitofemoral nerve (G), lateral cutaneous nerve of the thigh (L), obturator nerve (O), femoral nerve (F), lumbosacral trunk (L). The sacral plexus forms on the anterior belly of the piriformis muscle and is formed by the lumbosacral trunk (L4-5) of the lumbar plexus, which enters the pelvis coursing medially to psoas major and unites with the ventral rami of the S1 to S4 nerve roots, which emerge from the anterior foramen of the sacrum. It forms a triangular shape with an inferiorly pointing apex. The anterior sacral rami give off six branches and then divide into anterior and posterior division, each giving off further branches.

The Anterior rami gives rise to the nerve to piriformis (S1-S2), the perforating cutaneous nerve (S2-S3), the posterior femoral cutaneous nerve (S1-S3), the parasympathetic pelvic splanchnic nerves (S2-S4), the pudendal nerve (S2-S4) and the perineal branch (S4). The anterior division of anterior rami gives rise to the nerve to quadratus femoris and inferior gemellus muscles (L4-S1), the nerve to internal obturator and superior gemellus muscles (L5-S2) and the tibial part (L4-S2) of the sciatic nerve (L4-S3). The Posterior division of anterior rami gives rise to the superior gluteal nerve (L4-S1), the inferior gluteal nerve (L5-S2) and the common peroneal part (L4-S2) of the sciatic nerve.

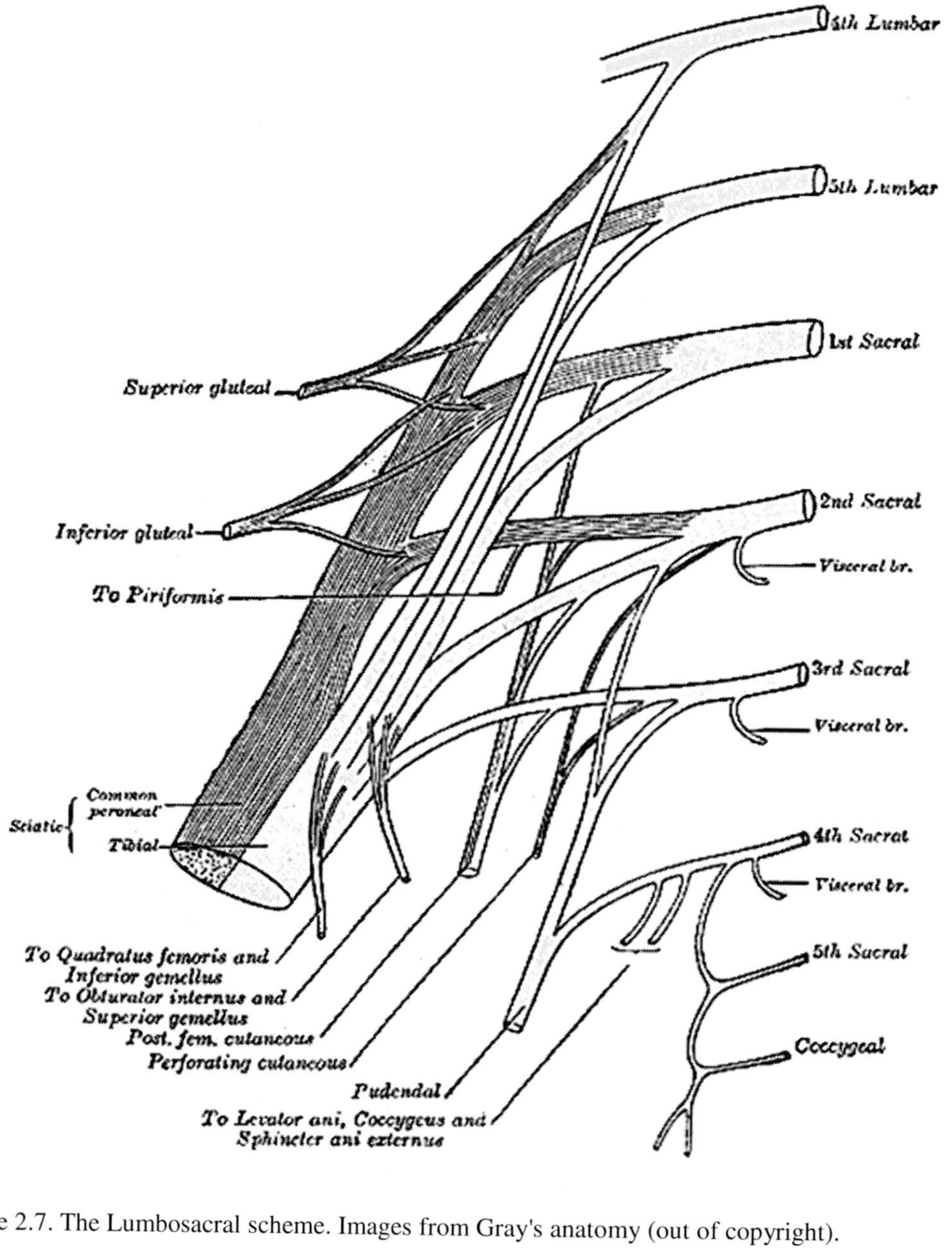

Figure 2.7. The Lumbosacral scheme. Images from Gray's anatomy (out of copyright).

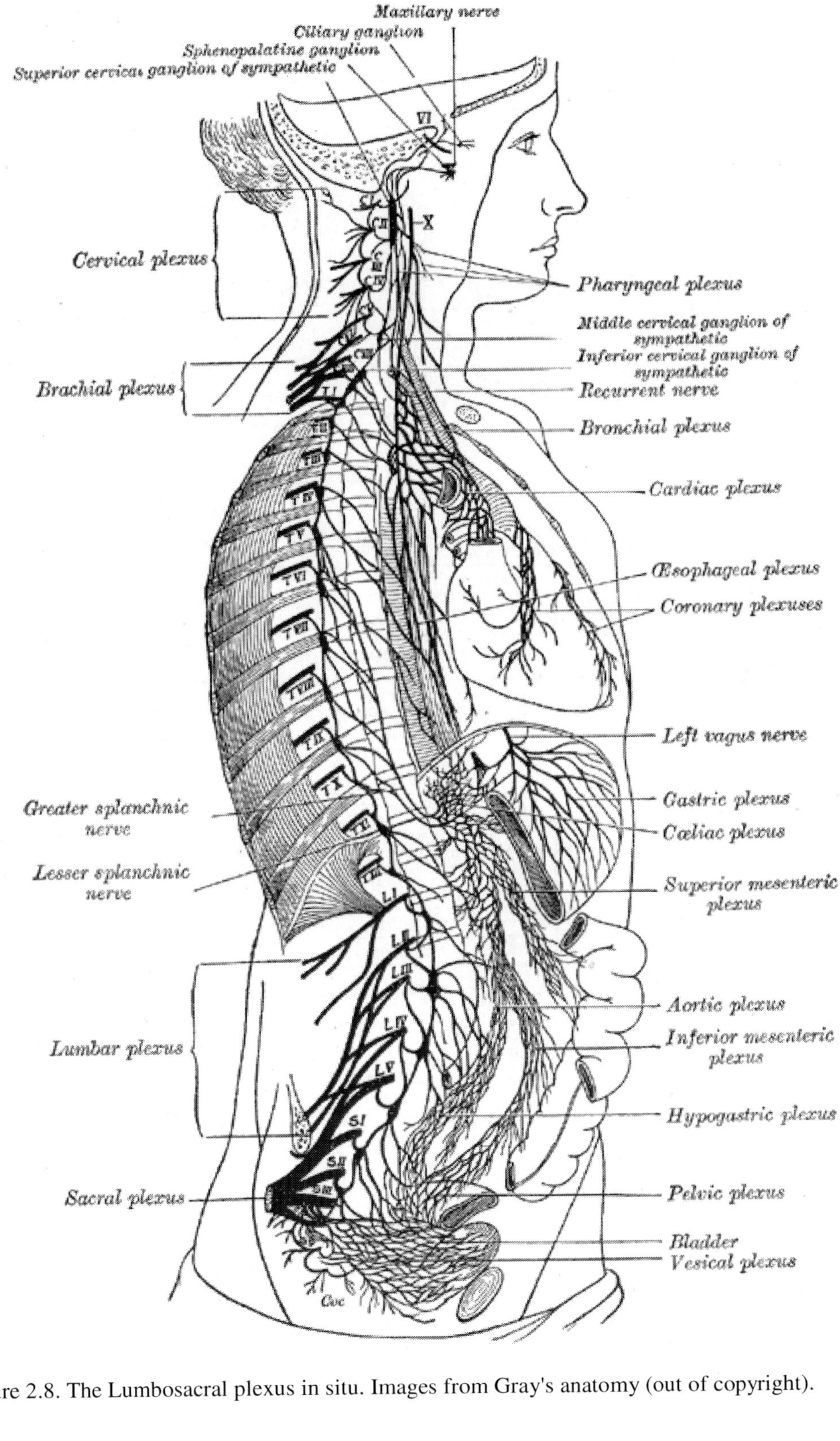

Figure 2.8. The Lumbosacral plexus in situ. Images from Gray's anatomy (out of copyright).

Table 2.2. Muscle Innervation of the Hip and Lower extremity

Nerve	Muscles	
Femoral	1	Iliopsoas
	2	Sartorius
	3	Quadriceps femoris
Obturator	1	Pectineus
	2	Adductor longus
	3	Adductor brevis
	4	Adductor magnus
	5	Gracilis
	6	Obturator externus
Superior gluteal	1	Gluteus medius
	2	Gluteus minimus
	3	Tensor of fascia lata
	4	Piriformis
Inferior gluteus	1	Gluteus maximus
Muscular branches	1	Obturator internus
	2	Gemelli
	3	Quadratus femoris
Sciatic (trunk)	1	Biceps femoris
	2	Semitendinosus
	3	Semimembranosus
Deep peroneal	1	Tibialis anterior
	2	Extensor digitorum longus
	3	Extensor halluces longus
	4	Extensor digitorum brevis
Superficial peroneal	1	Peroneus longus
	2	Peroneus brevis
Tibial	1	Posterior tibialis
	2	Flexor digitorum longus
	3	Flexor halluces longus
	4	Flexor digitorum brevis
	5	Flexor halluces brevis
	6	Gastrocnemius
	7	Plantaris
	8	Soleus
	9	Abductor halluces
Pudendal	1	Perineal muscles
	2	Anal sphincters

2.4.4. Entrapment Syndromes

The most common symptom is pain (frequently at rest, more severe at night, often with retrograde radiation causing more proximal lesion to be suspected) with tenderness at the point of entrapment. Brief compression of the peripheral nerve primarily affects myelinated fibers, and classically spares unmyelinated fibers. Acute compression compromises axoplasmic flow which can reduce membrane excitability. The issue of ischemia is more controversial in the etiology of the disease. The understanding of the different entrapment syndromes requires a detailed knowledge of the peripheral nerve course and important osseous and ligamentous obstacles. For the purpose of a short neuroanatomical review, these were distilled to a few key features per entrapment syndrome and are presented in table 2.3.

Table 2.3. Entrapment Syndromes

Occipital nerve entrapment	The Greater occipital nerve (the nerve of Arnold) is the sensory branch of C2 spinal nerve root. It is entrapped on exiting the Occipital Triangle. Pain in occiput usually with a trigger point near the superior nuchal line. Pressure here reproduces pain radiating up along back of head towards vertex. More common in women.	
Median nerve entrapment	**Arm**	Possible entrapment point is the Struther's ligament (supracondylar process of humerus).
	Forearm	The nerve passes between two heads of pronator teres and supplies this muscle. Entrapment in this site may occur from direct trauma or repeated pronation with tight hand-grip.
	Palm	The nerve passes through the carpal tunnel. In this location, entrapment and inflammation is the most common of the entrapment syndromes
Ulnar nerve entrapment	**Arm**	The nerve can be entrapped in the Struther's arcade / medial intermuscular septum.
	Forearm	The nerve can be entrapped at the postcondylar groove or the Osborne's fascia (Flexor carpi ulnaris band).
	Palm	The nerve can be entrapped at Guyon's canal
Axillary compression	**Axilla**	Crutch misuse; poor arm position during drunken sleep.
	Upper arm	The nerve can be compressed in the spiral groove of humerus or at the intermuscular septum.
Posterior interosseous neuropathy	May result from entrapment of the nerve at the arcade of Frohse (rare). Manifested by a marked extensor weakness of thumb and fingers (finger drop). It is distinguished from radial nerve palsy by less wrist extensor weakness (no wrist drop) as well as no sensory loss.	
Radial tunnel syndrome	AKA supinator tunnel syndrome, The "radial tunnel" extends from just above the elbow to just distal to it, and is composed of different structures. It contains the radial nerve and its two main branches. Repeated forceful supination / pronation may traumatize the nerve at this location. This injury may be mistakenly diagnosed as resistant "tennis elbow". This syndrome responds to nerve decompression.	
Meralgia Paresthetica	Originally known as Bernhardt-Roth syndrome, called "swashbuckler's disease". A condition caused by entrapment of the lateral femoral cutaneous nerve (LFCN) of the thigh, where it enters the thigh though the opening between the inguinal ligament and its attachment to the anterior superior iliac spine. Manifest with burning dysesthesias in the lateral aspect of the upper thigh, occasionally just above the knee, usually with increased sensitivity to clothing (hyperpathia).	
Common peroneal nerve	Entrapment may occur as the nerve crosses the fibular neck or penetrates peroneus longus. Entrapment produces weak ankle dorsiflexion (foot drop) due to anterior tibialis palsy, weak foot eversion and sensory impairment in areas innervated by deep & superficial peroneal nerve. Occasionally, only the deep peroneal nerve is involved, resulting in foot drop with minimal sensory loss.	
Tarsal tunnel	Entrapment of posterior tibial nerve may occur in the tarsal tunnel, posterior & inferior to the medial malleolus. The nerve may be trapped at the retinacular ligament. Entrapment may cause toes clawing (weakness of intrinsic foot muscles).	

2.5. Functions of the Spinal Cord

1) **A receptive sensory function:** the Spinal cord receives primary sensory input from receptors in skin, skeletal muscle, tendons [SS (somatosensory) Fibers], and from thoracic, abdominal, pelvic viscera [VS (Viscerosensory) fibers]. Via multisynaptic relays, much of this information is conveyed to higher levels of the neuroaxis.
2) **An effector motor function**: SM (Somatomotor) fibers, innervates striated muscle, VM (visceromotor) fibers (also termed parasympathetic fibers), after synapsing in peripheral ganglia, innervate smooth muscle, cardiac muscle and glandular epithelial.
3) **Autonomic reflex function: SS** fibers entering the dorsal root and gray mater horn influence ventral horn motor neurons either directly or indirectly via interneurons, producing involuntary movements (the spinal reflex arc).
4) **A conduit to higher centers**: Ascending and descending fibers within the spinal cord, designated to various locations of the neuroaxis are housed in the spinal cord.

2.6. Development and Embryology of the Spinal Cord

Formation of the neural tube consists of 3 successive stages of development:

I. The Neural plate. It results from thickening and differentiation of ectoderm overlying the notochord. The ectoderm of the plate is called neuroectoderm and will give rise to the central nervous system, consisting of the brain and spinal cord. The plate is wider at its cephalic end than at its caudal end, and is formed in humans, before the appearance of the first somite or about day 18 of development (refer to figure 2.9).
II. The neural groove and neural folds. The lateral edges of the neural plate elevate to form the neural folds. The neural groove develops as a result of invagination of the neural plate along its central axis, between the neural folds (about day 18).
III. The neural tube. The neural folds move together, fuse by the end of week 3, and convert the plate into a tube (also called the neurula stage). The ectoderm thus is separated from the nervous tissue to form the surface ectoderm.

The 3 stages (plate, groove and folds, and tube) all coexist at the same time in different regions of the embryo. Closure of the neural groove at about day 21, in humans, takes place near the fourth somite (future cervical region), which is in the middle portion of the embryo, and progresses toward both its cephalic and caudal ends. Two orifices at the ends of the neural tube persist for a relatively short period of time and are called the anterior and posterior neuropores. They temporarily form open connections between the neural tube lumen and the amniotic cavity. The anterior neuropore indicates the area of the lamina terminalis and closes about day 25 or the 18-to-20-somite stage.

When the neural folds fuse and, before the neural groove closes completely, some neuroectodermal cells detach themselves from the region where the neural tube borders on the ectoderm (lateral edges of the neural plate). These groups of cells are not incorporated into the neural tube, but form a neural crest over the tube. Crests are distinct from both the neural tube as well as the overlying ectoderm after the neural groove is closed. They form longitudinal tracts which extend from the middle brain regions of the neural tube to its caudal end. The neural crests soon fragment into segments that give rise to the primordia of the ganglia. The segmentation corresponds to that of the somites, with each ganglionic primordium corresponding to a muscle primordium. The ganglia later give rise to general sensory innervation, and the corresponding level of the spinal cord gives motor innervation to the muscles.

The neural tube is composed of precursor cells, forming the ventricular layer that will give rise to ependymal cells, neuroblasts, glia cells (these will form the mantle layer – the intermediate one). The mantle layer consists of four rostro-caudally oriented columns of neuroblasts, forming the paired alar plates (dorsally) and the paired basal plates (ventrally). These are separated from each other by the sulcus limitans. Neurons of the alar plate differentiate into sensory neurons. These form tract neurons and interneurons of the dorsal horn. The Neurons originating from the basal plate form the motor neurons and interneurons of the ventral horn. This embryological distinction is also evidently clear and important when discussing the brainstem (chapter 3). In between these areas, an intermediate zone (intermediate gray) exists. This is a region between dorsal and ventral spinal cord horns, originates from both alar and basal plates. This zone will give rise to visceromotor (VM) and viscerosensory (VS) derivatives. The Marginal layer contains gliablasts and out-growing processes of Mantle layer Neuroblasts. The descending axons of neurons found in the Brainstem/cortex, form the tracts (become myelinated).

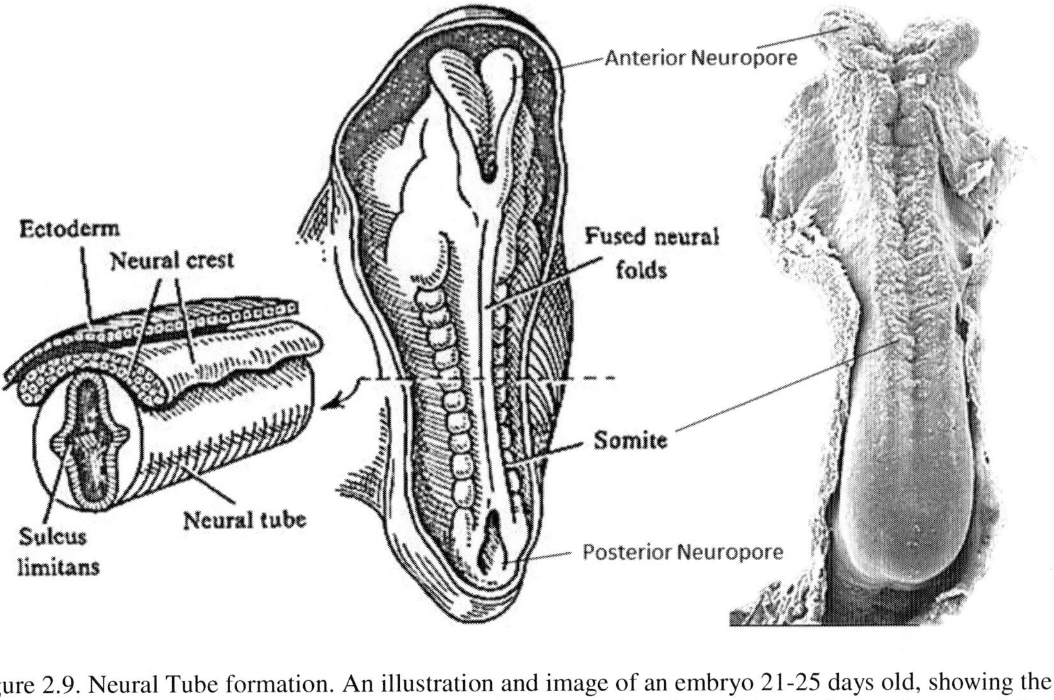

Figure 2.9. Neural Tube formation. An illustration and image of an embryo 21-25 days old, showing the neural folds bordering the anterior neuropore, the formation of somites with neural tube closure and the neural crest (the axial section). Taken with permission from www.Radiopaedia.org.

2.7. Spinal Cord Vasculature

2.7.1. Arterial Supply to the Spinal Cord

Blood supply to the spinal cord arises from branches of the vertebral artery and spinal radicular artery. The vertebral artery (VA) gives off the anterior spinal artery, running in the ventral aspect of the cord, supplying its anterior 2/3. The posterior spinal arteries may arise from the VA or may also arise from PICA (posterior inferior cerebellar artery). These supply the dorsal 1/3 of the spinal cord. The spinal arteries form a spinal arterial plexus surrounding the cord (termed as corona arteria). Refer to figures 2.10-2.12 for an overview of the arterial blood supply to the spinal cord. The anterior spinal artery develops as a longitudinal vessel connecting transversely oriented segmental arteries. It is located on the ventral surface of the cord, adjacent to the ventral median fissure of the spinal cord. It varies in size, more or less based on the amount of gray matter at the given segment. As such, its size is substantially larger in the cervical and lumbar segments, as compared with slender mid-thoracic size. Note that one end of the ASA has limited to no capacity to support the other should its dominant radiculomedullary supply fail.

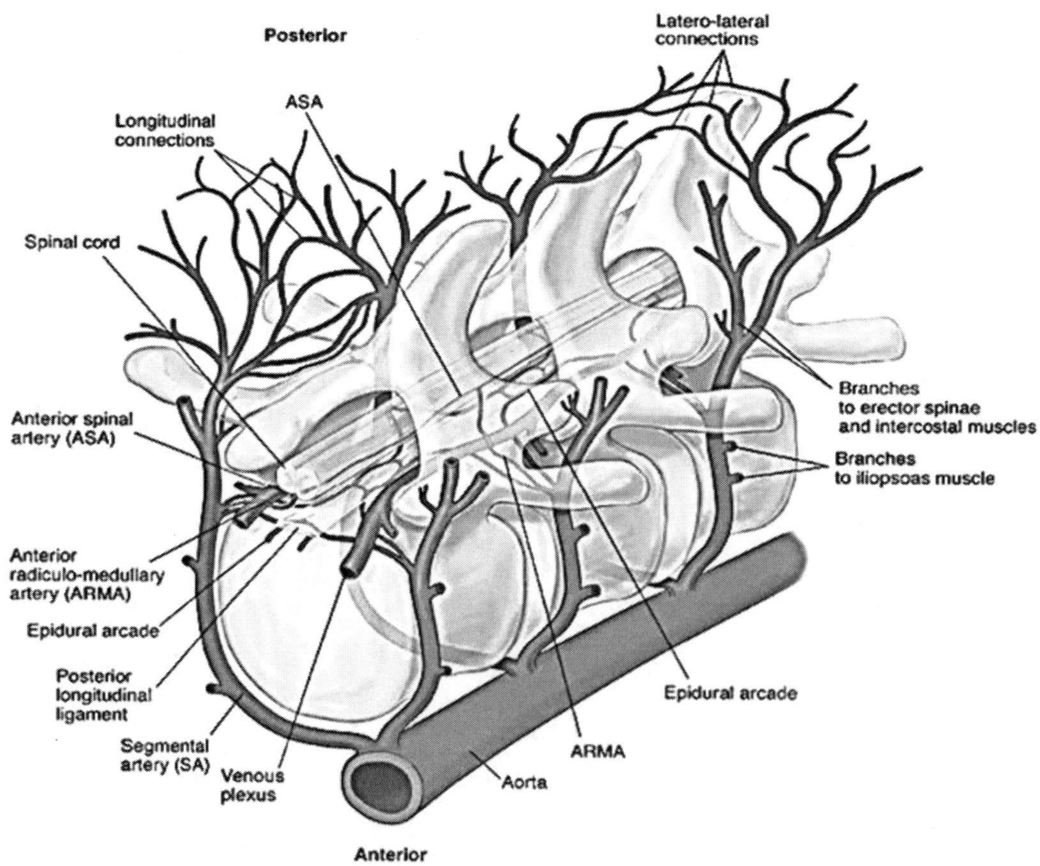

Figure 2.10. Spinal cord vascular supply, an overview.

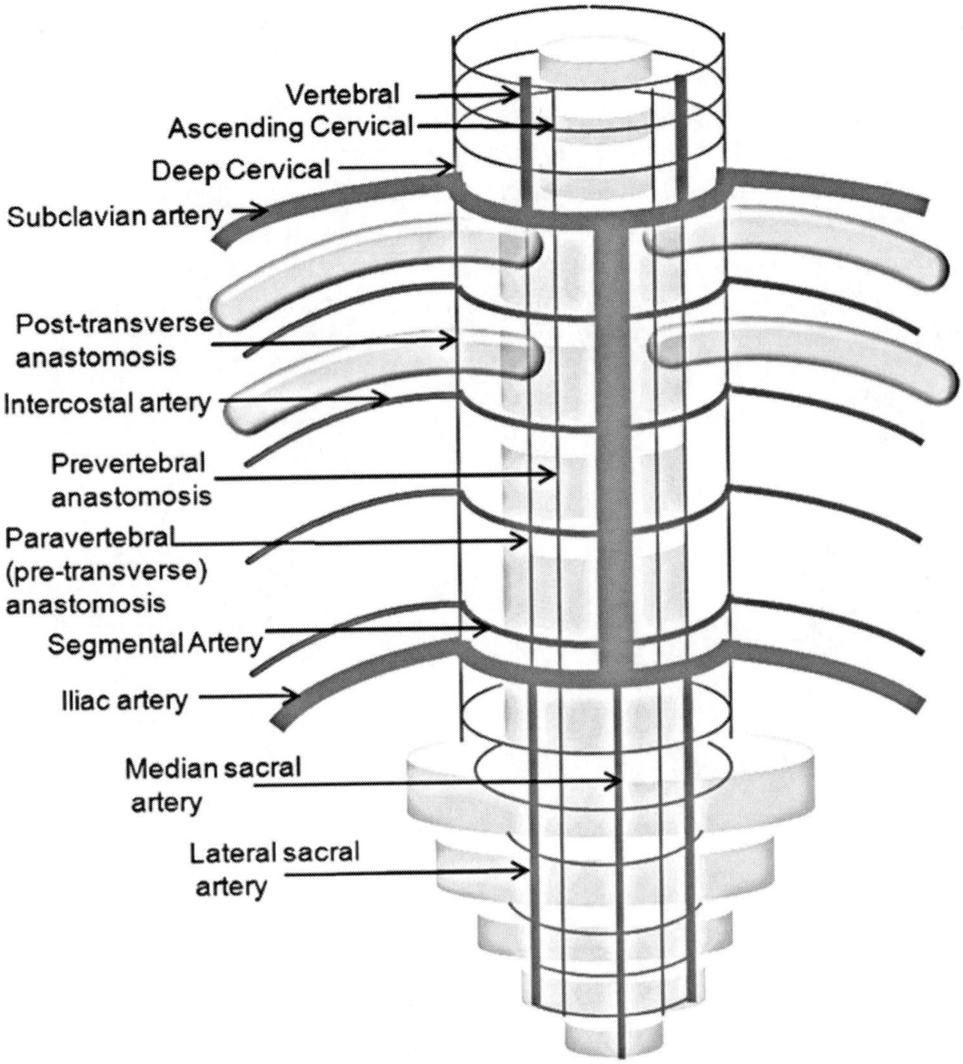

Figure 2.11. Somatotopic organization of the vertebrospinal arterial vasculature, highlighting segmental vascular organization of the vertebrospinal axis and homologous longitudinal anastomoses along its entire length. Shown are the numerous longitudinal vessels existing throughout the vertebrospinal axis, often with the same vessel going by several different names, for historical reasons (i.e., the lateral spinal, pre-transverse, and deep cervical arteries). The segmental arrangement is particularly modified in the cervical region, where longitudinal vessels are dominant (VA most obviously). It is important however to recognize the existence of segmental vessels connecting the three dominant cervical longitudinal arteries (ascending cervical, vertebral, and deep cervical). Taken with permission from www.neuroangio.org.

Thirty-one segmental branches of aorta enter the spinal canal (radicular arteries), yet most of these supply the dura and only about six to ten such arteries reach deeper to supply the spinal cord as radiculomedullary arteries, arising at different levels. Radiculomedullary arteries at the cervical region may arise from the VA (mostly at the C3 levels), from the deep cervical arteries (at the C6 level) or from the costocervical trunk (at the C8 level). The larger cervical and lumbar ASA segments are associated with larger radiculomedullary arteries to supply them — the famous artery of lumbar enlargement (Adamkiewicz), and the less well known (radiculomedullary) artery of the cervical enlargement, known as the artery of Lazorthes. The Lazorthes most commonly arises from lower cervical vertebral artery, though not infrequently from deep cervical or supreme intercostal vessels also. The Adamkiewicz (Arteria radicularis anterior magna) comes off between T9 and T12 in 75% of cases, more commonly on the left (75-80%). It is the main arterial supply for the spinal cord from T8 to the conus Medullaris. The spinal cord at the midthoracic level suffers a relative paucity of blood supply, in terms of a major radiculomedullary arterial supply to the anterior spinal artery. Due to its tenuous vascular supply, it is sometimes referred to as a watershed zone, namely a region most in danger of insults and infarcts in cases of hypoperfusion or hypotension.

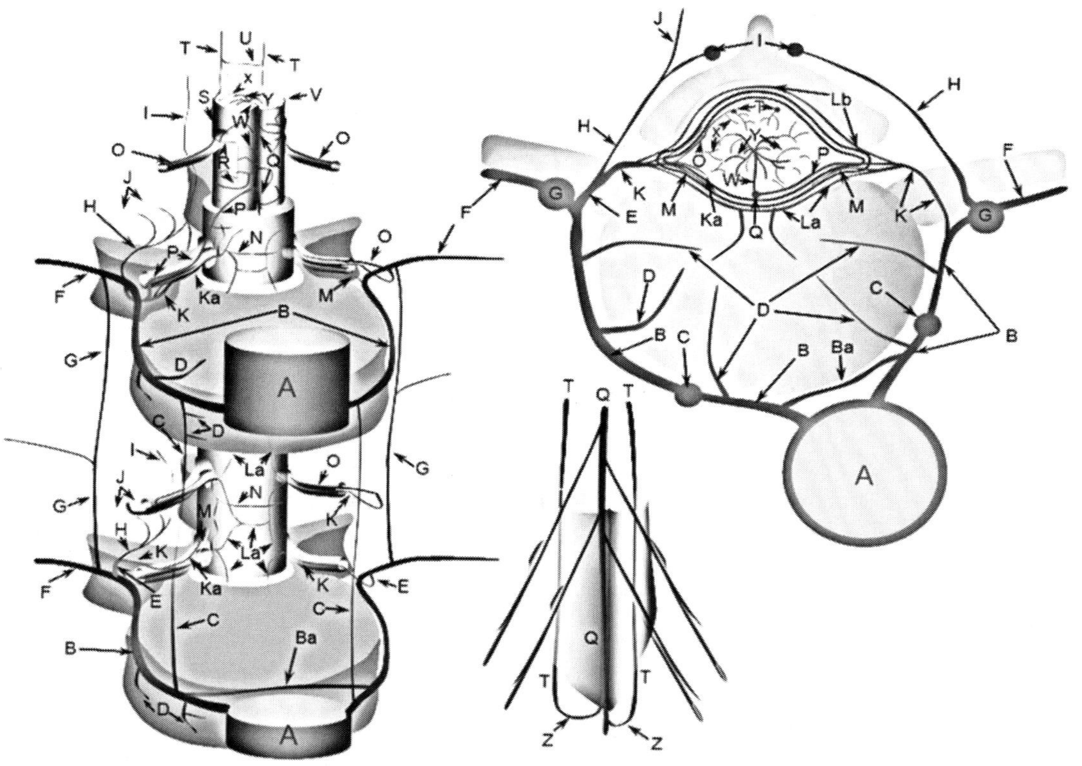

Figure 2.12. A diagram showing the arterial anatomy of the spinal elements. A – aorta; B – segmental artery; Ba – intersegmental arterial anastomosis; C – prevertebral anastomotic network; D – direct vertebral body feeding arteries; E – dorsal spinal artery; F – intercostal/muscular artery; G – pretransverse anastomotic network; H – dorsal division of the dorsal spinal artery; I – post-transverse anastomotic network; J – muscular branches of the post-transverse anastomotic network; K – ventral division of the dorsal spinal artery; Ka – radicular artery; La – ventral epidural arcade; Lb – dorsal epidural arcade; M – nerve root sleeve dural branch of the ventral division dorsal spinal artery; N – dural branch of the ventral division dorsal spinal artery; O – radiculopial artery; P – radiculomedullary artery; Q – anterior spinal artery; R – mesh-like pial arterial network; S, T – posterior spinal artery; U, V – pial arterial network (a.k.a. vasocorona) anastomoses between anterior and posterior spinal arterial systems, W – sulco-commissural artery, X – rami perforantes of the peripheral (centripetal) system, Y – central (centrifugal) system of sulcal arteries, originating from pial network of the cord; altogether, the pial network and rami perforantes (R+Y) are called the vasocorona or corona vasorum; Z – rami cruciantes (a.k.a. crux vasculosa, a.k.a. rami anastomotici arcuati). Taken with permission from www.neuroangio.org.

2.7.2. Venous Drainage of the Spinal Cord

Broadly speaking, the vertebral venous system can be divided into three components. These are the intradural (extramedullary and intramedullary veins), the extradural (epidural) and the intraossesous/paraspinal veins. Classically, the names used more commonly are anterior external, anterior internal, posterior internal, and posterior external venous plexuses, corresponding to intradural and extradural networks. The epidural venous plexus (refer to figures 2.10 and 2.13) are termed **Batson's plexus.** This venous plexus system has no valves. Thus, an elevated intra-abdominal pressure (due to a tumor mass, abscess or other causes) can cause a retrograde reflux of blood carrying metastatic cells or pelvic infections to the spinal canal and cord.

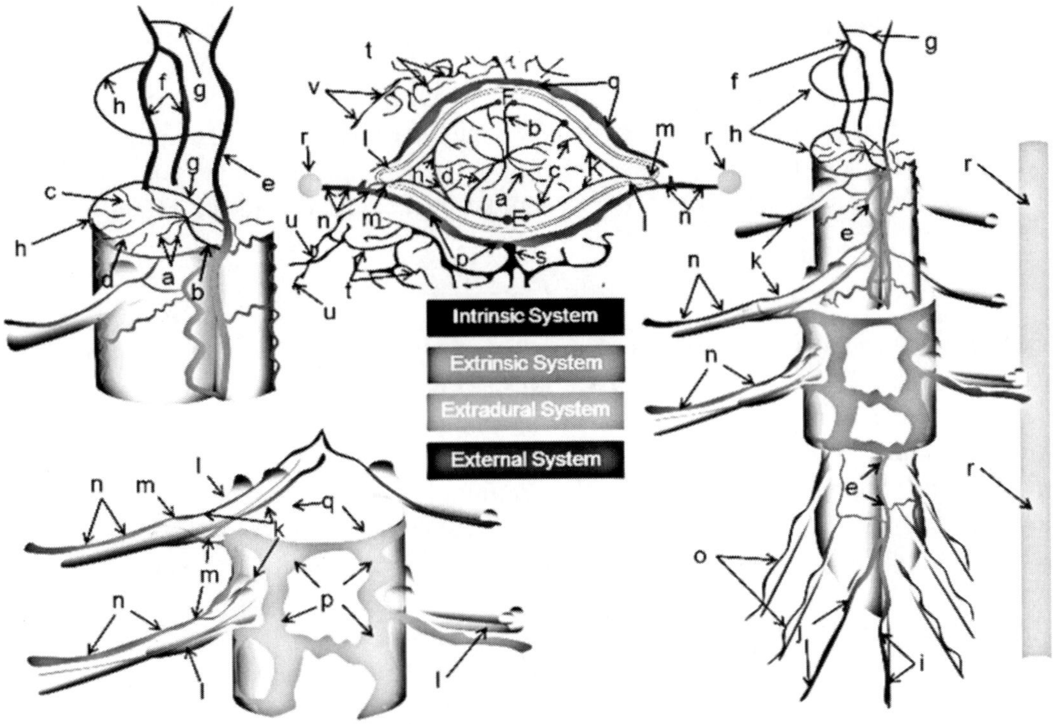

Figure 2.13. Venous drainage architecture of the spinal cord. a –centripetal network of veins, predominantly draining the gray matter into: b – central (sulcal) veins of the intrinsic system; c – peripheral (radial, a.k.a. marginal) centrifugal veins of the intrinsic system; d – venous anastomosis between the centripetal and centrifugal systems; e – anterior (ventral) median vein; f – posterior (dorsal) median vein; g – transmedullary anastomosis between dorsal and ventral median venous systems; h – extrinsic surface anastomosis between dorsal and ventral median veins; i – vein of filum terminale; j – dominant radicular vein of the cauda equina; k – radicular vein (this is the weak link between the cord venous system and the extradural space); l – nerve root sleeve; m – shallow angle of radicular vein piercing the dura of the nerve root sleeve; n – intervertebral vein; o – radicular veins of the cauda equina; p – anterior epidural (a.k.a. ventral intrinsic) venous plexus; q – posterior epidural (a.k.a. dorsal intrinsic) venous plexus; r – ascending spinal (lumbar) vein; s – basivertebral vein, draining the intravertebral body venous plexus (t); u – anterior extrinsic venous plexus surrounding the surface of the vertebral body; v – posterior extrinsic venous plexus on the surface of the lamina /posterior elements, also participating in drainage of the paraspinal muscles. Taken with permission from www.neuroangio.org.

The veins are a capacitance network. As much as 75% of the intracranial blood pool at any given time is situated in the veins. The same probably holds true for the spinal cord, if not more. The intramedullary and extramedullary systems are highly redundant and therefore fail only under extreme circumstances. The weakest link (locus minore resistante), and therefore site of pathology, are the radiculomedullary veins bridging the two systems across the dura. These veins are relatively fewer, and have no secondary support network across the thick dura mater. Thrombosis of these veins is the immediate proximal cause of venous hypertension experienced by patients with spinal dural fistulas.

2.8. Gross Anatomy of the Spine and Coverings

2.8.1. Spinal Meninges

All three protective coverings termed the meninges are continuous from the intracranial cavity to the spinal canal. The most external one, the dura mater, forms the spinal dural sac. The dural sac is attached cranially to the rim of foramen magnum, and is closed caudally. The dural sac is anchored to the coccyx by a bandlike thickening termed the Filum terminale externum. The dural sac is separated from the vertebral bodies and laminae by the epidural space.

The spinal cord is attached to the dural sac via the two types of structures formed by a thickened arachnoid mater. The arachnoid mater, composed as it does in the intracranial cavity, of membranous and weblike layers, forms a few thickenings, adhering the underlying pia and spinal cord to the dural sac. As shown in figures 2.14-2.17, these are the denticulate ligament (limiting rotational movement of the spinal cord relative to the dural sac and vertebral column) and the filum terminale internum, extending caudally from the conus medullaris (the tapering end of the spinal cord) to terminates in the coccyx. The subarachnoid space and the cerebrospinal fluid (CSF) within are continuous with the so named intracranial space.

An enlarged part of the subarachnoid space is present at the L2-S5 vertebral column region, where in the adult no spinal cord is present, only the spinal nerve roots and CSF. This region is termed as the lumbar cistern and is frequently tapped for CSF access in clinical practice.

Since during normal development, the vertebral column and muscles develop much more than the spinal cord, this size discrepancy results in the absence of spinal cord below the L2 level in the normal adults. The spinal canal at this level is occupied by the spinal nerves existing the spinal cord (now ending physically at the L2 level), but leave the spinal canal at the original embryological level. This arrangement has resulted in these spinal nerves termed as the "horse tail" (Caude equine). The pia mater is intimately attached to the surface of the cord, as it does to the brain.

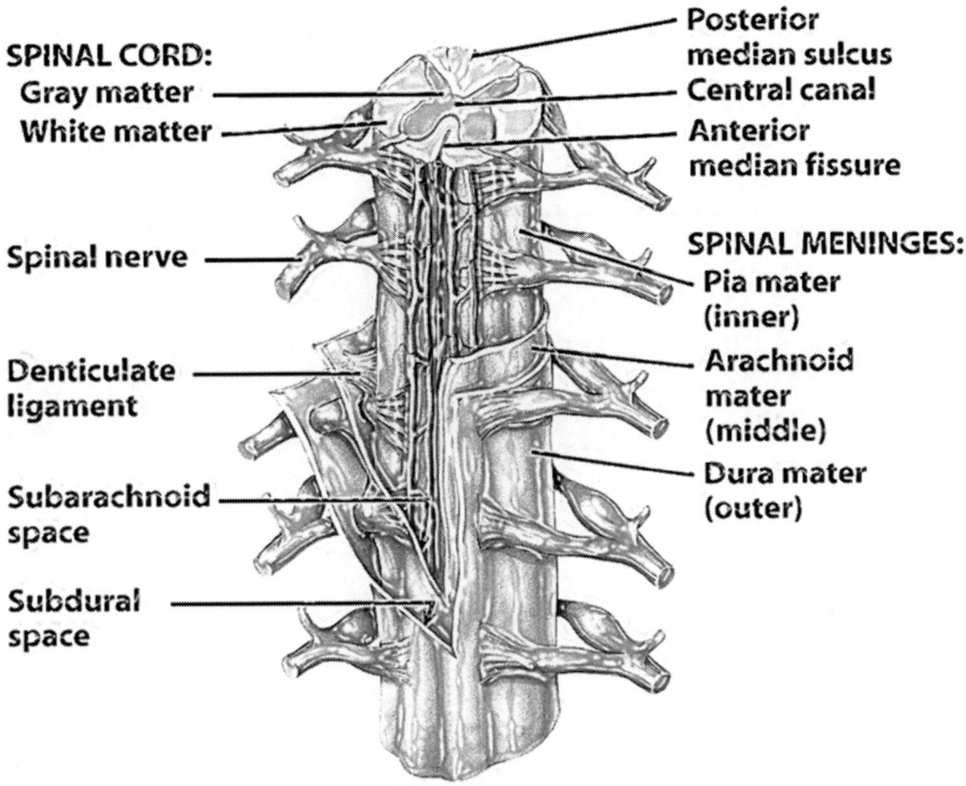

Figure 2.14. An illustration of an anterior view of the spinal cord. Notice the meningeal coverings, the denticulate ligament and the origin of the ventral and dorsal spinal nerve roots.

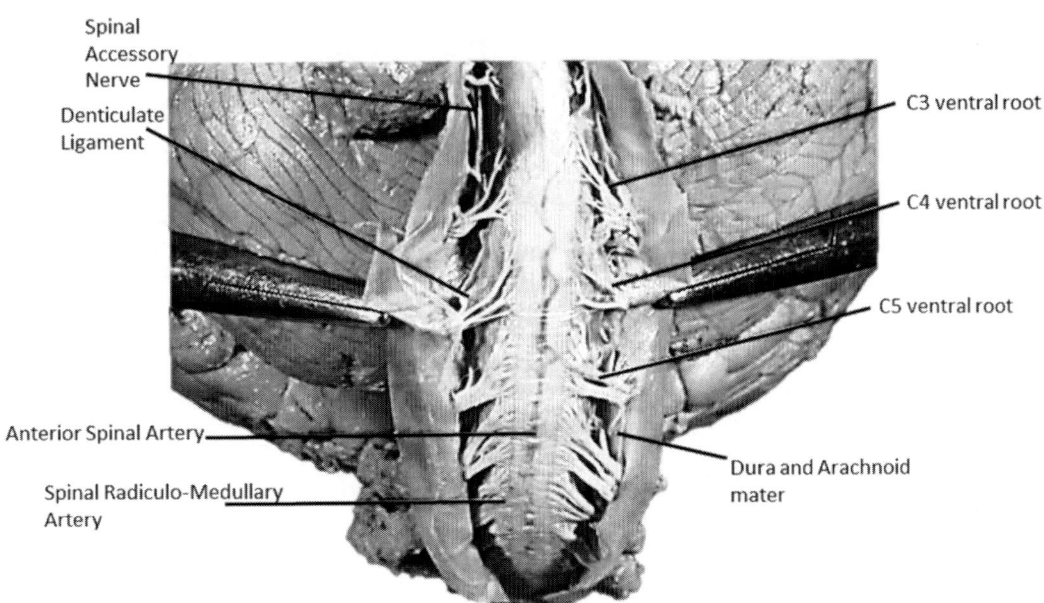

Figure 2.15. Anterior View of the cervical spinal cord.

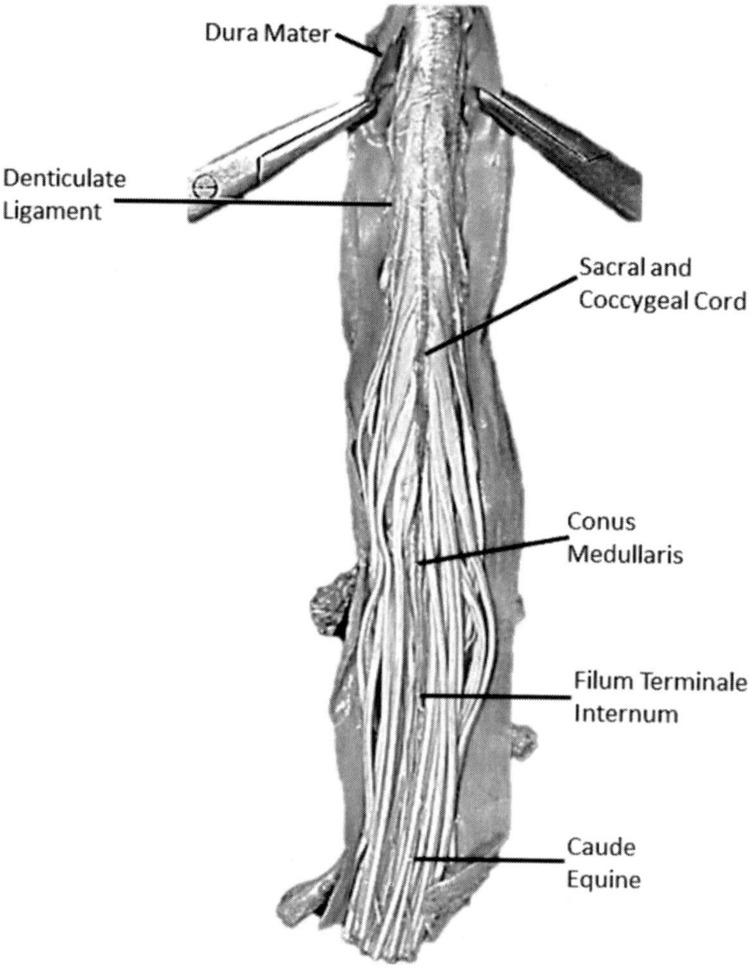

Figure 2.16. Anterior View of the lumbosacral spinal cord and Caude equine.

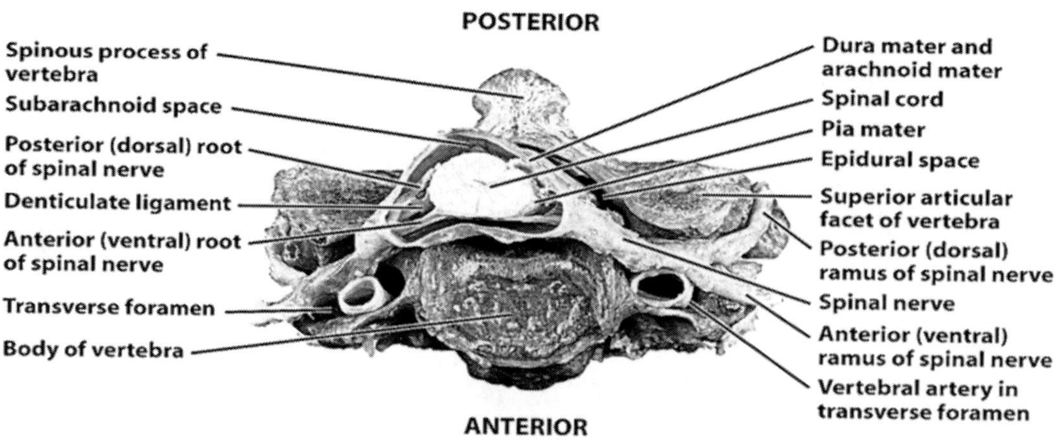

Figure 2.17. An axial section at the level of C4 vertebra, showing the spinal meninges and related spaces.

2.8.2. Surface Features of the Spinal Cord

The spinal cord spans the spinal canal from the level of foramen magnum to the L1~L2 lumbar vertebrae level (in the adult, refer to the neuro-embryology and 2.8.1 for details). The spinal cord consists of eight cervical segments, twelve thoracic segments, five lumbar segments, five sacral segments and one coccygeal segment. This should not be confused with the osseous bony vertebrae, numbered similarly to some extent (except in the cervical region where there are only seven cervical vertebrae, and in the Sacrum considered in osteology as a single bone). Each spinal level is specified by the intervertebral foramina through which the dorsal and ventral roots exit the vertebral canal. The spinal cord has cervical and lumbar enlargements, serving upper & lower limbs. As shown in figure 2.18, the spinal cord has several indentations and grooves throughout its length in addition to specific regional unique features discussed later. These grooves are detailed next.

The **Posterior median sulcus** separates the dorsal portion of the cord into 2 halves. It contains a delicate layer of pia (the posterior median septum). The **posterior lateral sulcus** runs the full length of the cord, representing the entry point of the spinal nerve's dorsal root (Sensory fibers). The **posterior intermediate sulcus and septum** are found in the cervical and upper thoracic regions, between the posterolateral and posteromedian sulci. The **antero-lateral sulcus** marks the exit point for the spinal nerve's ventral Root (motor fibers). The **antero-median fissure** is a prominent space dividing the ventral part into halves. It contains pia strands and more importantly, the sulcal branches of the anterior spinal artery.

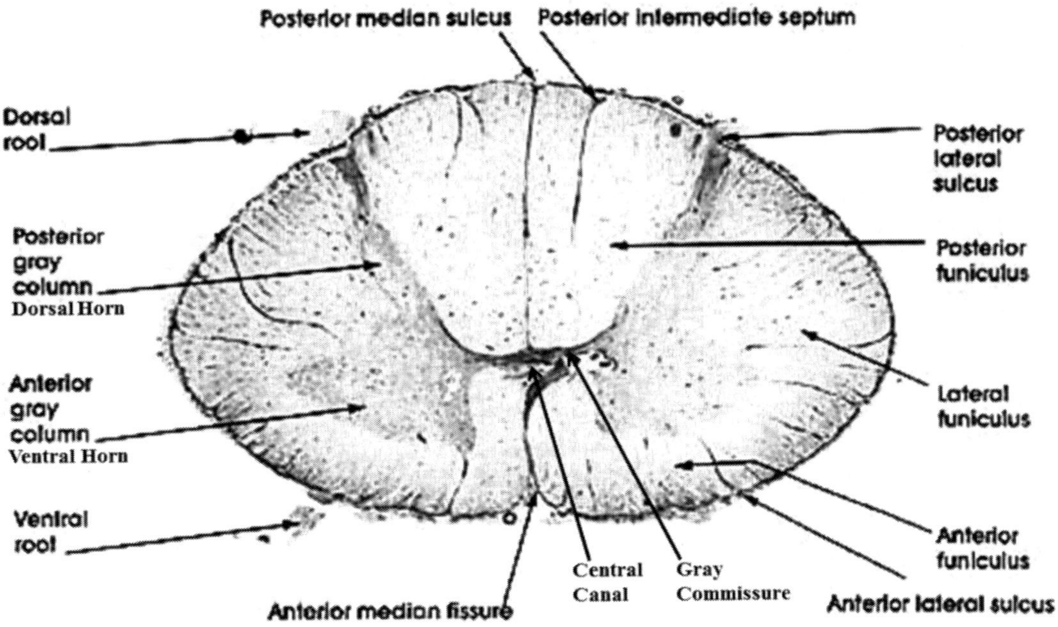

Figure 2.18. A transverse section through the spinal cord showing the different surface markings.

2.8.3. Gross Anatomy of the White Matter

The spinal cord white matter is divided into three regions, each composed of many different tracts (fasciculi, discussed later). Refer to figure 2.18. The **posterior (Dorsal) funiculus** lies between the posterior-median septum and the medial edge of dorsal horn. In the cervical levels of the spinal cord, it consists of the gracile and cuneate fasciculi (also termed as dorsal columns, discussed later). The **lateral funiculus** lies between the postero-lateral and the antero-lateral sulci, and contains clinically important ascending and descending tracts like the lateral corticospinal tract (also termed the pyramidal tract) and the anterolateral system (ALS, also termed the spinothalamic tract). The **anterior (ventral) funiculus** lies between the anterolateral sulcus and the ventromedian fissure. Its content includes the reticulospinal and vestibulospinal fiber tracts, portions of ALS (i.e., the spinothalamic tract), the anterior (ventral) corticospinal tract (i.e., the pyramidal tract) and the Medial longitudinal fasciculus (a composite bundle).

The **anterior spinal white commissure**, by definition a white matter bundle connecting mirror locations on both sides of the cord, is located on the ventral midline, separated from the central canal by a Narrow band of small cells (the so called gray commissure). The **dorsolateral fasciculus** (also termed as the "tract of Lissauer"), is a small bundle of lightly myelinated and unmyelinated fibers, capping the dorsal horn. These are located at the border of the posterior and lateral funiculi and function as part of the ALS (spinothalamic tract, discussed later).

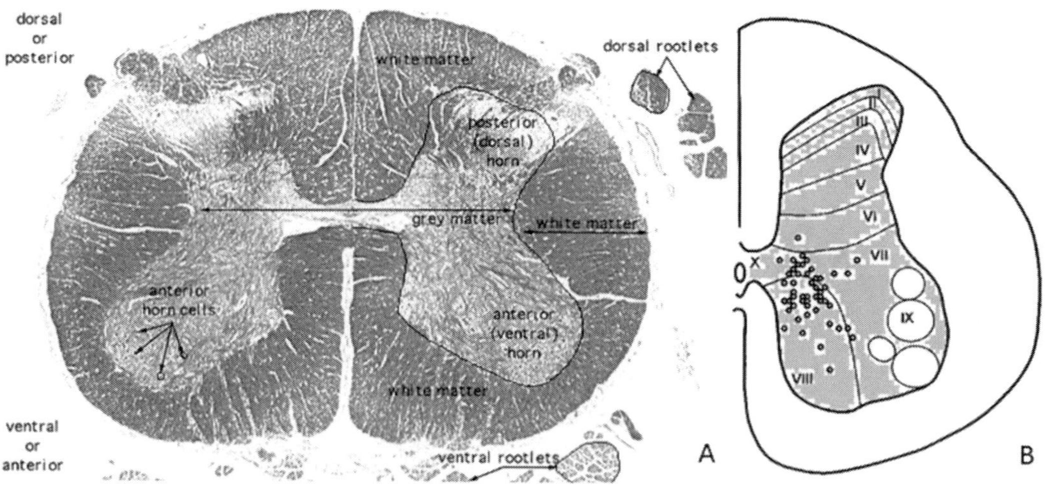

Figure 2.19. Gross Anatomy of the Gray Matter. A, cross section delineating the different gray matter regions. B, Rexed Laminae (refer to text).

2.8.4. Gross Anatomy of the Gray Matter

The center of the spinal cord is composed of a column of gray matter (i.e., cell bodies and dendrites) in the shape of a butterfly. This butterfly of gray matter is divided to two identical sides, controlling ipsilateral body. Within each side, the gray matter is divided into a ventral (anterior) horn (cell columns), a dorsal (posterior) horn (cell columns), and a lateral (intermediate) horn (cell columns) which is unique to the T1-L2 and S2-S4 spinal cord segments (these are substantially smaller columns, carrying VM and VS functions discussed later). The spinal cord gray matter has a bilateral symmetrical structure, the right and left sides are separated by the central canal, a remnant of the neural tube, which is continuous with the fourth ventricle and subarachnoid space. The two sides of the spinal cord are connected by the gray commissure (discussed previously).

This anatomical division of the spinal cord gray matter has functional meaning as well. The ventral horn contains cell bodies of motor neurons and their efferent fibers. The dorsal horns contain cells involved in processing sensory information, and are the targets of afferent sensory fibers entering the cord through the dorsal root. The lateral horn contains cell bodies of ANS (sympathetic and parasympathetic) neurons (refer to figure 2.19).

The Rexed laminae comprise a system of ten layers of grey matter (I-X), identified in the early 1950s by Bror Rexed to label portions of the grey columns of the spinal cord. Similar to the Brodmann areas (discussed in chapter 7), these are defined by their cellular structure rather than by their location, but the location still remains reasonably consistent. The distribution of cells and fibers within the gray matter of the spinal cord exhibits a pattern of lamination. The cellular pattern of each lamina is composed of various sizes or shapes of neurons (cytoarchitecture) which led Rexed to propose a new classification based on 10 layers (laminae). This classification is useful since it is related more accurately to function than the previous classification scheme which was based on major nuclear groups. Refer to table 2.4 for a detailed description of the laminae. Generally speaking, laminae I-IV are concerned with exteroceptive sensations, whereas laminae V and VI are concerned primarily with proprioceptive sensation and act as a relay between the periphery to the midbrain and the cerebellum. Laminae VIII and IX form the final motor pathway to initiate and modulate motor activity via α, β and γ motor neurons, which innervate striated muscle. All visceral motor neurons are located in lamina VII and innervate neurons in autonomic ganglia.

Table 2.4. The Rexed Laminae

Lamina	Other Name	Functions
I	Posteromarginal nucleus	A thin layer of cells that cap the tip of the dorsal horn with small dendrites and a complex array of nonmyelinated axons. Cells in lamina-I respond mainly to noxious and thermal stimuli. Lamina I cell axons join the contralateral spinothalamic tract
II	Substancia gelatinosa	Tightly packed interneurons. This layer responds to noxious stimuli while others respond to non-noxious stimuli. The majority of its neurons receive information from sensory dorsal root ganglion cells as well as descending dorsolateral fasciculus (DLF) fibers. They send axons to Rexed laminae III and IV (fasciculus proprius). Lamina-II is believed to be important for the modulation of sensory input.
III, IV	Fasciculus proprius	Variable cell sizes. Axons of these neurons bifurcate several times and form a dense plexus. Cells contain dendrites of cells from laminae IV, V and VI. Most of the neurons in lamina III function as propriospinal (interneuron) cells. Some of the cells project to the thalamus via the contralateral and ipsilateral spinothalamic tract.
V	Its neurons receive monosynaptic information from $A\beta$, $A\delta$ and C axons which also carry nociceptive information from visceral organs. Many of its cells project to the brain stem and thalamus via the contralateral and ipsilateral ALS.	

Table 2.4. (Continued)

Lamina	Other Name / Functions
VI	Is a broad layer which is best developed in the cervical and lumbar enlargements. Lamina VI divides also into medial and lateral parts.
VII	This region is also known as the zona intermedia (or intermediolateral nucleus). Its shape and boundaries vary along the length of the cord. Lamina VII neurons receive information from Rexed lamina II to VI as well as visceral afferent fibers, and they serve as an intermediary relay in transmission of visceral motor neurons impulses. The dorsal nucleus of Clarke forms a prominent round oval cell column from C8 to L3. The large cells give rise to uncrossed nerve fibers of the dorsal spinocerebellar tract (DSCT). Cells in laminae V to VII, which do not form a discrete nucleus, give rise to uncrossed fibers that form the ventral spinocerebellar tract (VSCT). Cells in the lateral horn of the cord in segments T1 and L3 give rise to preganglionic sympathetic fibers to innervate postganglionic cells located in the sympathetic ganglia outside the cord. Lateral horn neurons at segments S2 to S4 give rise to preganglionic neurons of the sacral parasympathetic fibers to innervate postganglionic cells located in peripheral ganglia.
VIII	This lamina includes an area at the base of the ventral horn, but its shape differs at various cord levels. In the cord enlargements, the lamina occupies only the medial part of the ventral horn, where descending vestibulospinal and reticulospinal fibers terminate. The neurons of lamina VIII modulate motor activity, most probably via γ motor neurons which innervate the intrafusal muscle fibers.
IX	This lamina is composed of several distinct groups of large α motor neurons and small γ and β motor neurons embedded within this layer. Its size and shape differ at various cord levels. In the cord enlargements the number of α motor neurons increase and they form numerous groups. The α motor neurons are large and multipolar cells and give rise to ventral root fibers to supply extrafusal skeletal muscle fibers, while the small γ motor neurons give rise to the intrafusal muscle fibers. The α motor neurons are somatotopically organized
X	Neurons surround the central canal and occupy the commissural lateral area of the gray commissure, which also contains decussating axons.

2.8.5. Regional Characteristics

All spinal levels have dorsal, lateral and ventral funiculi in terms of white matter, and dorsal and ventral gray matter horns. Their shape and proportion vary between major spinal regions. As illustrated in figure 2.20, the cervical (C4-T1) and lumbosacral (L1-S2) cord shows prominent dorsal and ventral horns (due to abundance of sensory input and motor output to the limbs). At the thoracic level, the dorsal and ventral horns are smaller. The cervical spinal cord is oval, having large amount of white matter (since the full component of ascending and descending tracts are present at this level). Horns (dorsal and ventral) are small at the C1-C3 segment level, but large at C4-C8 level (due to participation of the C4-C8 cord in upper extremity innervation).

The thoracic spinal cord is round, showing small horns. From cephalad to caudal direction, a progressive decrease in white matter is seen in the funiculi. A few unique structures to this segment include Clarke's dorsal nucleus, located at the medial aspect of Rexed lamina VII. Its axons project to the cerebellum. The lateral horn, also part of lamina VII, is unique at this segment as well. It is a protrusion into the lateral funiculus formed by the intermediolateral cell column (at times seen from c7-c8 level). These are preganglionic sympathetic neurons, whose axons will terminate at peripheral ganglia, the paravertebral sympathetic chain).

The Lumbar spinal cord is round, having large horns and less white matter than higher levels. The Sacral spinal cord is round and smaller than in the lumbar segment, consisting mainly of gray matter, with a thin shell of white matter. Intermediate gray matter of S2-S4, contains Preganglionic parasympathetic cell Bodies (Sacral VM nucleus, AKA Onuf's nucleus).

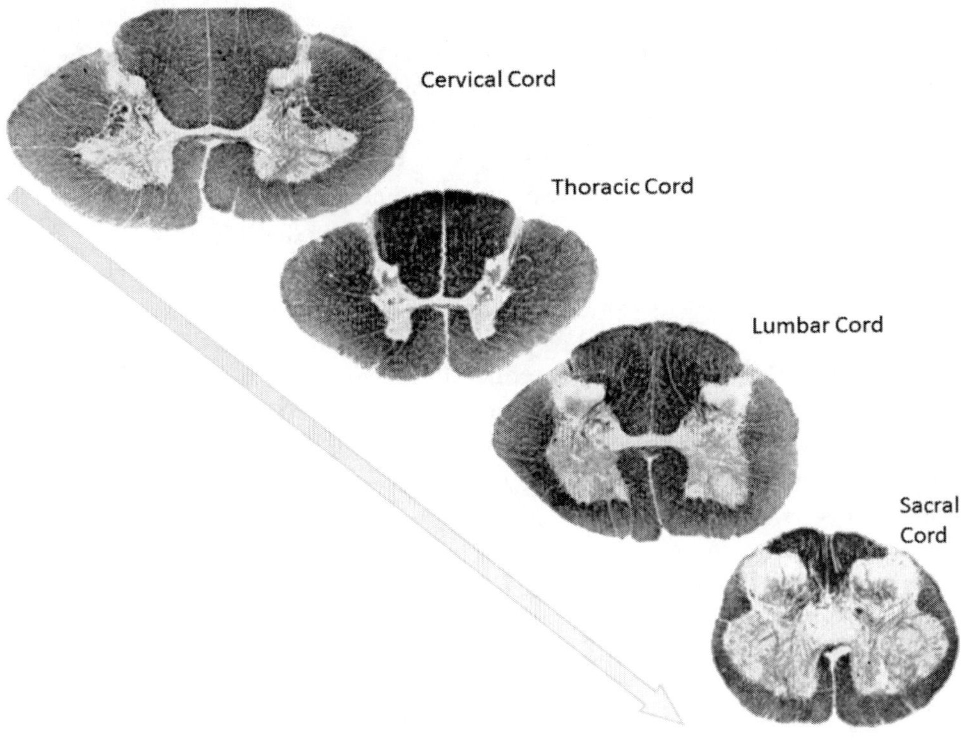

Figure 2.20. Regional Characteristics of the spinal cord at different levels.

2.9. Important Pathways and Tracts

The white matter bundles and fascicles within the spinal cord serve one of two functions. It may be a part of a long ascending or descending tract, linking this spinal cord region to higher levels of the neuroaxis conducting the information. Some descending fibers modulate the transmission of nociceptive information in dorsal horn, while others influence the activity of motor neurons. White matter fibers may be propriospinal fibers as well, projecting from one spinal level to another, forming the anatomical basis for intraspinal reflexes. In any event, the taxonomy of tracts is simple and predictive. The tract name should incorporate the origin and destination of the neural information, ordered according to the direction of information transfer. Thus, the spinothalamic tract, by virtue of its name only, implies that the information conducted in it is originating from the spinal cord and destined to the thalamus. As such, it is an ascending tract. Being an ascending tract, as a general rule, implies that the information is sensory in nature. Similarly, the bulbospinal tract is originated in the brainstem (bulbar part), destined to reach the spinal cord carrying descending information. Descending information, as a general rule, is motor in nature.

2.9.1. Ascending Tracts

2.9.1.1. Dorsal Funiculus Tracts - The Dorsal Columns

These are the Gracile, cuneate fasciculi (central processes of heavily myelinated fibers), conveying proprioceptive, tactile and vibratory information from ipsilateral body. The name refers to its location in the posterior (dorsal) funiculus. The fibers of the gracile tract originate below the level of the sixth thoracic vertebra, whereas the fibers of the cuneate tract originate above the level of the sixth thoracic vertebra. This somatotopic arrangement with the lower parts of the body represented more medially, is unique. As discussed later, in most other spinal tracts, the upper parts of the body are represented medially with progressively lower parts of the body as we progress laterally in the tract. Injury to the tract on one side results in an ipsilateral loss of proprioception, discriminative touch, vibratory sense, below the level of the lesion.

The peripheral sensory neuron (also termed first neuron in pathway) has its cell body in the dorsal root ganglion, dendrite in the periphery in close proximity to the receptor and its axon entering the spinal cord through the dorsal root. This axon (still belonging to the first neuron) then ascends with no processing to the so named nuclei located in the medulla oblongata (gracile and cuneate Nuclei). It is here that the first synapse occurs. The second neuron, now belonging to a broad white matter band called the medial lemniscus than decussates (crosses the midline in a symmetric manner) and ascends contralaterally to reach the thalamus (the VPL nucleus, discussed later). A second synapse occurs here, from which the third neuron ascends to reach the primary somatosensory cortex, located at the post-central gyrus. Refer to figure 2.21a, 2.22 for an illustration of the path.

2.9.1.2. Lateral Funiculus Tracts

2.9.1.2.1. Posterior and Anterior Spinocerebellar Tracts

These tracts are located on the lateral surface of the cord white matter (lateral funiculus), meeting at the level of the denticulate ligament. The posterior spinocerebellar tract has fibers that arise from the Clarke's nucleus (Rexed lamina VII at the T1-L2 cord levels). The anterior spinocerebellar tract has fibers that arise from the cells of Rexed lamina V-VIII and from large ventral horn neurons (spinal border cells) at the lumbosacral level. These tracts carry unconscious proprioception information from muscles and joints of the lower extremity to the cerebellum. Refer to figure 2.22.

2.9.1.2.2. Antero-Lateral System (The Spinothalamic Tract)

This important tract is located in the ventrolateral area of the lateral funiculus (refer to figure 2.21b, 2.22). This pathway system encompasses those regions of white matter that were divided into the anterior & lateral spinothalamic tracts. This tract contains spino-thalamic fibers, spino-mesencephalic fibers, spino-hypothalamic fibers and spino-reticular fibers. The first order neuron entering the cord through the dorsal horn synapses at the dorsal root ganglion almost immediately or shortly after entering the spinal cord. The short distance span these fibers travel before synapsing is manifested anatomically by the existence of the Dorsolateral Fasciculus (also termed as the "tract of Lissauer", refer to 2.8.3 and Table 2.4).

Upon synapsing, the second order neuron decussates in the white commissure and ascends contralaterally in the ALS tract to reach the thalamus (VPL nucleus discussed later). From there, the third order neuron ascends to reach the primary somatosensory cortex, located at the post-central gyrus of the parietal lobe. The ALS (spinothalamic tract) conveys nociceptive, thermal, and touch information. An injury to the tract at the spinal cord level will result in loss of these sensory modalities contralaterally, one to two segments below the lesion. This tract is somatotopically organized, in a way that the lower portions of the body are represented dorsolaterally, progressively more ventromedially as we ascend in the body.

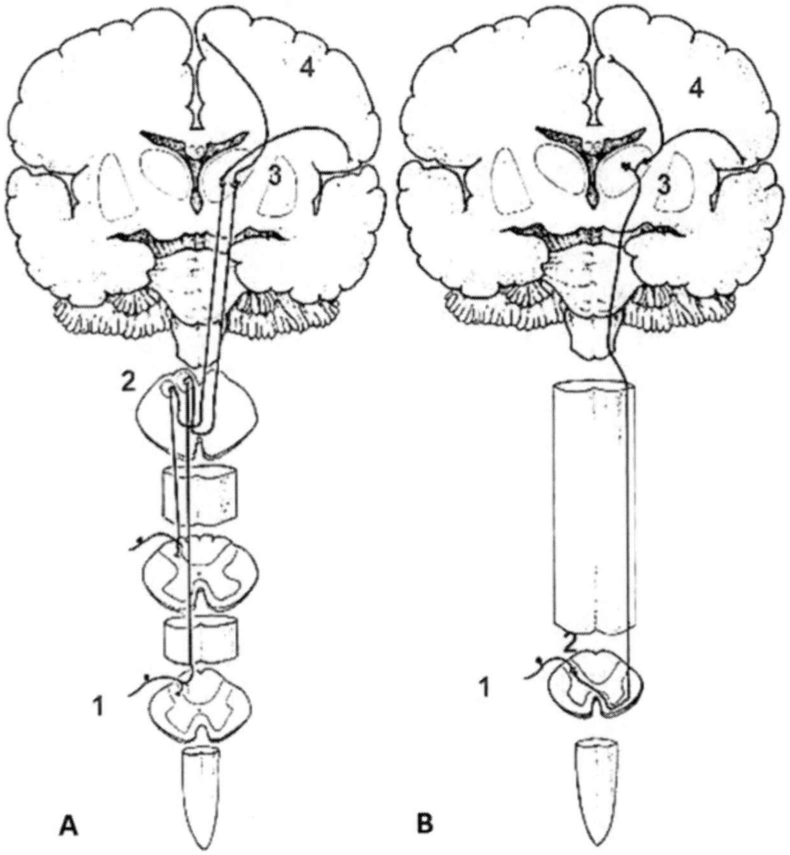

Figure 2.21. Ascending tracts. A, The dorsal columns. 1-First sensory neuron entering the dorsal column through the dorsal root ascending ipsilaterally. 2-the gracile / cuneate nucleus of lower medulla oblongata, first synapse occur, next the second neuron decussates (the so called sensory decussation) and ascends contralaterally as the medial lemniscus to reach the thalamus. 3-Thalamus, VPL nucleus for information from the body. 4-Primary somatosensory cortex, post-central gyrus of the parietal lobe. B, The Spinothalamic tract. 1-First sensory neuron entering the dorsal column through the dorsal root enter and synapse shortly after entering the cord (within 1-2 segments). 2-Second order neurons than decussate to ascend in the contralateral ALS. 3-VPL nucleus of the thalamus. 4-Primary somatosensory cortex, post-central gyrus of the parietal lobe.

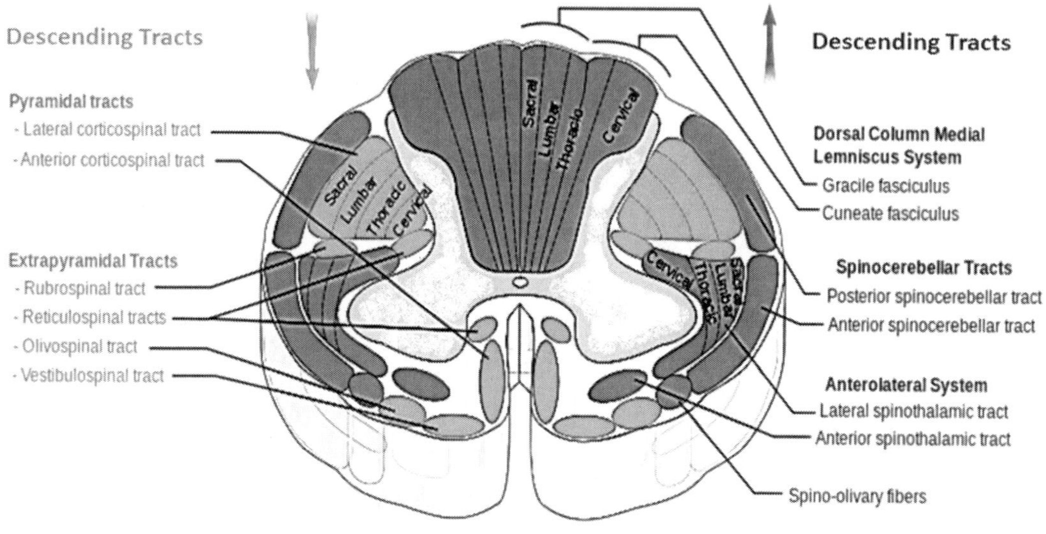

Figure 2.22. Summery of Ascending (Sensory) and Descending (Motor) Tracts.

2.9.1.3. Ventral (Anterior) Funiculus Tracts

In the ventral column (funiculus) there are four prominent tracts. The **paleospinothalamic** tract (or anterior spinothalamic tract), carries pain, temperature, and information associated with touch to the brain stem nuclei and to the diencephalon. The **spinoolivary** tract carries information from Golgi tendon organs to the cerebellum. The **spinoreticular** tract and the **spinotectal** tract. Intersegmental nerve fibers traveling for several segments (2 to 4) and are located as a thin layer around the gray matter is known as fasciculus proprius, spinospinal or archispinothalamic tract. It carries pain information to the brain stem and diencephalon (refer to table 2.4, figure 2.22).

2.9.2. Descending Tracts

The descending tracts originate from different cortical areas and from brain stem nuclei. The descending pathway carry information associated with maintenance of motor activities such as posture, balance, muscle tone, and visceral and somatic reflex activity.

Descending upper motor neurons (UMN) pathways arise from the cerebral cortex and brainstem. These are divided according to location in the spinal cord into **Lateral and medial motor systems.** The lateral systems synapse on the more lateral groups of ventral horn motor nerves. These include the lateral corticospinal tract and the rubrospinal tract. The

Medial motor systems are located in the anteromedial cord column (Funiculus) and synapse on medial ventral horn motor neurons. These include the anterior corticospinal tract, the vestibulospinal tract, the reticulospinal tract and the tectospinal tract.

2.9.2.1. Important Descending Tracts in the Lateral Funiculus

2.9.2.1.1. The Lateral Corticospinal Tract

This tract, also termed the pyramidal tract (due to the pyramidal process it creates at ventral medulla oblongata) arises from the cortex primary somatomotor center, located at the pre-central gyrus of the frontal bone. The first UMN then descends through the brainstem. It passes through the internal capsule, crus cerebri (middle portion) and ventral Pons and Medulla oblongata (details discussed at the specific chapters). At the medulla oblongata spinal cord junction, most fibers converge to form this tract, but some remain to form the anterior corticospinal tract (lateral to the anterior-median fissure). Nerve fibers are somatotopically arranged in a way that fibers originating from the leg areas of cortex and destined to reach lower motor neurons (LMN) in the lumbosacral levels are located more laterally in the tract, while those destined to reach LMN in the cervical levels of the cord, from arm areas of cortex, are more medially located. This tract functions to influence spinal motor neurons (especially the distal muscles). Refer to figure 2.23 for an illustration.

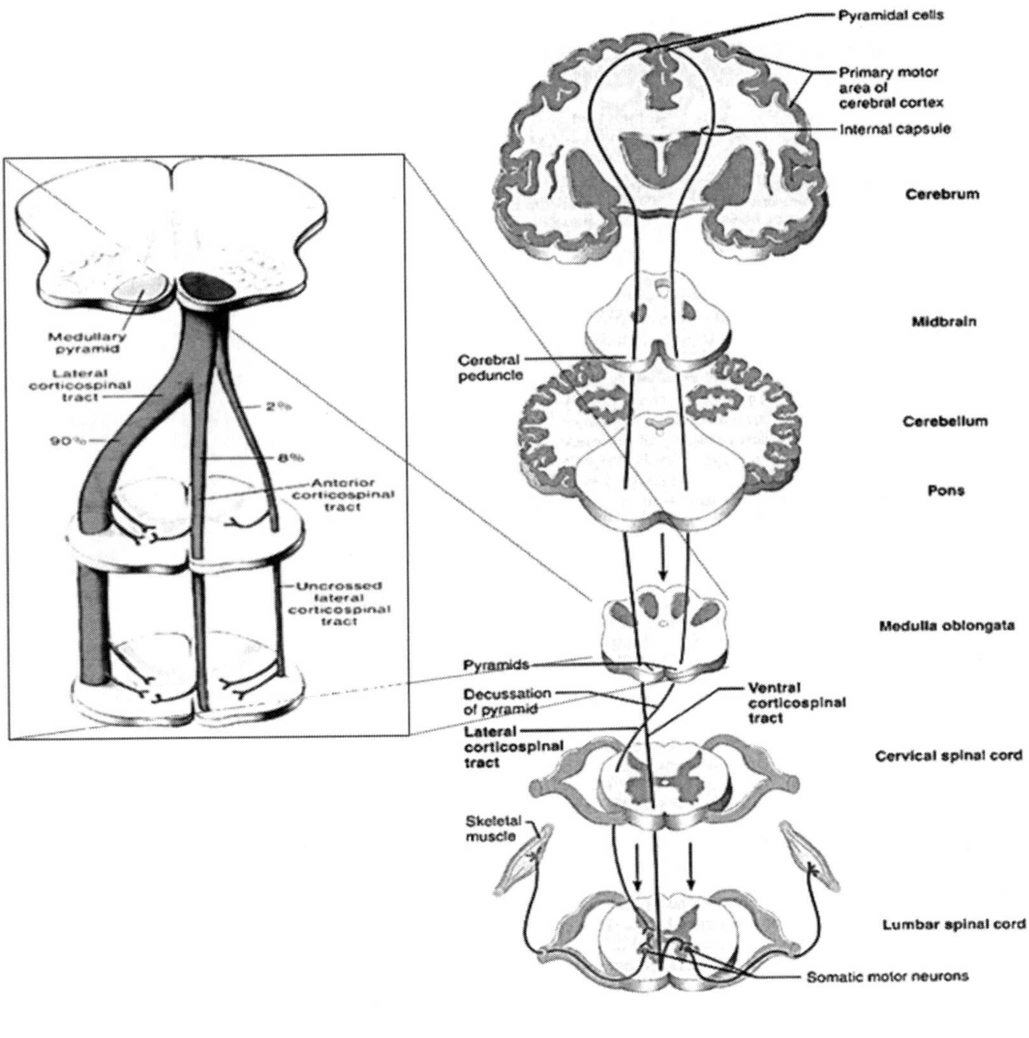

Figure 2.23. The Corticospinal (Pyramidal) Tract. Refer to the text.

2.9.2.1.2. The Rubrospinal Tract

The rubrospinal tract is a part of the lateral indirect extra-pyramidal tract. Fibers arise from the red nucleus of midbrain, descending with the lateral corticospinal tract fibers (located just anterior to these). It is one of the pathways for the mediation of voluntary movement. The tract is responsible for large muscle movement as well as fine motor control, and it terminates primarily in the cervical spinal cord, suggesting that it functions in upper limb but not in lower limb control. It primarily facilitates flexion in the upper extremities (see decorticate posture).

2.9.2.2. Important Descending tracts Diffusely Arranged

The **reticulospinal tract** originates from the medullary reticular formation. At the spinal level, these fibers are uncrossed. It is an extrapyramidal motor tract that descends from the reticular formation in two tracts to act on the motor neurons supplying the trunk and proximal limb muscles. It is involved mainly in locomotion and postural control, although it does have other effects as well. This tract influences muscle tone, mediates autonomic functions, modulates pain impulses and was found to influence blood flow to lateral geniculate nucleus of the thalamus.

The **fastigiospinal tract**, originating from the so named nucleus of cerebellum is crossed at the spinal level, terminating on motor neurons. The **raphespinal tract** originates from the raphe nucleus of the brainstem and descends bilaterally in the dorsal lateral funiculus. It modulates transmission of nocicpetive information at the spinal level. The **Hypothalamospinal tract** influences the activity of the intermediolateral cell column. Its fibers descend through the lateral brainstem and spinal cord.

2.9.2.3. Important Descending Tracts in the Anterior Funiculus

The **reticulospinal** tract fibers arise from the pontine reticular formation of brainstem. The **lateral vestibulospinal** tract fibers arising from Lateral vestibular nuclei. The lateral part of the vestibulospinal tract is composed of fibers originating in the lateral, superior, and inferior vestibular nuclei (primarily the lateral). It projects ipsilaterally down to the lumbar region of the spinal cord. There it helps to maintain an upright and balanced posture by stimulating extensor motor neurons in the legs. It also innervates muscles of the trunk, thus additionally aiding in body posture. The lateral vestibular nuclei receive input from cerebellum, particularly the vestibulocerebellum, or the flocculi and nodulus. The cerebellum aids in coordinating postural adjustments. The **Anterior corticospinal** tract (discussed previously, see figure 2.23) has uncrossed fibers, most of which cross in the ventral white commissure before terminating on medial Motor neurons to axial muscles.

The **medial longitudinal fasciculus (MLF),** discussed in great detail in the section on the brainstem, is composed of a few fiber tracts. The **medial vestibulospinal** tract (from the so named nucleus)**, the tectospinal** tract (exists on in cervical levels of the cord) and the **interstitiospinal tract** (arising from the interstitial nucleus of rostral midbrain), which also extends to the lower cord, to terminate in lamina VII-VIII.

2.10. Neuroanatomy of Micturition and the Lower Urinary Tract

2.10.1. Central Nervous System Control of Micturition

2.10.1.1. Cortex, Basal Ganglia, and Cerebellum Control of Micturition

The Antero-medial portion of the frontal lobes of the cerebral cortex and cingulate gyrus are involved in the voluntary initiation of micturition and inhibition of reflex voiding activity. In general, cortical input is inhibitory on micturition reflexes. Lesions resulting from tumors, aneurysms, or cerebrovascular disease remove the cortical inhibition, which results in increased excitatory input to the brainstem, facilitation of the micturition reflex, and the clinical appearance of urinary frequency and urgency.

2.10.1.2. Pons Control of Micturition

Although the process of micturition involves anatomic regions throughout the CNS and PNS, the center of this reflex can be localized to the pontomesencephalic reticular formation. The pontine micturition center (PMC), or Barrington's nucleus, functions as a switch to regulate bladder capacity and coordinate bladder and external sphincter activity. Descending spinal efferent pathways from the PMC to the sacral cord motor centers are located in the reticulospinal tracts.

2.10.1.3. Spinal Cord Control of Micturition

The primary excitatory input to the bladder is the parasympathetic preganglionic neurons located in the intermedio-lateral gray matter of the sacral cord in segments S2-4. Sympathetic preganglionic neurons are located in antero-medio-lateral gray matter of thoracolumbar cord in segments T9-L1. Sensory and proprioceptive afferents ascend through the posterior columns of the cord. Somatic centers innervating the external sphincter and pelvic floor musculature are localized at Onuf's nucleus within the anterior horn of the sacral cord at the spinal cord level S2-4.

2.10.2. Peripheral Nerves Control of Micturition

Preganglionic sympathetic pathways from the T9 to L1 segments of the spinal cord pass through the spinal roots to the sympathetic chain ganglia, prevertebral ganglia in the superior hypogastric and pelvic plexuses, and the short adrenergic neurons in the bladder and urethra. Sympathetic nerves course vertically along the anteromedial portion of the vertebral bodies in the sympathetic chain and form plexuses at the celiac, superior hypogastric, and inferior hypogastric branches of the aorta. Dissection of the retroperitoneum, particularly around the great vessels, can disrupt the pelvic sympathetic innervation.

Parasympathetic nerves travel through the sacral spinal nerve roots and form the pelvic splanchnic nerves. The pelvic nerves coalesce with the sympathetic nerves in the pelvic plexus. Injury to the parasympathetic nerves can occur during rectal surgery, uterine surgery, and dissection posterior to bladder. Efferent somatic stimulation of the external sphincter begins in the ventral horn of the sacral cord (Onuf's nucleus) and travels via the pudendal nerves. Somatic input travels via the pudendal nerve in Alcock's canal in the perineum and innervates the striated sphincter and the pelvic floor. Injury can occur as a result of pelvic fracture or perineal surgery.

2.10.3. Summary and Implications

Micturition is organized as a series of "on-off" reflexes at various levels of the neuraxis. Voluntary voiding occurs as a result of sudden relaxation and opening of the bladder outlet and external sphincter coordinated with detrusor contraction of adequate magnitude. The normal micturition event is coordinated at the level of the pons via ascending and descending spinal pathways to ensure opening of the bladder outlet just before the onset of voluntary detrusor contraction. Depending on the specific neurological lesion, voiding reflexes may be facilitated (resulting in urgency and frequency) or suppressed (resulting in urinary retention). Storage and evacuation of urine should occur at low pressure. When high pressure exists within the urinary tract, regardless of the cause, consequences include urinary tract infections, stones, upper urinary tract deterioration, and eventual renal failure.

2.11. Clinical Correlation

2.11.1. Definitions

Tetraplegia (Quadriplegia) is the impairment or loss of motor and/or sensory function in the cervical segments of the spinal cord due to damage of neural elements within the spinal canal. It results in impairment of function in the arms as well as in the trunk, legs and pelvic organs. It does not include brachial plexus lesions or injury to peripheral nerves outside the neural canal.

Paraplegia refers to the impairment or loss of motor and/or sensory function in the thoracic, lumbar or sacral (not cervical) segments of the spinal cord, secondary to damage of neural elements within spinal canal. With paraplegia, arm functioning is spared, but depending on the level of injury, the trunk, legs and pelvic organs may be involved. The term is used in referring to cauda equine and conus medullaris injuries, but not to lumbosacral plexus lesions or injury to peripheral nerves outside the neural canal.

Quadriparesis / paraparesis. The use of these terms is discouraged, as they describe incomplete lesions imprecisely. Instead, the ASIA Impairment Scale (table 2.5) and the muscle strength grading scale (table 2.6) provide a more precise approach.

UMN versus LMN injury. These concepts have been introduced previously. The damage to either UMN or LMN presents very differently. The ventral horn LMN cell bodies are under constant tonic inhibition by the UMN. Thus, damage to the UMN results in disinhibition of the LMN, manifesting spasticity. On the other hand, normal LMN firing levels are required for muscle viability and mass. Hence, a LMN injury results among other presentations with muscle atrophy and uncontrolled minimal contractions (fasciculations). Refer to table 2.7 for a comparison between the two syndromes.

Neurological level of injury refers to the most caudal segment of the spinal cord with normal sensory and motor function on both sides of the body. In fact, the segments at which normal function is found often differ by side of body and in terms of sensory vs. motor testing. Thus, up to four different segments may be identified in determining the neurological level. These are the sensory level for right and left sides and the motor level for right and left sides.

Incomplete injury. If partial preservation of sensory and/or motor functions is found below the neurological level and includes the lowest sacral segment, the injury is defined as incomplete. Sacral sensation includes sensation at the anal mucocutaneous junction and deep anal sensation. The test of motor function is the presence of voluntary contraction of the external anal sphincter upon digital examination.

Complete injury. This term is used when there is an absence of sensory and motor function in the lowest sacral segment.

Zone of partial preservation (ZPP). This term refers to those dermatomes and myotomes caudal to the neurological level that remain partially innervated. When some impaired sensory and/or motor function is found below the lowest normal segment, the exact number of segments so affected should be recorded for both sides as the ZPP. This term is used only with complete injuries.

Table 2.5. The ASIA impairment Scale

A	Complete	No motor or sensory function preserved in segments S4-S5
B	Incomplete	Sensory but not motor function preserved below the neurologic level
C		Motor function preserved below the neurologic level (>1/2 of key muscles have a grade <3)
D		Motor function preserved below the neurologic level (<1/2 of key muscles have a grade ≥3)
E	Normal	

Table 2.6. Muscle Strength Grading Scale

Grade	Strength		
0	No contraction (total paralysis)		
1	Flicker or trace contraction (fasciculations, palpable or visible)		
2	Active movement with gravity eliminated		
3	Active movement against gravity		
4	Active movement against resistance	4-	Slight resistance
		4	Moderate resistance
		4+	Strong resistance
5	Normal strength (against full resistance)		

Table 2.7. Comparing UMN and LMN Paralysis

Parameters	UMN* Paralysis	LMN+ Paralysis
Possible Etiologies	Stroke, spinal cord injury	Herniated disc, nerve entrapment, polio
Muscle Tone	Initially flaccid than spastic (with clasp-knife resistance)	Flaccid
Tendon Reflexes	Hyperactive, clonus	Absent
Pathologic Reflexes (Babinski, Hoffman)	Present (after days-weeks)	Absent
Muscle Manifestations	Spasms may occur and very mild atrophy of disuse	Fibrillations, fasciculations, atrophy within days-weeks.

*upper motor neuron, +lower motor neuron

2.11.2. Physical Neurological Examination

The basic physical neurological examination has two components (sensory and motor), which are separately described. Further, the neurological examination has both required as well as optional, elements. The required elements are used in determining the sensory motor and neurological levels, in generating scores to characterize sensory or motor functioning and in determining completeness of the injury. The optional measures, though not used in scoring, may add to a specific patient's clinical description. When the patient is not fully testable, i.e., when a key sensory point or key muscle is not testable for any reason, the examiner should record `NT' (not testable) instead of a numeric score. The required portion of the sensory examination is completed through the testing of a key point in each of the 28 dermatomes on the right and on the left sides of the body. At each of these key points, two aspects of sensation are examined, the sensitivity to pin prick and to light touch. Appreciation of a pin prick and of light touch at each of the key points is separately scored on a scale (refer to table 2.8). In addition to bilateral testing of these key points, the external anal sphincter should be tested through insertion of the examiner's finger. Perceived sensation should be graded as being present or absent. This information is needed in determining completeness/ incompleteness of injury.

The required portion of the motor examination is completed through the testing of a key muscle (one on the right and one of the left sides of the body) in the 10 paired myotomes. Each key muscle should be examined in a rostral-caudal sequence. Table 2.9 summarizes the key motor and sensory landmarks according to spinal root level together with actions to be tested, assigned reflexes and sensory dermatome. This knowledge serves as the basic medical knowledge required from any medical doctor before stepping foot in the emergency room or ward.

Table 2.8. Sensory Grading Scale

Grade 0	Absent
Grade 1	Impaired (partial / altered)
Grade 2	Normal

Table 2.9. Key motor and sensory landmarks

Level	Muscle	Action to test	Reflex	Sensory dermatome
C2				Occipital protuberance
C3				Supraclavicular fossa
C4	Diaphragm	Tidal volume, vital capacity, FEV1		Top of acromio-clavicular joint
C5	Biceps, deltoid	Flex elbow, abduct arm	Biceps	Lateral antecubital fossa
C6	Wrist extensors	Cock up wrist	Supinator	Thumb, dorsal surface, proximal phalanx
C7	Triceps	Extend elbow	Triceps	Middle finger, dorsal surface, proximal phalanx
C8	FDP	Grasp		Little finger, dorsal surface, proximal phalanx
T1	Hand intrinsics	Abduct little finger		Medial (ulnar) side of antecubital fossa
T2-9	Intercostals	Use sensory level, abdominal reflexes & Beevor's sign		T2 – apex of axilla, T4 – nipple line,
T9-10	Upper abdominals			T10 - umbilicus
T11-12	Lower abdominals			T12 – mid inguinal ligament
L2	Iliopsoas	Hip flexion	Cremasteric	Mid- anterior thigh
L3	Quadriceps	Knee extension	Knee jerk	Medial femoral condyle
L4	Tibialis anterior	Ankle dorsiflexion	Medial hamstrings	Medial malleolus
L5	EHL	Dorsiflex big toe		Dorsum foot at 3rd metatarsal phalangeal joint
S1	Gastrocnemius	Plantar-flexion of foot	Achilles	Lateral heel
S2	Flexor digitorum, flexor halluces			Popliteal fossa in midline
S3	Bladder, bowel, anal sphincter			Ischial tuberosity
S4-5				Perianal region

2.11.3. Clinical Syndromes

There are many different clinical syndromes involving spinal cord injuries. For tutorial purposes, we have selected a few demonstrative syndromes, whose clinical presentation relies heavily on anatomical localization and details. Generally speaking, although holds true in general, the promise that a detailed anatomical knowledge assists directly in the clinical diagnosis is more valid for the spinal cord than any other segment of the CNS. Refer to table 2.10 and figures 2.24-2.27.

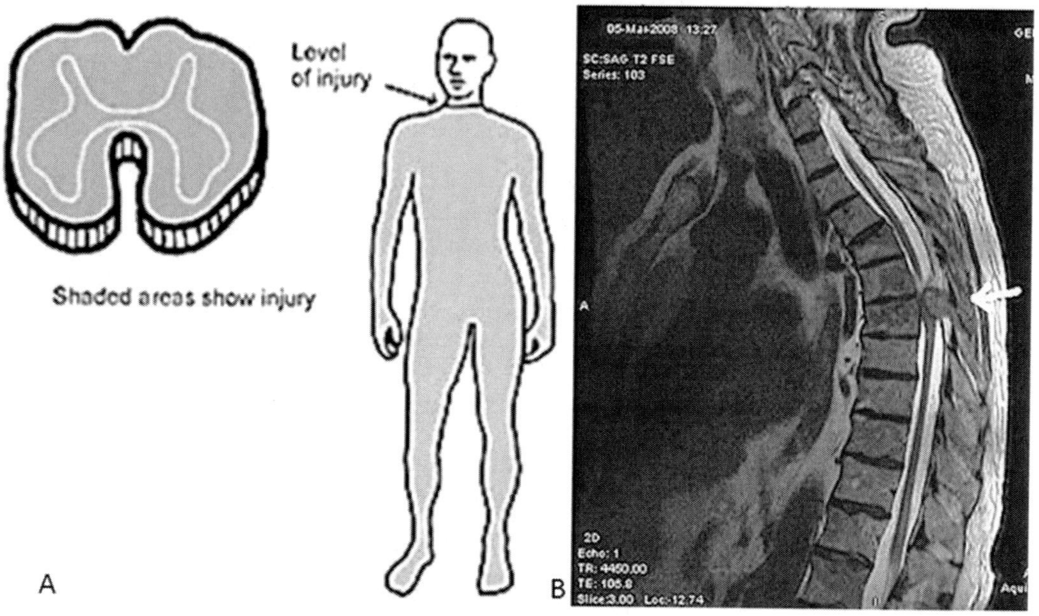

Figure 2.24. Complete Spinal Cord Injury. A, A diagram showing the cord area and affected body regions. B, a lower injury, an upper thoracic mass compressing on the posterior spinal canal obliterating completely this cavity and resulting in paraplegia.

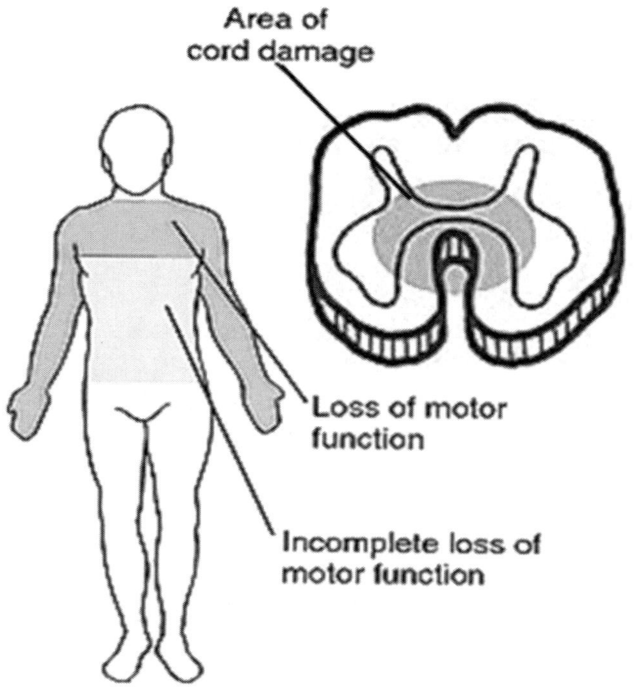

Figure 2.25. Central Cord Syndrome.

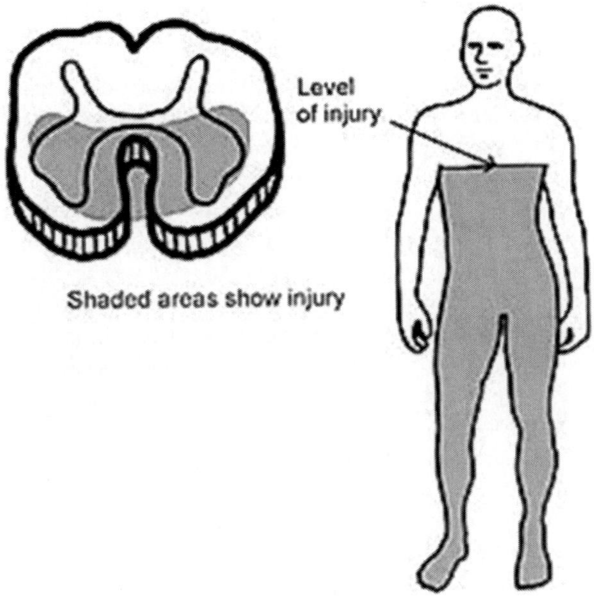

Figure 2.26. Anterior Cord Syndrome. Refer to the Text.

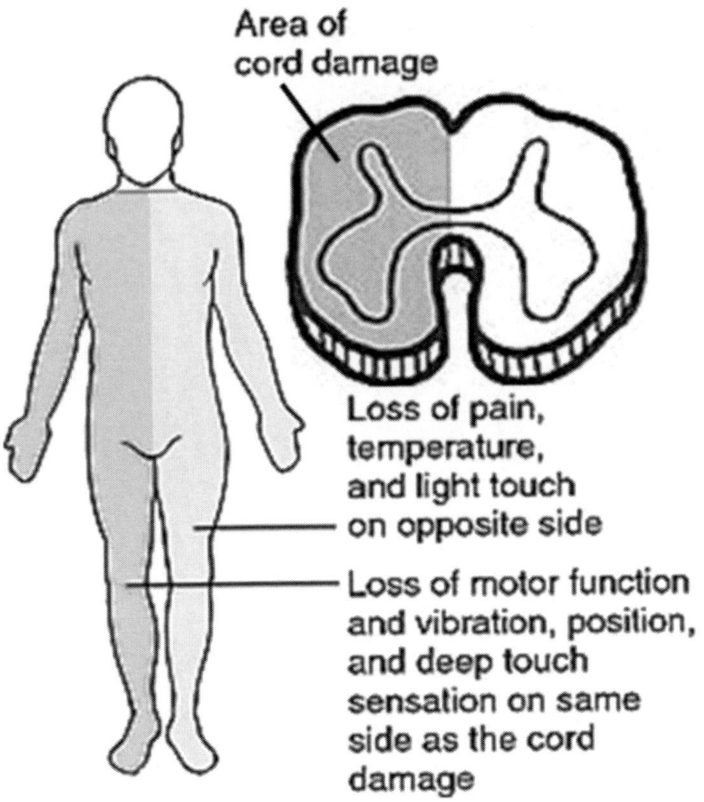

Figure 2.27. Brown-Sequard syndrome. Refer to text.

Table 2.10. Clinical Syndromes in Spinal Cord Injury

Transverse cord lesion		All sensory and motor pathways are interrupted (Figure 2.24).
Central cord syndrome	A lesion occurring almost exclusively in the cervical region that produces sacral sensory sparing and greater weakness in the upper limbs than in the lower limbs (Figure 2.25).	
	Small lesions	Damage to spinothalamic fibers, crossing the anterior commissure, causes bilateral regions of suspended sensory loss to pain and temperature (termed sensory dissociation). When in cervical region, classical cape distribution.
	Larger lesions	Anterior horn cells are damaged, producing LMN. The corticospinal tract is also affected causing UMN signs. Dorsal columns and ALS may be involved.
Posterior cord	Dorsal (Posterior) Columns are affected (due to trauma, compression, Multiple sclerosis, B12 deficiency, Tabes dorsalis).	
Anterior cord	A lesion that produces variable loss of motor function and of sensitivity to pain and temperature while preserving proprioception (sensory dissociation). Damage to anterior horn may cause LMN weakness. (Figure 2.26).	
Brown-Sequard syndrome	Hemicord lesion, producing an ipsilateral motor weakness, ipsilateral proprioceptive loss and contralateral loss of sensitivity to pain and temperature (because of the different levels of decussation of the dorsal columns versus the ALS).	
Conus Medullaris syndrome	Injury of the sacral cord (conus) and lumbar nerve roots within the spinal canal, which usually results in an areflexic bladder, bowel and lower limbs. Sacral segments may occasionally show preserved reflexes (bulbocavernosus and micturition reflexes). It is an UMN syndrome.	
Cauda Equine syndrome	Injury to the lubosacral nerve roots within the neural canal resulting in areflexic bladder, bowel and lower limbs. It is LMN injury (Figure 2.27).	

Chapter 3

The Brainstem and Cranial Nerves

3.1. Abstract

The brainstem is the most feared part of the nervous system for the aspiring, short in time, medical student. It's seemingly endless details and out of rule cases poses a formidable task. This chapter aims at a layer like description of brainstem anatomy, dessicating the complex inner architecture to mention only the clinically important tracts and nuclei while maintaining an understanding of the overall arrangement. For this aim, the chapter starts with a focused embryological description, followed by an overview of the brainstem. The gross anatomical description is followed by a sections part. This is followed by a synopsis of cranial nerves subchapter, presenting again the key internal architectural points. The synopsis contains a short description of each cranial nerve, its central nuclei and tracts as well as its peripheral course. Eye movements and pupillary Control are discussed in this frame as well. Next an overview of the brainstem vascular supply, with relevant clinical implications is presented.

3.2. Neuro-Embryology of the Brainstem

The brainstem is formed by the myelencephalon (fifth vesicle), the metencephalon (fourth vesicle), and the mesencephalon (third vesicle). The cerebellum is derived from and is attached to the brainstem. In the brainstem, the gray and white matter is not in the same orientation to each other as they are in the spinal cord. Cephalization, the process through which these suprasegmental structures are found, begins in the brainstem. Primary brain vesicle development reveals how these changes occur. A key point in following the brainstem development is the realization that there is always a roof plate derived from the dorsal part of the neural tube and a floor plate from its ventral part. The plates and their lateral boundaries delineate the cavities of the neural tube (the future ventricles and interventricular communications). The myelencephalic cavity, the fourth ventricle, remains in communication with the spinal central canal at its caudal end, and with the mesencephalic cavity via the metencephalic cavity.

The derivatives of the third, fourth, and fifth vesicles consist of gray and white matter. The gray matter, derived from the alar and basal plates, includes segmental nuclei (similar to the medullary centers, these are nuclei of cranial nerves as well as autonomic nuclei) and suprasegmental structures (indicating cephalization). These structures are relay or association centers and head up the spinal cord even though they are integrated into a motor system (the extrapyramidal tract), they are derived in whole or in part from the alar plates which, even in the spinal cord, give rise to the synaptic relay and association centers. White matter is formed from myelinated tracts which thicken the marginal layer ventrally or just pass through the gray nuclei. These form different tract types. Segmentary association tracts (making the brainstem a functionally homogeneous whole) connect it to its subjacent and suprajacent structures.

Cerebro-medullary or medullo-cerebral pathways use the brainstem only as a crossover. Brainstem pathways, like the geniculate tract, connect the cerebral cortex to the nuclei of the cranial nerves.

The external shape of the cephalic portion of the neural tube changes markedly with the appearance of brain vesicles and the development of cervical and cephalic flexures. Despite these changes, some morphologic characteristics seen in the spinal cord are recognizable in most of the brain vesicles.

Distinct basal and alar plates, representing the motor and sensory areas respectively, are seen on each side of the midline in most of the brain vesicles. The sulcus limitans, which forms the boundary line between the alar and basal plates in the cord, is present in the rhombencephalon and mesencephalon, where it also forms the divider between sensory and motor areas.

The myelencephalon is the most caudal brain compartment, extending from the first spinal nerve to the pontine flexure, giving rise to the medulla oblongata. The medulla oblongata differs from the cord in that its lateral walls rotate around an imaginary long axis in the floor plate (refer to figure 3.1), like opening a textbook, and as a result, the roof plate stretches and becomes a single layer of cells covering an enlarged central cavity called the fourth ventricle.

The lateral wall structures are similar to that of the spinal cord; one sees alar and basal plate's derivatives separated by the sulcus limitans. The basal motor plate of the myelencephalon, like the spinal cord, contains the motor nuclei, but these are divided into 3 groups. These groups are a medial somatic efferent group, an intermediate special visceral efferent group and a lateral general visceral efferent group.

The medial somatic efferent group forms the cephalic continuation of the anterior horn cells containing the motor neurons which innervate striated muscle (derived from myotomes in the cephalic region). The intermediate special visceral efferent group extends into the metencephalon and forms the special visceral efferent motor column which contains motor neurons supplying striated muscles derived from the mesenchyme of the pharyngeal or branchial arches.

The lateral general visceral efferent group contains the neurons whose axons grow out as preganglionic fibers to synapse in the parasympathetic ganglia supplying involuntary muscles of the heart, respiratory tract, and intestinal tract as well as innervating the salivary glands. In the myelencephalon, this group is represented by the dorsal nucleus of the vagus (X) and the inferior salivatory nucleus which, by way of the cranial nerve IX (glossopharyngeal), innervates the parotid gland (discussed later).

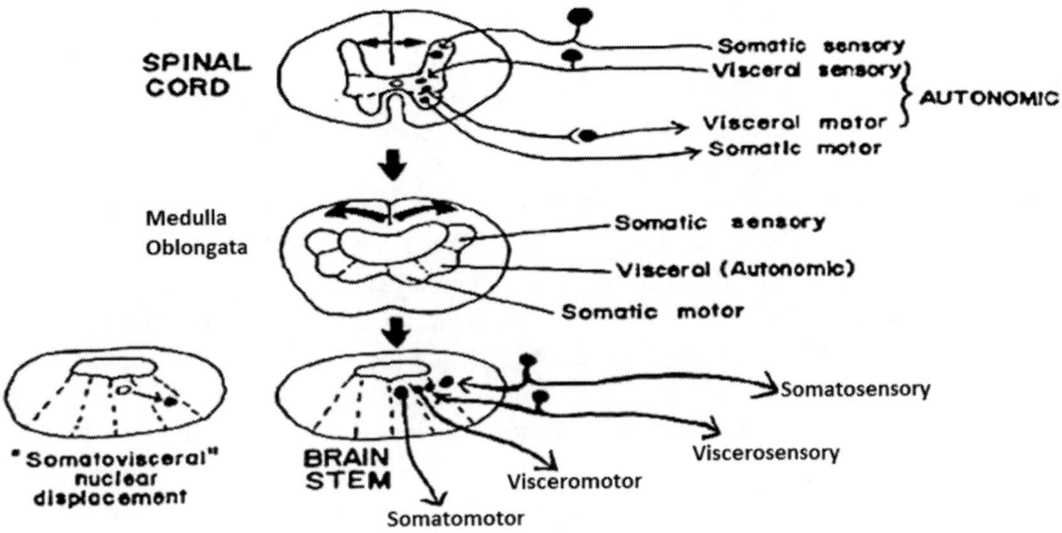

Figure 3.1. The development of the brainstem. The transition from the spinal cord to the brainstem. A process of "fanning out" occurs. Derivatives of the Alar plate forming the ventral horn (motor) cells of the spinal cord gray matter, become the medial columns of the brainstem (still motor in function). Derivatives of the Basal plate forming the dorsal horn (sensory) cells of the spinal cord gray matter, become the lateral columns of the brainstem (still sensory in function). Refer to text.

3.3. Overview of the Brainstem

The brainstem connects the cerebrum to the spinal cord and the cerebellum. It is the source and target for 10 cranial nerves (III to XII, discussed later). Among the many essential functions it performs, it had dedicated centers (nuclei or diffuse networks) performing all basic life functions. These include respiratory control centers, blood pressure and heart beat regulation centers, areas controlling the level of consciousness, areas controlling different advanced reflexes, like the eye and neck movements, mastication, sucking etc. Balance, audition and many visual related functions are also localized to the brainstem. In addition, through direct conduits (i.e., the cranial nerves) it receives raw sensory information and transmits motor control, both to skeletal muscles and to the internal organs.

3.3.1. Basic Organization of the Brainstem

There are two ways to look at the brainstem functionally, as either stacks of structures put one on top of another by evolution (the horizontal or axial organization), or as longitudinal columns facing different anatomical surfaces. A full understanding requires us to be able to view the different structures using both organization methods and hence a short description of both is given. Figure 3.2 presents the longitudinal organization whereas many other sections of the chapter present different axial views of the brainstem. We start our description with the axial view of the brainstem.

The medulla oblongata is the most caudal portion of the brain, with which the spinal cord merges. Foramen magnum demarcates the location of the pyramidal decussation and the transition from spinal cord to medulla. The Medulla enlarges in diameter as it ascends rostrally (to the pons). The Pons-medulla junction (the pontomedullary junction) is represented by the caudal edge of the middle inferior cerebellar peduncles, and ventrally it is represented by the caudal edge of the basilar pons. Cranial nerves VIII-XII emerge at the medulla, leaving at different medullary landmarks (or the lateral pontomedullary junction for CN-VIII). The pons (ventral metencephalon) is the rostral continuation, spanning from the Ponto-medullary junction to a line drawn from the exit of CN-4 (Dorsally), to rostral edge of basilar pons (which is bulbous in shape). Cranial nerves V-VIII emerge from the pons. Cranial nerve V (the trigeminal nerve) emerges from mid-lateral pons, whereas cranial nerves VI-VIII emerge from the ventral aspect of the ponto-medullary junction.

The cerebellum, although a part of the metencephalon, it is not a part of the brainstem, regarded as a separate entity. It is joined to the brainstem by three paired bundles, the cerebellar peduncles (superior, middle, inferior). The midbrain extends rostrally from the pontomidbrain junction to join the diencephalon (thalamus). This junctions is defined by a line drown from the posterior commissure (dorsally) to the caudal edge of the mammillary bodies ventrally. CN III (oculomotor) exits the ventral aspect of the midbrain at the inter-peduncular fossa whereas CN IV (the trochlear nerve) exits the dorsal aspect, below the inferior colliculus, being the only cranial nerve exiting the brainstem at its dorsal surface.

The longitudinal organization of the brainstem, divides it to three columns: The basilar surface, the roof (or tectum) and the tegmentum (located between the two layers). Refer to figure 3.2. The tegmentum and the continuous central portion of the medulla oblongata contain ascending and descending tracts, relay nuclei, nuclei of cranial nerves. Some important pathways include the posterior columns medial lemniscus system, the anterolateral system (the spinothalamic tract), the medial longitudinal fasciculus (MLF), cerebellar relay nuclei and tracts and cranial nerve nuclei and roots. The reticular formation with its diffuse cellular arrangement (discussed later) is located mainly in the tegmentum.

The roof (Tectum) is formed by the quadrigeminal plate at midbrain level (a name given to the superior and inferior colliculi pair) and CN.IV, by the cerebellum and roof of the fourth ventricle at the pons level and by the tela choroidea and choroid plexus at the medulla oblongata level. The basilar surface is formed by the crus cerebri (pes pedunculi) at the midbrain level, basilar pons and CN-V at the pons level and by the pyramids processes at the medulla oblongata level.

3.3.2. Surface Landmarks of the Brainstem

Discussing the surface landmarks with regards to the brainstem is the simplest of tasks in studying the brainstem. A few very discernable surface gross anatomical features need mentioning and recognition. Refer to figures 3.3-3.8 for details. Starting from the dorsal surface, a few important markings are to be mentioned at the midbrain level. The quadrigeminal plate (corpora quadrigemina) composed of the two superior and two inferior colliculi (related in function to the visual and auditory systems respectively). Each is continued laterally with its connection (or the anatomical proof of its connection) to the thalamus via the brachium of the superior colliculus and the brachium of the inferior colliculus. The fourth cranial nerve (the trochlear) arises below the inferior colliculus, being the only cranial nerve emerging from the dorsal surface of the brainstem.

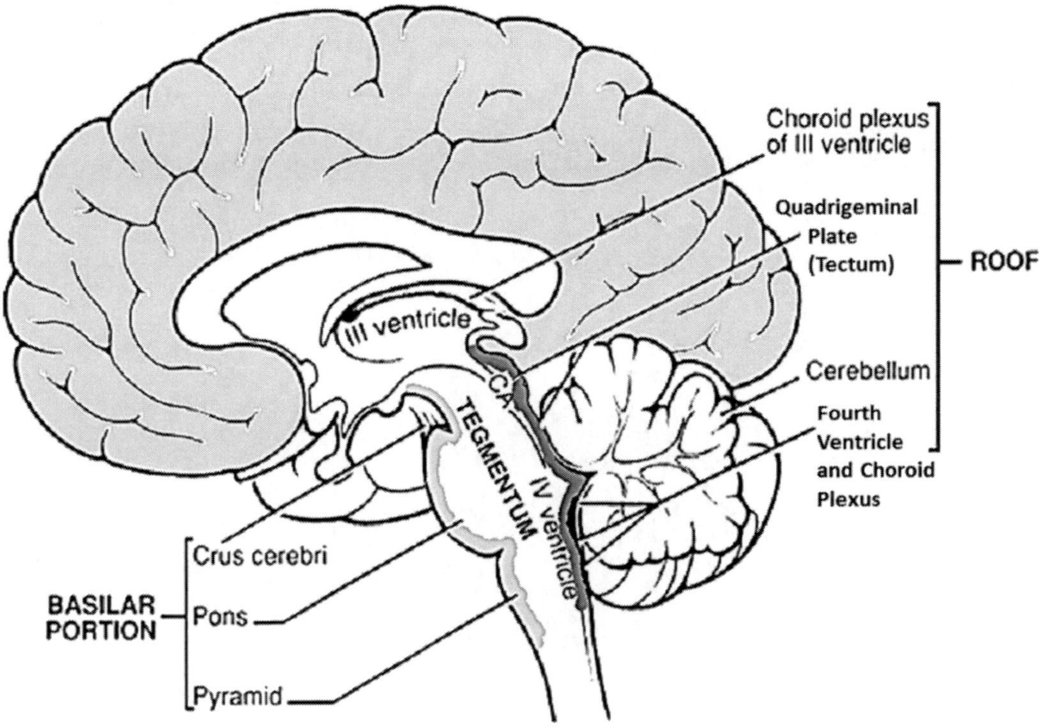

Figure 3.2. The longitudinal organization of the Brainstem. Light Gray – Basilar aspect, Dark Gray – the Tectum (Roof), White – Tegmentum. Refer to text.

At the ponto-medullary level, the dorsal surface is composed of the three cerebellar peduncles and different markings on the floor of the fourth ventricle, being the dorsal brainstem. These markings can be subdivided into longitudinal sulci and different elevations. The median sulcus runs in the midline splitting the brainstem into its two halves. Lateral to it, on both its sides, is the sulcus limitans (an important structure in the understanding of alar and basal plate derivatives and the segregation of motor and sensory nuclei columns mentioned earlier and discussed in greater details later). The different elevations are segregated according to their position relative to these sulci. Medial to the sulcus limitans we can find the vagal trigone (trigonum Vagi), hypoglossal trigone (trigonum Hypoglossi) and the facial colliculus (actually formed by the fibers of the seventh cranial nerve hooking around the abducens nucleus. Lateral to sulcus limitans we can find the vestibular areas, as well as other structures.

The ventral (basal) surface of the brainstem is marked by the cerebral peduncles (crus cerebri) at midbrain level. The fossa between these peduncles (the interpenducular fossa) serves as the exit point for the third cranial nerve (oculomotor). The ventral surface of the pons is smooth, continuous laterally with the formation of the cerebellar peduncles. At mid-pons, the fifth cranial nerve (trigeminal) leaves at the lateral aspects of the ventral pons. The ponto-medullary junction is a discernable fissure sharply demarcating the border between these structures and houses the exit of several cranial nerves. From medial to lateral these are the sixth seventh and eighths cranial nerves. The ventral aspect of the medulla is unique for the median triangular shaped longitudinal ridge, mimicking a pyramid (hence its names, the pyramids). It houses the tracts of the corticospinal tract that because of this ridge is also known as the pyramidal tract. Lateral to the pyramids a small elevation termed appropriately as the olive can be seen, and the fissue surrounding it from adjacent structures is the pre-olivary and post-olivary sulci. The post-olivary sulcus is the exit point for cranial nerves IX-XI, whereas the pre-olivary sulcus is the exit point for CN-XII (the hypoglossal nerve).

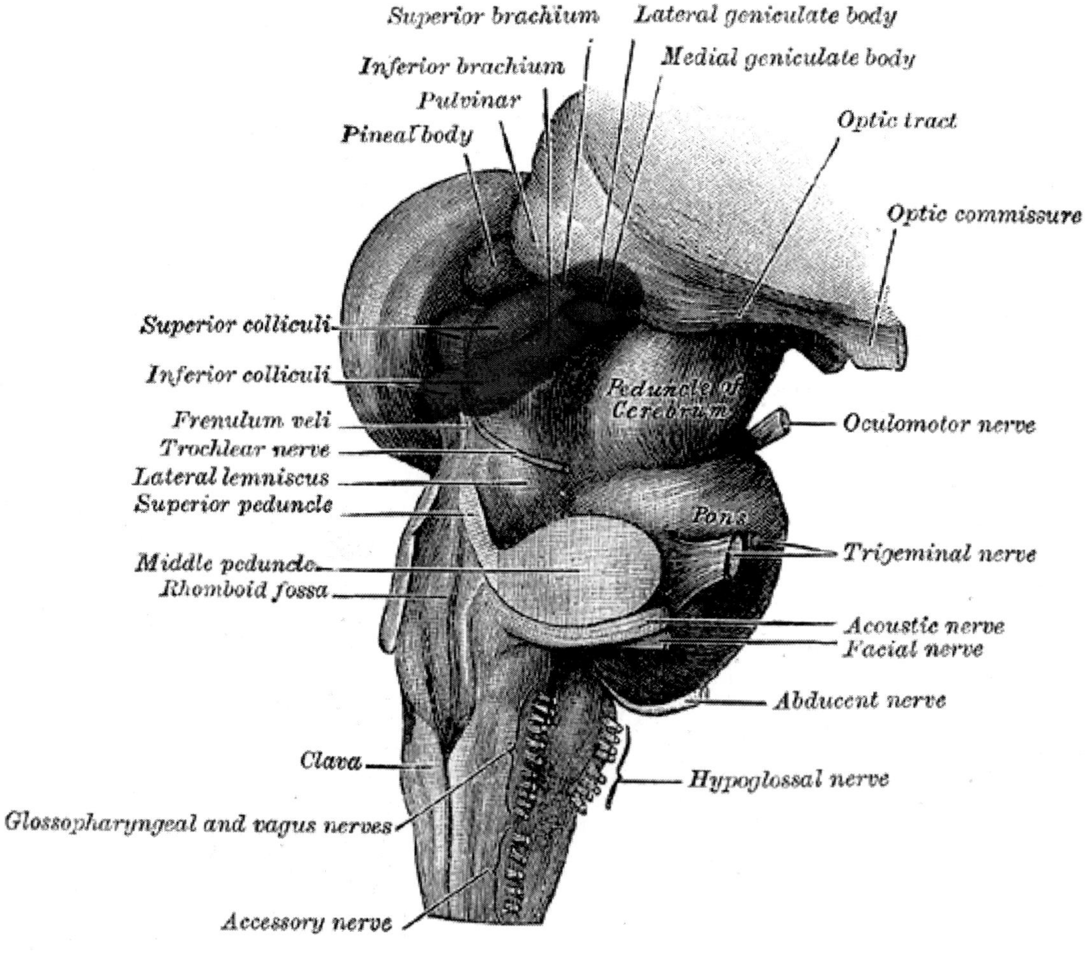

Figure 3.3. Gross anatomy of the brainstem, oblique view. Brainstem Images from Gray's anatomy (out of copyright).

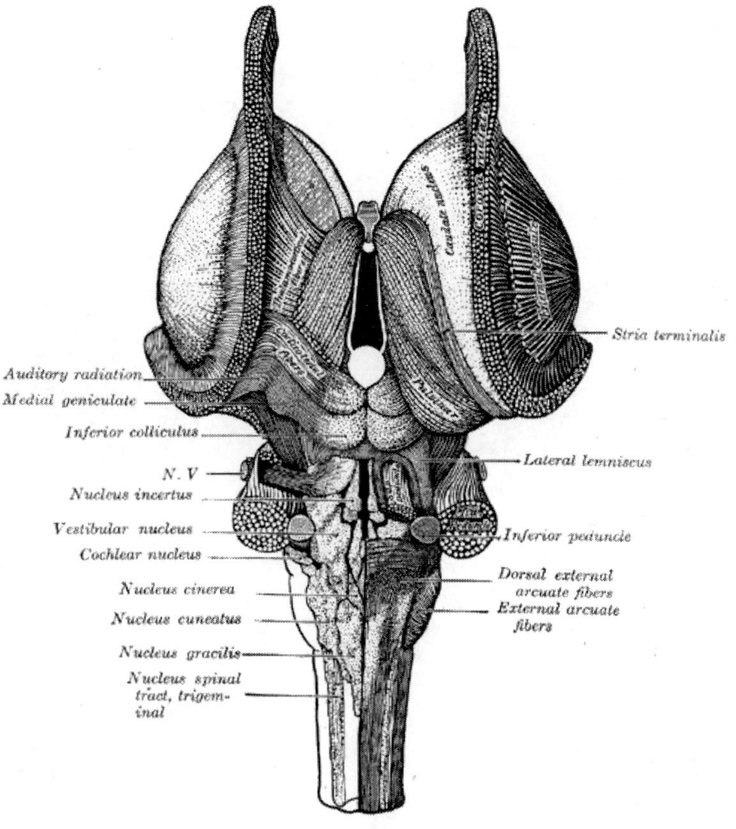

Figure 3.4. Gross anatomy of the brainstem, dorsal view. Brainstem Images from Gray's anatomy (out of copyright).

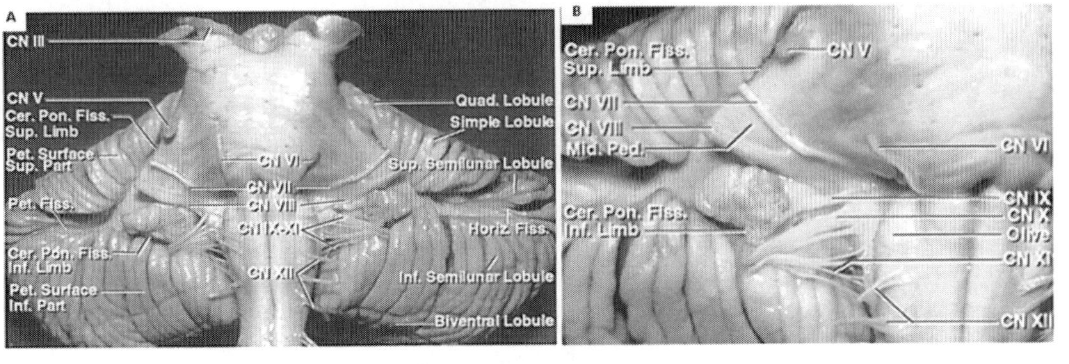

Figure 3.5. Gross anatomy of the brainstem, ventral view (petrosal surface). A, The petrosal surface of the cerebellum faces forward toward the petrous temporal bone and is the surface that is retracted to surgically expose the cerebellopontine angle. B, Enlarged view. The petrosal fissure extends laterally from the apex of the cerebellopontine fissure. The abducens nerve arises in the medial part of the pontomedullary sulcus rostral to the medullary pyramids. The facial and vestibulocochlear nerves arise just rostral to the foramen of Luschka near the flocculus at the lateral end of the pontomedullary sulcus. The hypoglossal nerves arise anterior to and the glossopharyngeal, vagus, and accessory nerves arise posterior to the olives. Choroid plexus protrudes from the foramen of Luschka behind the glossopharyngeal and vagus nerves. Ant., anterior; Cer.Med., cerebellomedullary; Cer.Pon., cerebellopontine; CN, cranial nerve; Fiss., fissure; Horiz., horizontal; Inf., inferior; Pet., petrosal; Post., posterior; Quad., quadrangular; Suboccip., suboccipital; Sup., superior; Tent., tentorial. Taken with permission from the Rhoton Collection.

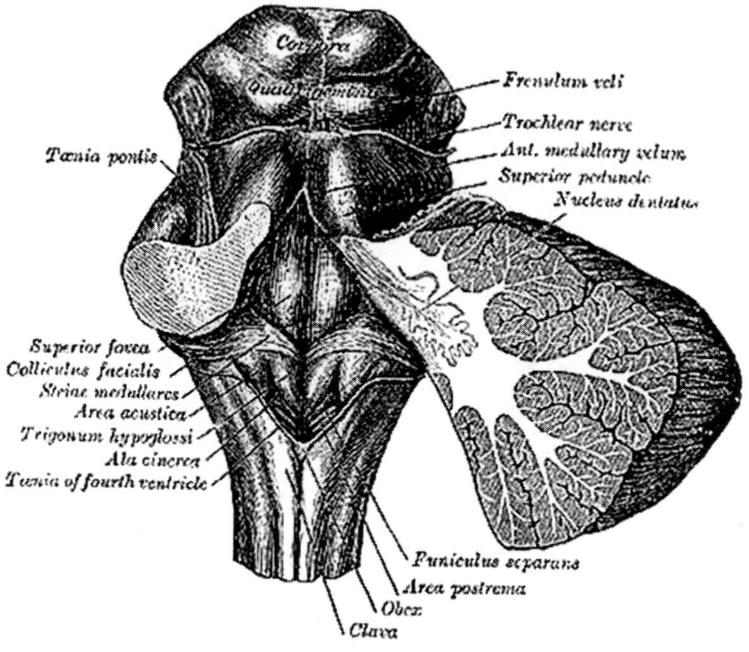

Figure 3.6. Gross anatomy of the brainstem, dorsal view. Corpora quadrigemina is shown with the cerebellum partially removed Brainstem Images from Gray's anatomy (out of copyright).

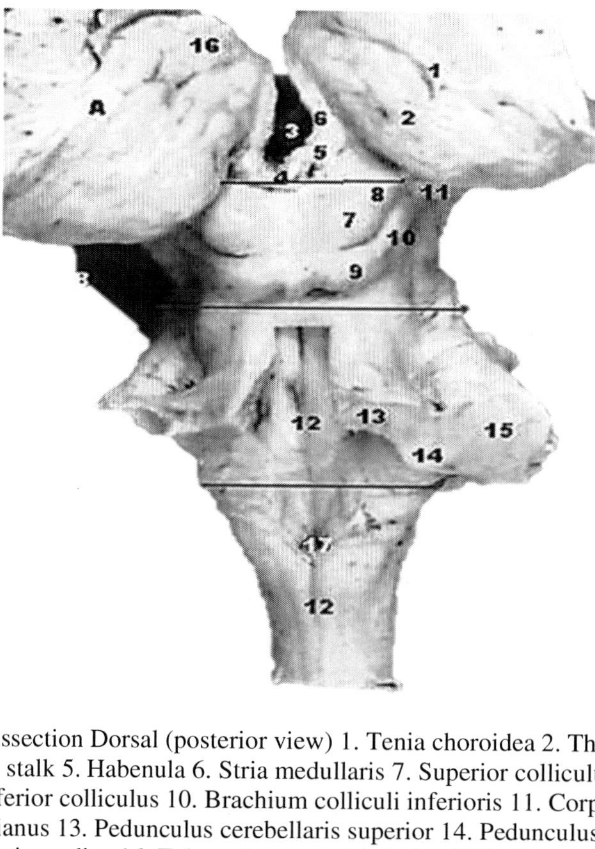

Figure 3.7. Brainstem dissection Dorsal (posterior view) 1. Tenia choroidea 2. Thalamus 3. 3rd ventricle 4. Pineal gland stalk 5. Habenula 6. Stria medullaris 7. Superior colliculus 8. Brachium colliculi superioris 9. Inferior colliculus 10. Brachium colliculi inferioris 11. Corpus geniculatum mediale 12. Sulcus medianus 13. Pedunculus cerebellaris superior 14. Pedunculus cerebellaris inferior 15. Pedunculus cerebellaris medius 16. Tuberculum anterius thalami 17. Obex, area postrema A: thalamus. Taken with permission from www.Radiopaedia.org.

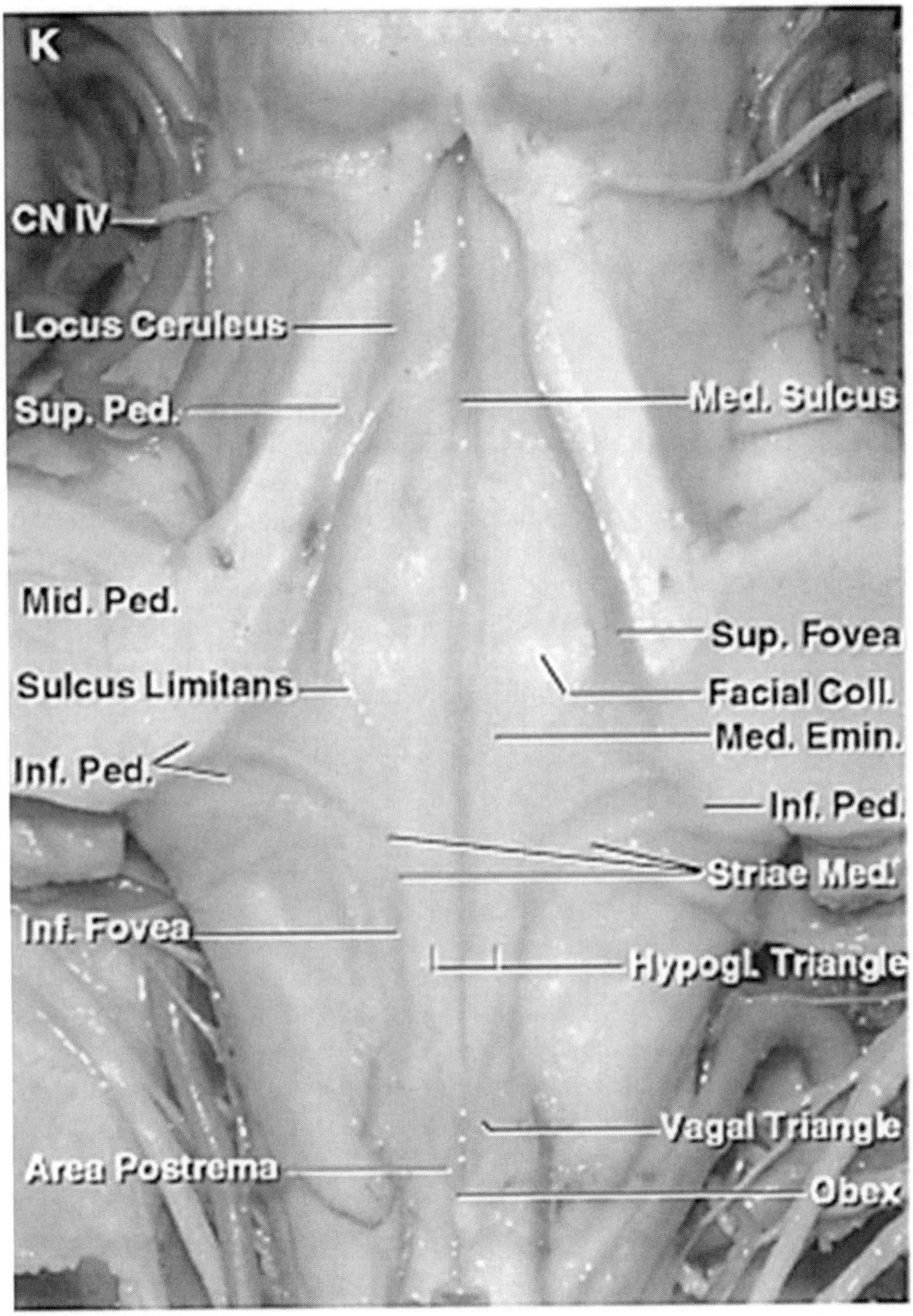

Figure 3.8. Enlarged view of the floor of the fourth ventricle. The median sulcus divides the floor longitudinally in the midline. Each half of the floor is divided longitudinally by an irregular sulcus, the sulcus limitans, which deepens lateral to the facial colliculus and hypoglossal triangles to form the superior and inferior foveae. A darkened area of cells, the locus ceruleus, is located at the rostral end of the sulcus limitans. The stria medullaris crosses the floor at the level of the lateral recess. The hypoglossal and vagal nuclei and the area postrema are stacked one above the other in the lower part of the floor to give the configuration of a pen nib and, thus, the area is referred to as the calamus scriptorius. Taken with permission from the Rhoton Collection.

3.4. The Ventricular Spaces of the Brainstem

The cerebral aqueduct is a narrow channel (1~3mm diameter), connecting the 3rd and 4th ventricles (the cavity of the diencephalon and the Rhombencephalon). It is located in the midbrain and contains no choroid plexus. Its walls are formed by continuous mantle of cells, the so named peri-aqueductal gray (PAG, important in pain modulation, limbic functions and consciousness, discussed in later chapters). Some common developmental abnormalities of the aqueduct involve septae, webs or forking of the aqueduct or congenital aqueductal stenosis (which may manifest in early childhood as a clinically overt hydrocephalus syndrome, but at times remains silent to be discovered incidentally during adulthood).

The fourth ventricle is the cavity of the rhombencephalon, whose rostral portion lies between the pons and cerebellum, and its caudal part is in the medulla. It communicates with the subarachnoid space via the three foramina: **Magendie foramina** located at the caudal roof of the fourth ventricle and opening into the cerebello-medullary cistern, **Luschka foramina** located at end of the lateral recesses of the ventricle, opening into the subarachnoid space at the cerebellopontine angles and the **lateral recesses** which are horn-shaped widening of the ventricle extending around the brainstem at pontomedullary junction. The roof of the fourth ventricles is formed mainly by anterior (Superior) medullary velum rostrally, by the tela choroidae caudally (thin membrane) and a small part of the cerebellum (at the midline). The walls of the fourth ventricle are formed from rostral to caudal by the superior, middle and inferior cerebellar peduncles respectively and by the attachment of the tela choroidae to the medulla. The tela choroidae arises from the inferior cerebellum to attach to the V-shaped edges of the medullary portion of the ventricle space. The choroid plexus is suspended from the inner surface of the tela, and partly protrude through foramina of Luschka.

The rhomboid fosse floor of the fourth ventricle, as explained previously is divided to halves by the median sulcus (deep), and each half is traversed longitudinally by the sulcus limitans. Several elevations are shown, formed by the underlying CN nuclei structures. Medial to the sulcus limitans (between it and the median sulcus), the hypoglossal and vagal trigons represent so named underlying nuclei. The facial colliculus (located superior to these) represents the abducens nucleus and the internal genu of the facial nerve (facial nerve fibers hooking around the abducens nucleus). Lateral to the sulcus limitans, different more diffuse structures can be identified, including the vestibular area, locus ceruleus etc.

3.5. Cranial Nerve Nuclei and Their Functional Components

As discussed in chapter two, the different fibers comprising the nerves, are classified on the basis of origin or common structural and functional components. These are segregated into motor versus sensory fibers. Within the motor group of fibers, we distinguish general somatic efferants (GSE, Somatomotor), general visceral efferants (GVE, Visceromotor) and special visceral efferants (SVE, also termed somatovisceral), a term given to those cranial nerves innervating muscles originating from the pharyngeal arches. The sensory fibers are segregated into general somatic afferent (GSA, somatosensory), general visceral afferent (GVA, Viscerosensory) and special visceral afferent (SVA) referring to special senses like the vestibular, auditory and taste functions. Refer to table 3.1 for a summary overview of the different fiber components each cranial nerve holds and respective names.

Initially the cell columns forming the alar and basal plate's derivatives extend throughout the brainstem. The primitive cell columns retain its relative position as it differentiates, but it may become discontinuous as the individual nuclei derived from the same column are formed. Motor nuclei of cranial nerves arise from basal plate neuroblasts while nuclei receiving primary sensory input (i.e., sensory cranial nerves nuclei), are derived from alar plate. The sulcus limitans, persisting from embryonic time, separates structures derived from the basal and alar plates. The transition from the spinal cord to the medulla (as discussed previously), is accompanied by a 90 degrees rotation of the column orientation, a form of fanning out process. Ventral horn cells become medially situated whereas dorsal horn spinal cells become laterally situated. Thus, in the brainstem, all motor columns (basal plate derivatives) are located medially and alar plate derived sensory columns are located laterally. Refer to figure 3.9-3.11 and table 3.1.

Skeletal muscles supplied by the motor nuclei of the basal plate originates from occipital myotomes (for the tongue), or mesenchyme (for the orbit), and thus are defined as GSE. These are cranial nerves III, IV, VI, XII. These form the most medial column. Lateral to this column, a second cell (nuclei) population whose axons synapse in peripheral ganglia (innervate Smooth muscle and glands), are termed GVE. These are the dorsal motor vagal nucleus, inferior salivatory nucleus, superior salivatory nucleus and the Edinger-Westphal (oculomotor Visceromotor) nuclei.

A third nuclei column group located between these column and slightly more ventrally are the ambiguus, facial and trigeminal motor nuclei, innervate muscles arising from pharyngeal arches (not myotomes), and thus defined as SVE.

Sensory nuclei columns, derivatives of the alar plate are segregated into two columns. Nerve fibers transmitting sensory input via CN-VII, IX, X contains both SVA fibers (taste) and GVA (touch, vibration, temperature, pain). These form the solitary tract, ending in the solitary nucleus. The vestibulocochlear nerve (CN-VIII) transmits signals of balance, equilibrium and hearing. CN-VIII fibers end in the vestibular and cochlear nuclei of the medulla oblongata and the pons. Because of the unique origin of the CN-VIII receptors, the functional component associated with them is SSA.

GSA fibers (i.e., somatosensory) from the face, parallel to the functions of the dorsal columns medial lemniscus system and the spinothalamic tracts discussed in chapter two for sensation from the rest of the body, are conveyed by different aspects of the trigeminal nucleus and tract. The trigeminal nucleus is a continuous column of cells from the cervical spinal cord-medullary junction to the midbrain. It is subdivided to three functional regions. The spinal trigeminal nucleus, which begins at the spinal cervical cord and reaches up to the caudal pons, is subdivided into pars caudalis, pars interpolaris and pars oralis. The spinal trigeminal nucleus is analogous to anterolateral system (so conveying pain and temperature sensations).

Thus, spinal trigeminal tract is analogues to Lissauer's tract. The chief trigeminal nucleus is analogous to posterior columns system, with its mesencephalic portion receiving the proprioceptive information from the face.

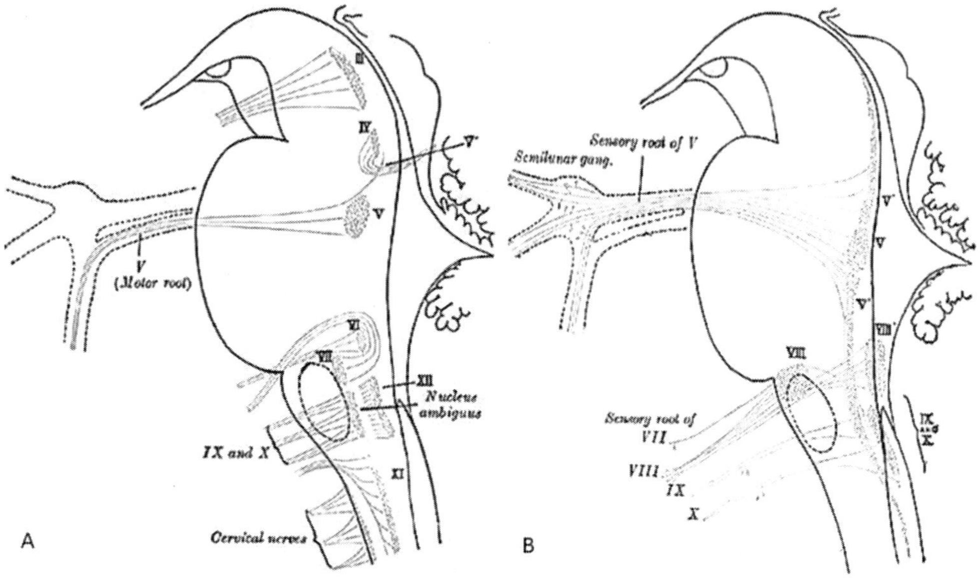

Figure 3.9. Brainstem with schematic nuclei. A, Motor nuclei columns. B, Sensory nuclei columns. Images from Gray's anatomy (out of copyright).

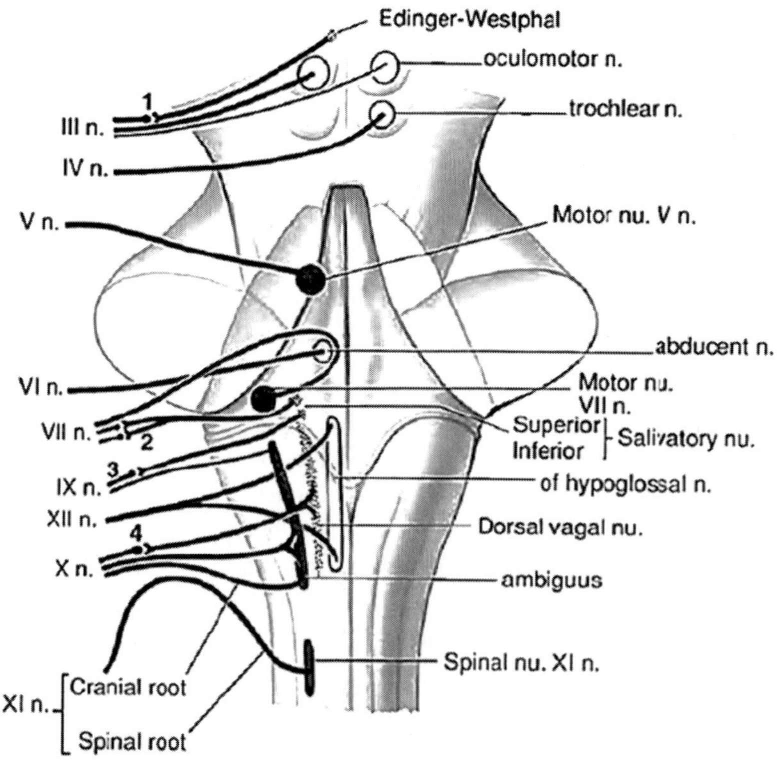

Figure 3.10. Brainstem with schematic Motor nuclear columns. Images from Gray's anatomy (out of copyright).

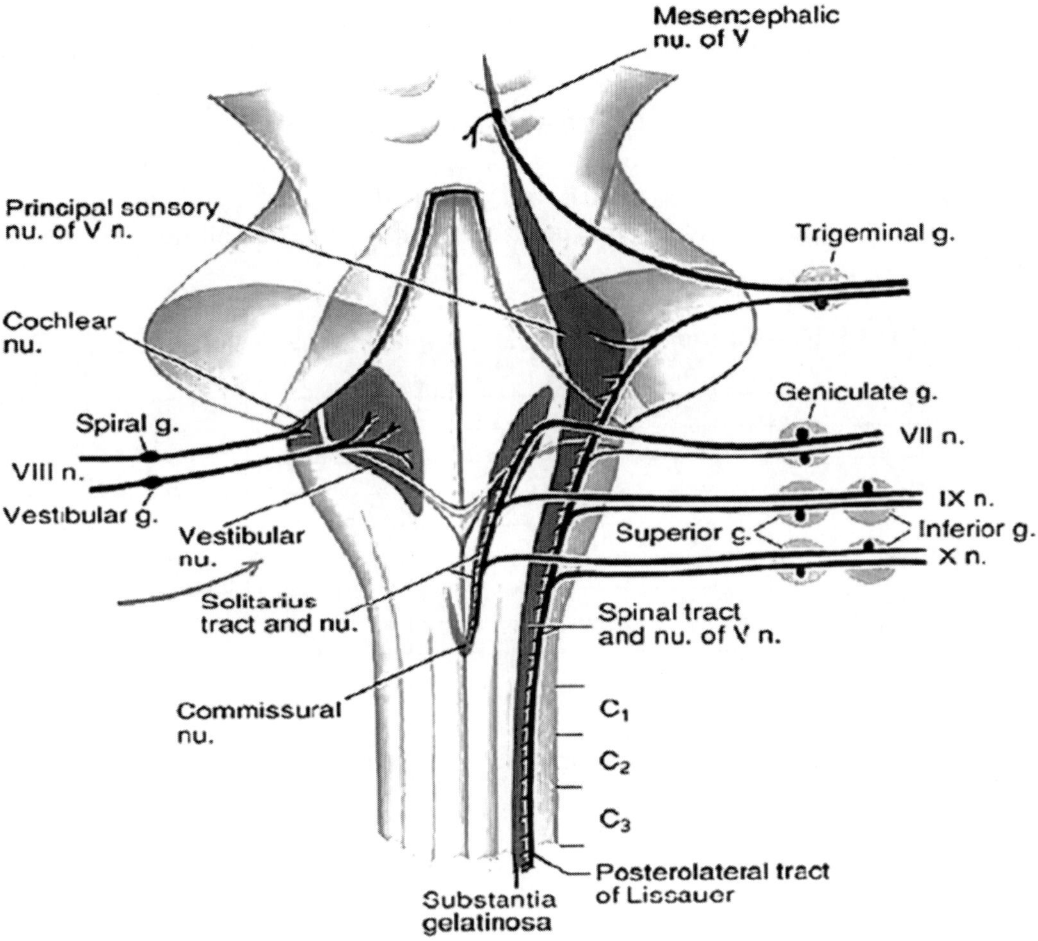

Figure 3.11. Brainstem with schematic Sensory nuclear columns and peripheral destinations. Images from Gray's anatomy (out of copyright).

3.6. Brainstem – Internal Structures

3.6.1. Cerebellar Circuitry

The neuroanatomy of the cerebellum will be discussed separately (chapter 6), yet a few relevant points merit mentioning. Ataxia is a clinical term referring to the characteristic uncoordinated wavering movement whose etiology is cerebellar dysfunction. That is, by describing a patient's gait or walk as atactic, one also describes the neuroanatomical location of the lesion. Special care should be given to understanding both anatomy and the clinical unique features of ataxia versus other gait and walking disturbances. Ataxia refers to a broad based (because of instability) gait, at times also described as a magnetic gait (where feet seem glued to the floor). This should be distinguished from apractic gait (simulating an infant learning to walk where the steps are not even in height or distance). Ataxia typically occurs ipsilaterally to the side of the lesion, since cerebellar circuits tend to decussate twice before reaching the lower motor neuron.

The first decussation occurs upon existing from the cerebellum through the superior cerebellar peduncle (which contains mainly cerebellar outputs). This decussation occurs in the midbrain, at the inferior colliculi level. Fibers next proceed to the red nucleus (nucleus rubrum, discussed later) or rostrally. Those ascending fibers, after synapsing elsewhere (discussed later) finally reach the primary motor cortex (pre-central gyrus). From there the information descends via the pyramidal tract, which decussates at the spino-medullary junction. Thus, the cerebellar information decussates twice to finally be ipsilateral to the side of the lesion.

Table 3.1. Cranial Nerves Functional Components and Related Nuclei

<table>
<tr><th colspan="3">Cranial nerves</th><th colspan="2">SM*</th><th>VM**</th><th>VS+</th><th>SS++</th></tr>
<tr><td rowspan="3">Sensory</td><td>I</td><td>Olfactory</td><td colspan="2"></td><td></td><td colspan="2" rowspan="2">Not in brainstem</td></tr>
<tr><td>II</td><td>Optic</td><td colspan="2"></td><td></td></tr>
<tr><td>VIII</td><td>Vestibulocochlear</td><td colspan="2"></td><td></td><td></td><td></td></tr>
<tr><td rowspan="4">Motor</td><td>III</td><td>Oculomotor</td><td colspan="2"></td><td></td><td></td><td></td></tr>
<tr><td>IV</td><td>Trochlear</td><td colspan="2"></td><td></td><td></td><td></td></tr>
<tr><td>VI</td><td>Abducens</td><td colspan="2"></td><td></td><td></td><td></td></tr>
<tr><td>XII</td><td>Hypoglossal</td><td colspan="2"></td><td></td><td></td><td></td></tr>
<tr><td rowspan="4">Mixed</td><td>V</td><td>Trigeminal</td><td rowspan="4">Somatovisceral</td><td>Motor trigeminal nucleus</td><td></td><td></td><td rowspan="4">CN-V</td></tr>
<tr><td>VII</td><td>Facial</td><td>Facial motor Nucleus</td><td>Superior Salivatory</td><td rowspan="3">Nucleus tractus solitarius</td></tr>
<tr><td>IX</td><td>Glossopharyngeal</td><td rowspan="2">Nucleus Ambiguus</td><td>Inferior Salivatory</td></tr>
<tr><td>X</td><td>Vagus</td><td>Dorsal motor vagal nucleus</td></tr>
</table>

*Somatomotor, **Visceromotor, +Viscerosensory, ++somatosensory.

Three white matter bands connect the cerebellum to the brainstem at the level of the pons. The superior peduncle as mentioned previously is the main output path for information from the cerebellum. The middle cerebellar peduncle is the largest, bulkier of the three, contains mainly cerebellar inputs arising from pontine nuclei, which receive input from the corticopontine fibers of the cerebral peduncles. The inferior cerebellar peduncle allows passage of input from the spinal cord (proprioceptive and other). A special form of ataxia, spinal ataxia, refers to the cervical spinal cord disconnection and lack of spinocerebellar proprioceptive information to the cerebellum via the inferior cerebellar peduncle as the etiology. This can be seen in different cervical pathologies, i.e., cervical canal stenosis, cervical myelopathy etc.

Palatal myoclonus is a rare, characteristic disorder having rhythmic clicking of the palate. The circuit damaged begins at the superior cerebellar peduncle, continues to the rostral (parvocellular) red nucleus, than to the central tegmental tract, next to the inferior olivary nucleus and finally to the Inferior cerebellar peduncle to enter the cerebellum.

3.6.2. Reticular Formation (RF) and Related Structures

It is a central core of nuclei that runs through the entire length of the brainstem. Continues rostrally with diencephalic structures and caudally with the intermediate spinal cord zone (Rexed lamina-VII). Its rostral aspect is shown to function to maintain an alert conscious state in the forebrain (part of the ARAS – ascending reticular activating system). Its caudal aspect functions with cranial nerve nuclei and spinal cord to carry out motor and reflex autonomic functions. It is that portion of the brainstem tegmentum in which clearly defined nuclei are not generally visible with conventional staining. Related structures include the PAG (periaqueductal gray matter, mentioned earlier, involved in pain modulation) and chemotactic trigger zones. The reticular formation projects to the entire neuroaxis diffusely. These widespread diffuse projections are essential in regulating attention, sleep-wake cycle, emotional balance etc.

The reticular formation has been functionally cleaved both sagittally and coronally. Refer to figure 3.12 for details. Traditionally the nuclei are divided into three columns: the median column (a.k.a. the raphe nuclei), the medial column (a.k.a. magnocellular nuclei, given to it because of larger size of the cells) and the lateral column (a.k.a. parvocellular nuclei, a name given to it because of smaller size of the cells). The original functional differentiation was a division of caudal and rostral, this was based upon the observation that the lesioning of the rostral reticular formation induces a hypersomnia in the cat brain. In contrast, lesioning of the more caudal portion of the reticular formation produces insomnia in cats. This study has led to the idea that the caudal portion inhibits the rostral portion of the reticular formation.

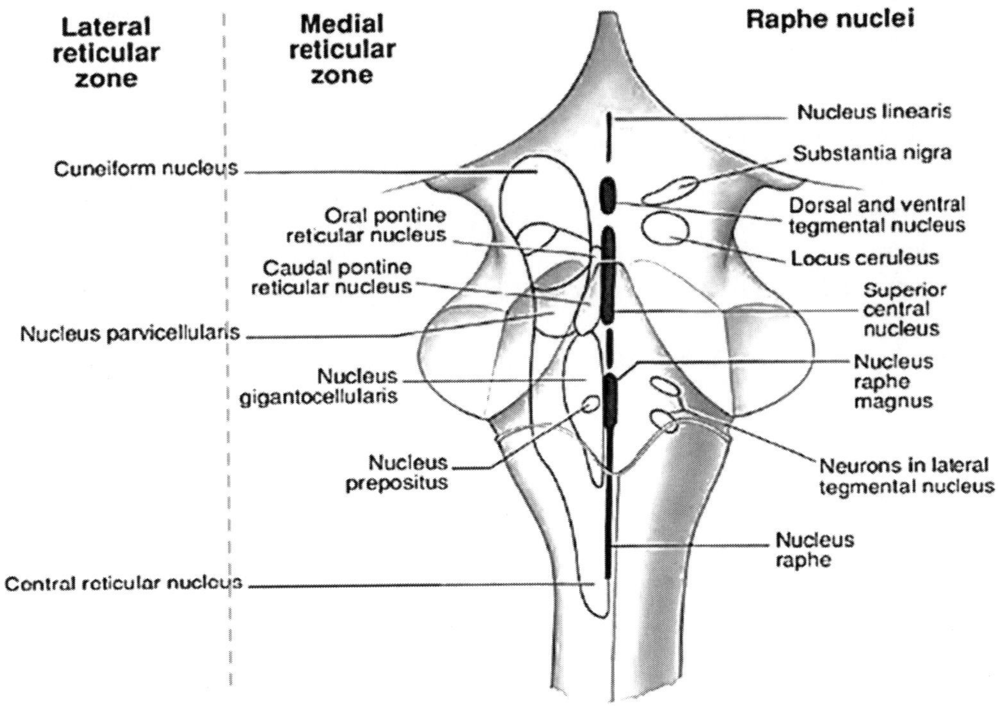

Figure 3.12.The longitudinal arrangement of zones of the brain stem reticular formation. The most lateral strips on both sides are the lateral zones. Along the midline is the median or raphe zone. In between is the paramedian or the medial zone. Refer to the text.

Sagittal division reveals more morphological distinctions. The raphe nuclei form a ridge in the middle of the reticular formation, and, directly to its periphery, there is a division called the medial reticular formation. The medial RF is large and has long ascending and descending fibers, and is surrounded by the lateral reticular formation. The lateral RF is close to the motor nuclei of the cranial nerves, and mostly mediates their function.

The Ascending reticular activating system (ARAS) is a functional subdivision of the reticular formation. It refers anatomically to the pontomesencephalic reticular formation which forms a circuit with certain thalamic nuclei, critical at maintaining consciousness. Its Name remains from the 1940's, although not all are ascending pathways and many systems are involved. Lesions causing coma must involve either the upper brainstem reticular formation (ARAS), result from dysfunction of extensive bilateral regions of cerebral cortex or lesions involving both thalami.

One should bear in mind that when discussing consciousness, we should specify which component of consciousness we are referring to. Consciousness is composed of content (dependent on systems mediating sensory, motor, memory and emotional functions) and level. The control of the level of consciousness involves three different anatomically unique processes (abbreviated as AAA). These are **alertness, attention and awareness.** Without breeching the scope of this book one should realize the conceptual difference between these elements, as a basis for understanding their different anatomical localization. Alertness depends on the proper functioning of the pontomesencephalic reticular formation (ARAS), the thalamus and the cortex. Attention maintenance uses similar circuits with fronto-parietal association cortex dominant influence, whereas awareness is subjective, personal, and poorly understood. Awareness is a multisynaptic process, involving among other structures, limbic and diencephalic structures as well.

3.6.3. Regional Sectional Anatomy

3.6.3.1. Medulla Oblongata

This section recapitulates previous text and structures, now in cross sections regional view. For practical purposes, this subchapter is arranged in bullet forms, for ease of memorizing.

Refer to figures 3.13-3.15. Important structures to note include:

a) The pyramids and the pyramidal (corticospinal tract) decussation.
b) Inferior olives – processing proprioceptive information from the spinal cord (spino-olivary tract), which is than forwarded to the cerebellum.
c) Dorsal Columns – Gracile and Cuneate nuclei. The medulla is the location of the first synapse of this tract. The secondary neuron than decussates (the so called sensory decussation), to form the medial lemniscus. While decussating, these fibers are referred to as the arcuate fibers.
d) The central gray, surrounding the central canal at spinal cord level is transformed to the floor of the fourth ventricle.
e) Spinal trigeminal tract, continuous with the Lissauer's tract of the spinal cord.

f) Posterior (dorsal) spinocerebellar tract, which enters the cerebellum through the inferior cerebellar peduncle.
g) Nuclei of cranial nerves CN-VIII – CN-XII.

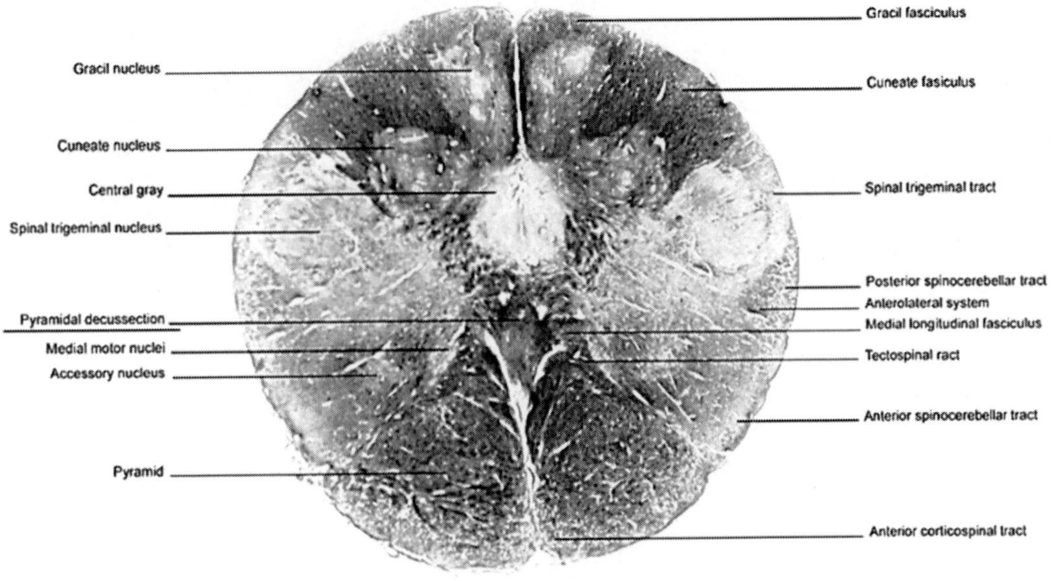

Figure 3.13. Medulla Oblongata, cross section at the level of the pyramidal (motor) decussation.

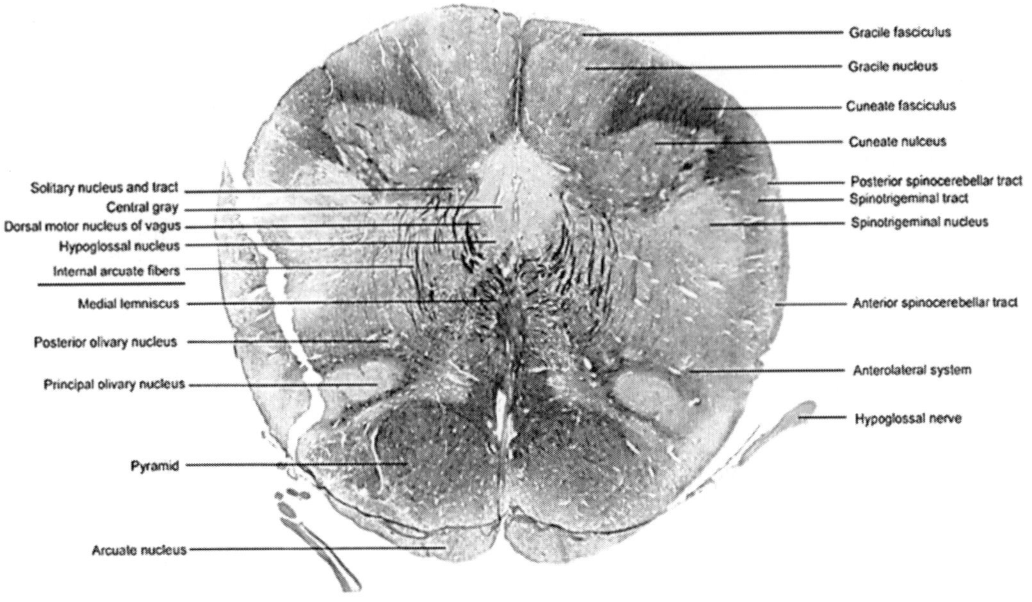

Figure 3.14. Medulla Oblongata, cross section at the level of the sensory decussation. The Gracile and Cuneatus nuclear output, i.e., the medial lemniscus, decussates above the pyramidal (motor) decussation. Upon decussation, it is termed as the arcuate fibers. Refer to text.

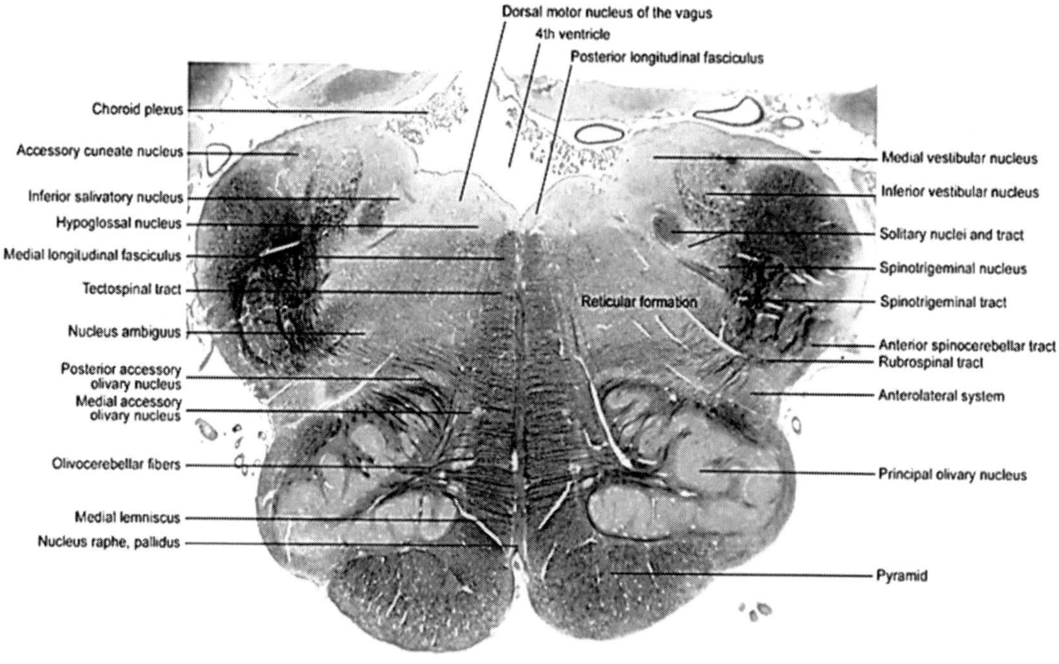

Figure 3.15. Medulla Oblongata, cross section at the level of the fourth ventricle, hypoglossal nucleus, olive, nucleus ambiguus etc. Refer to text.

3.6.3.2. The Pons

This section recapitulates previous text and structures, now in cross sections regional view. For practical purposes, this subchapter is arranged in bullet forms, for ease of memorizing.

Refer to figures 3.16-3.17. Important structures to note include:

a) Pontine nuclei. These convey relay information from descending cortical fibers to the cerebellum.
b) The lateral lemniscus. These are fibers originating in cochlear nuclei carrying auditory information and convey it to the inferior colliculi
c) The spinal lemniscus is composed of the anterolateral spinothalamic tract fibers as well as the spinotectal tract fibers.
d) Fibers entering the pons through the superior cerebellar peduncle.
e) Cranial nerves CN-V – CN-VIII nuclei.
f) The Facial colliculus formed by the CN-VII fibers looping around the abducens (CN-VI) nucleus.
g) The medial lemniscus rostral continuation.

3.6.3.3. The Midbrain

This section recapitulates previous text and structures, now in cross sections regional view. For practical purposes, this subchapter is arranged in bullet forms, for ease of memorizing.

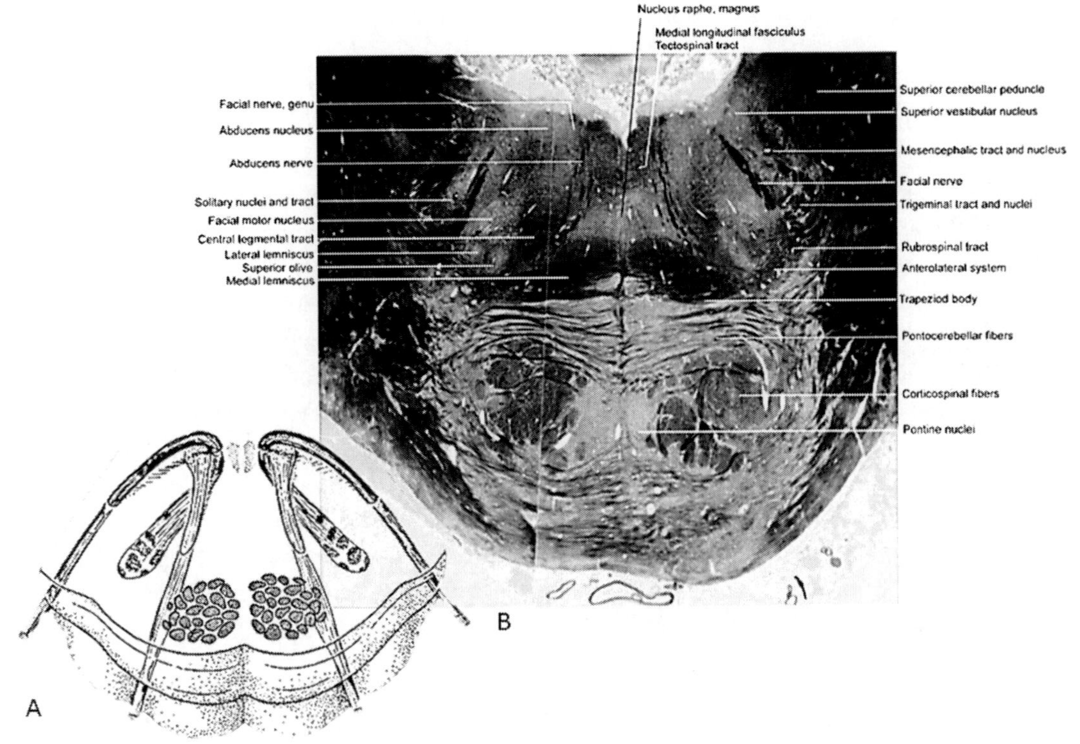

Figure 3.16. Pons, cross section at the level of the Facial colliculus. A, an illustration showing the concept that the facial colliculus is formed by the genu of the facial nerve (CN-VII) looping around the abducens (CN-VI) nucleus. B, Cross section. Refer to text.

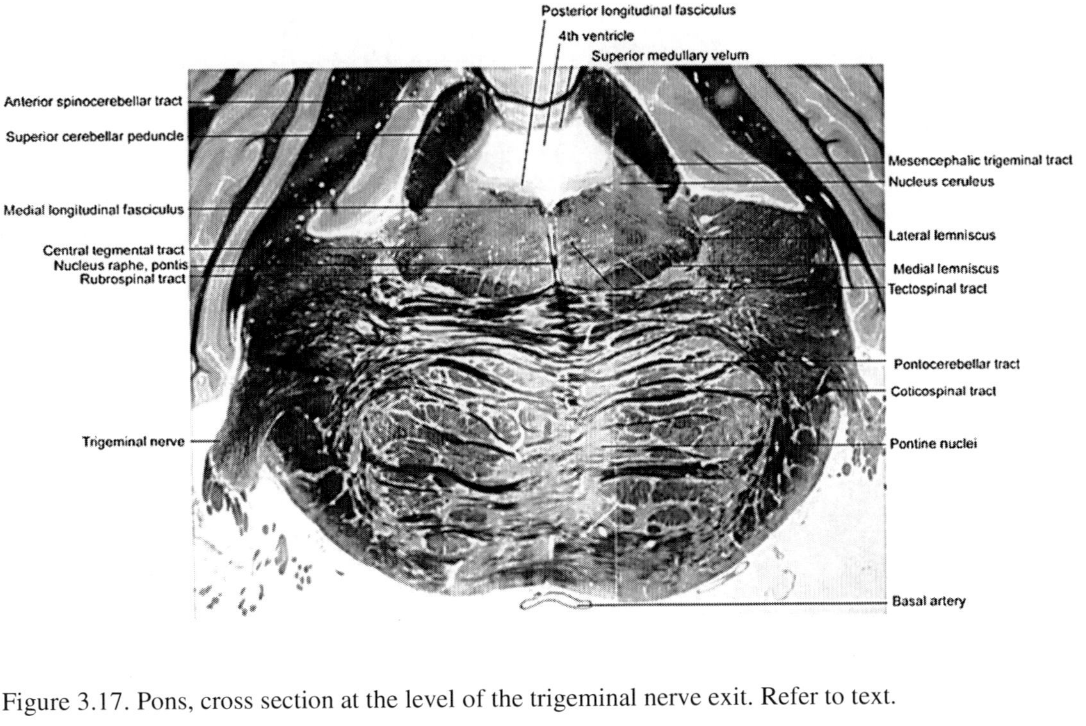

Figure 3.17. Pons, cross section at the level of the trigeminal nerve exit. Refer to text.

Refer to figures 3.18-3.21. Important structures to note include:

a) The cerebral peduncles. These are massive bundles of fibers descending from cerebral cortex to spinal cord and pons. About half descend to the spinal cord, forming the pyramids and corticospinal tract. The rest synapse on pontine nuclei.
b) Trigeminal tracts. Ascending fibers from the chief sensory and trigeminospinal nuclei ascend near the medial lemniscus.
c) Quadrigeminal bodies – dorsal region of midbrain (tectum). These are reflex centers involved in gaze and head direction. The superior colliculi are part of the visual reflex center, inferior colliculi are part of the auditory reflex center.
d) Red nucleus (Nucleus rubrum), it is an important motor relay. It forms the rubrospinal tract, and is involved in the motor circuitry. An important clinical distinction between decerebrate and decorticate pathological postures (discussed later) are made relative to it.
e) Substantia nigra. A dopaminergic center, contains important nuclei of the extrapyramidal motor system. Its autoimmune degradation is the etiological base for idiopathic Parkinson's disease. Together with the red nucleus it serves as part of the motor circuitry. Refer to figure 3.21.
f) Cranial nerves CN-III, CN-IV
g) The aqueduct and the PAG (periaqueductal gray).

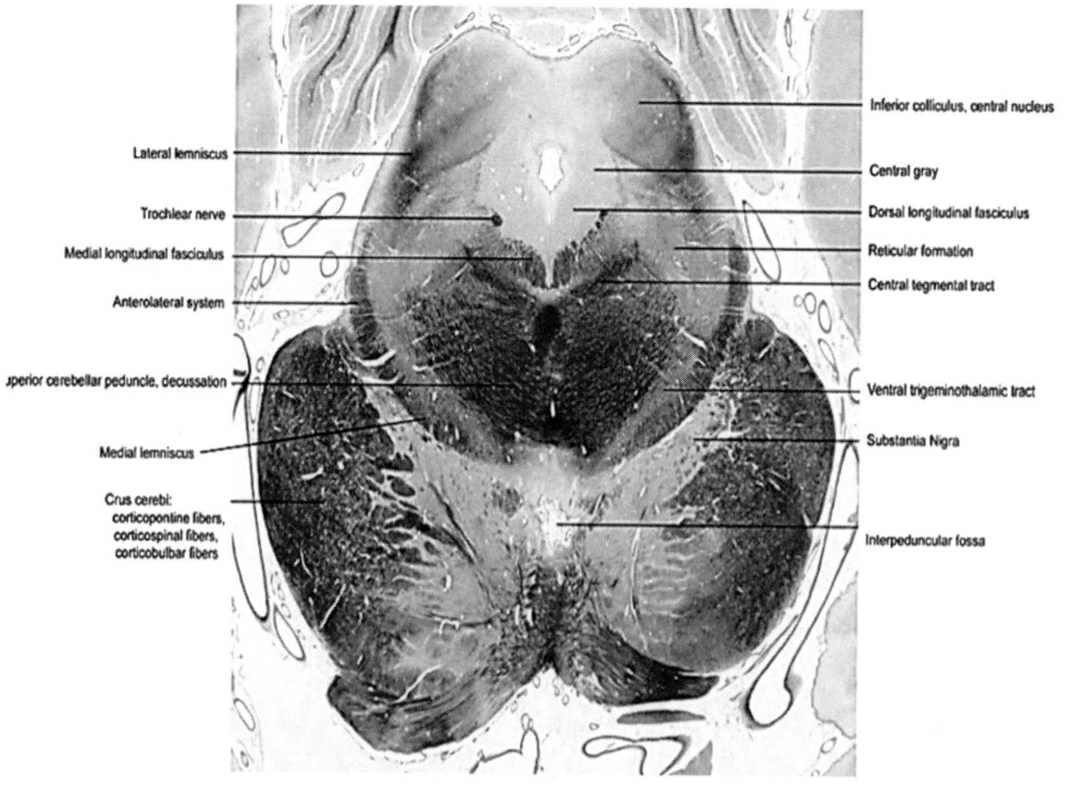

Figure 3.18. Midbrain. Cross section at the level of the trochlear nucleus and the inferior colliculus. Refer to text.

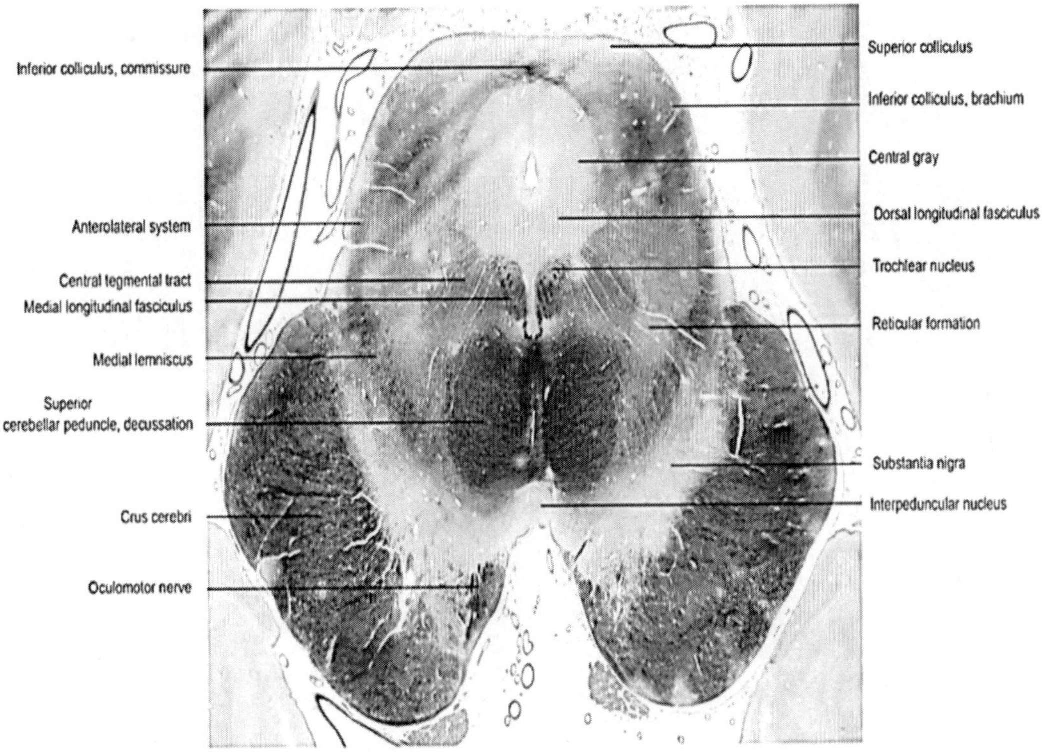

Figure 3.19. Midbrain. Cross section at the level of the superior peduncle decussation. Refer to text.

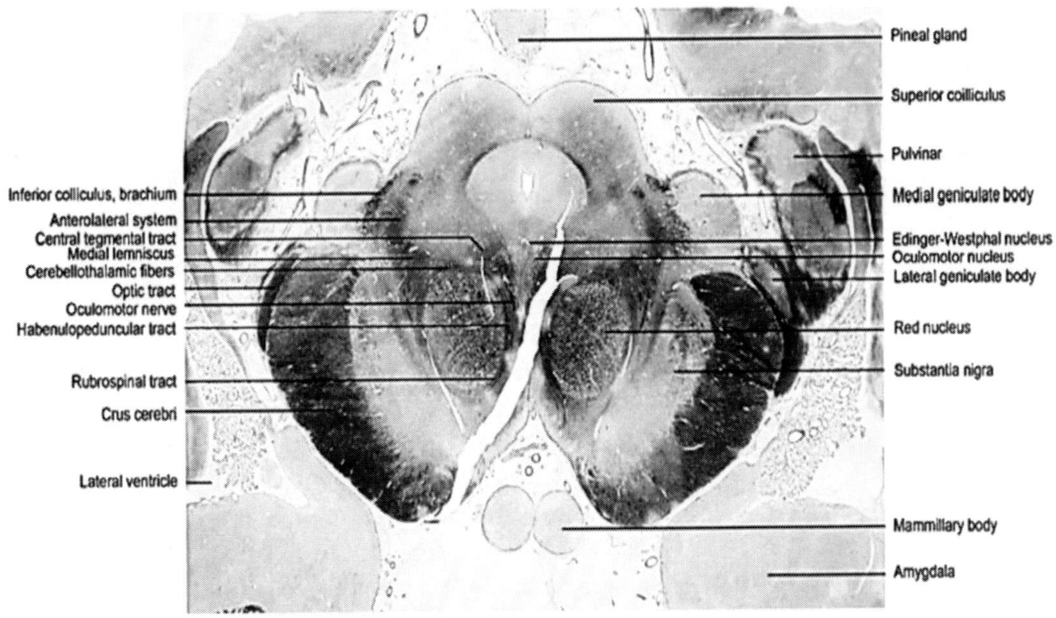

Figure 3.20. Midbrain. Cross section at the level of the superior colliculus, the oculomotor motor nucleus the Edinger-Westphal nucleus. Refer to text.

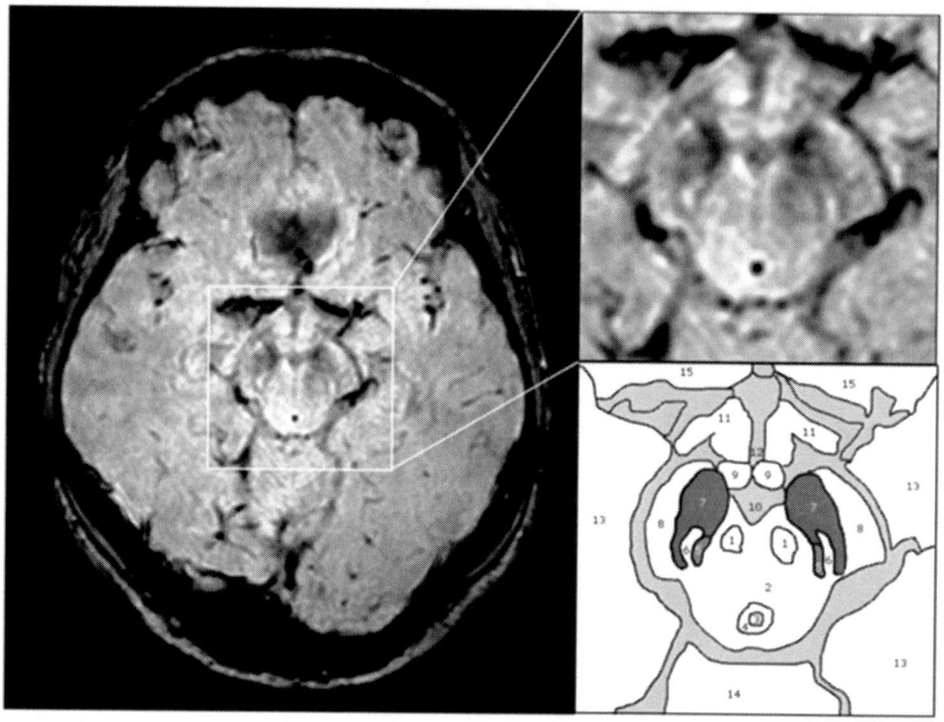

Figure 3.21. Substantia nigra anatomy on 3T SWI MRI. Anatomical structures: 1 red nucleus, 2 midbrain tegmentum, 3 aqueduct, 4 periaqueductal grey, 5 medial lemniscus, 6 nigrosome-1, 7 substantia nigra, 8 cerebral peduncle, 9 mammillary body, 10 inter-peduncular fossa, 11 optic radiation, 12 3rd ventricle, 13 temporal lobe, 14 cerebellum, 15 frontal lobe. Modified with permission from www.radiopaedia.org.

3.7. Synopsis - Cranial Nerves of the Brainstem

3.7.1. Motor Cell Columns and Nuclei

Motor nuclei are formed by the basal plates, which tend to form rostrocaudally oriented columns. These columns later become discontinuous (in line, but separated). The GSE column is most medial. It contains the CN-XII, VI, IV, III motor nuclei (refer to figures 3.9-3.10). There are a few shared characteristics to this column worth mentioning. All nuclei are located adjacent to the midline, anterior to the ventricular space. The motor neurons in these nuclei innervate skeletal muscles originating from head mesoderm in the occipital region (tongue muscles), and orbit from occipital myotomes, not from the pharyngeal arches.

Lateral and adjacent to the GSE column is the GVE column, the cranial part of the parasympathetic visceromotor system. Four nuclei form this column. These are the dorsal vagal motor nucleus (for CN-X), the inferior salivatory nucleus (for CN-IX), the superior salivatory nucleus (for CN-VII) and the Edinger-Westphal nucleus (for CN-III). All nuclei forming this column give rise to preganglionic axons that terminate in a peripheral ganglion (of which the Postganglionic fibers go to visceral structures).

The third column, located most laterally in the medulla and pontine tegmentum is the nucleus ambiguous, whose afferents travel on The CN-X, IX, together with the CN-VII motor nucleus and the CN-V motor nucleus. These four nuclei form a discontinuous column on the lateral part of the medulla, reflecting the differentiation of the basal plate in the brainstem. The muscles innervated by these lower motor neurons originate from the pharyngeal arches (I – mastication for CN-V, II – facial expression for CN-VII, III – Stylopharyngeus, for CN-IX, IV – constrictors of the pharynx, Vocalis, palatine muscles for CN-IX, CN-X). These are classified as SVE.

3.7.2. Sensory Cell Columns and Nuclei

Sensory nuclei of the brainstem arise from the alar plates. These are located (as discussed previously), lateral to the sulcus limitans. Three sensory nuclei form more or less three continuous cell columns in the lateral aspect of the brainstem. These are the solitary tract (nucleus tractus solitarius), the trigeminal sensory nucleus and the vestibular nucleus.

The solitary tract and nucleus are located most medially. It is the visceral afferent center of the brainstem. No matter what cranial nerve returns visceral information (VS or GVA) to the brainstem, the central processing of these primary afferent fibers always form the solitary tract, fibers terminate in the solitary nucleus. Visceral afferent information is conveyed on the CN-VII, IX, X, consisting of taste (**SVA**), and fibers conveying general visceral sensation (**GVA**). Most SVA reaches the rostral aspect of the nucleus, while most GVA reaches the caudal portion of it. Refer to figure 3.22 for an illustration of the solitary nucleus. The medial and spinal Vesitbular nuclei are posterior and adjacent to the solitary tract. These receive info only from CN-VIII complex, serving only the sense of hearing, hence termed SSA.

The trigeminal sensory nuclear complex forms a continuous column from the spinal cord-Medulla junction to rostral midbrain. It is divided to three separate segments. The spinal CN-V nucleus (subdivided to Pars caudalis, Pars Interpolaris, Pars Oralis) extends up to caudal pons. The principle (or chief) CN-V nucleus is located at mid-pontine level whereas the mesencephalic nucleus extends into the midbrain, located laterally to the PAG. As in the case of the solitary tract, the principle and spinal nuclei constitute the general sensory receiving center of the brainstem. Although GSA pain, thermal sensations enter the brainstem on 4 different CN (CN-V, CN-VII, CN-IX, CN-X), the central processes of these is in the spinal trigeminal tract, terminating in the medially adjacent spinal CN-V nucleus. In the medulla, the spinal CN-V tract is laterally adjacent to the spinal nucleus.

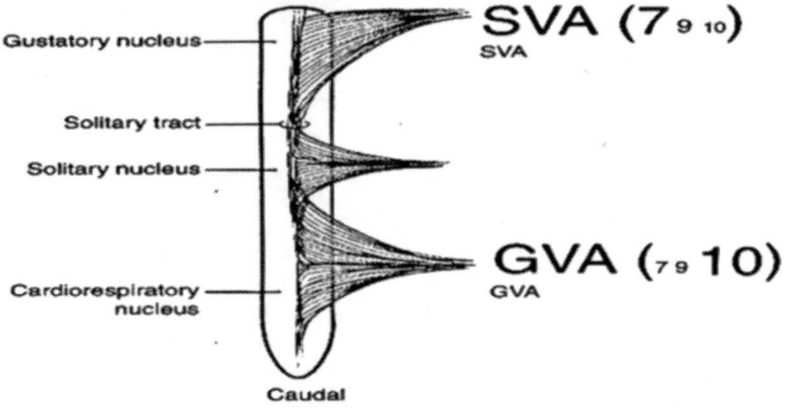

Figure 3.22. The Solitary Nucleus arrangement. Refer to text.

3.7.3. CN of the Medulla

3.7.3.1. CN-XII - Hypoglossal

The nucleus is internal to the hypoglossal trigone bulge at the floor of the fourth ventricle. Axons pass anterior along the lateral aspect of medial lemniscus, pyramid, exiting at the preolivary fissure. Fibers than continue through the hypoglossal canal, where the nerve receives hitch-hiking C1 nerve root fibers, which it distributes before reaching the tongue. The nerve proceeds to run behind the inferior ganglion of the vagus nerve, and then between the internal jugular vein and internal carotid artery until the occipital artery and its branch to sternocleidomastoid which hook over it (laterally). At this point the nerve runs forwards, with the carotid artery and uppermost loop of the lingual artery located medial to it. Its terminal branches supply all the muscles of the tongue except for palatoglossus. Refer to figure 3.23.

Branches:

a) A small meningeal branch that supplies some of the dura mater of the posterior cranial fossa (C1 fibers) which have traveled retrogradely along the nerve.
b) The superior root of the ansa cervicalis (C1 fibers) given off as the hypoglossal nerve lies between the internal jugular vein and internal carotid artery.
c) A nerve to thyrohyoid (C1 fibers) given off as the hypoglossal nerve lies on the loop of the lingual artery.
d) Nerve to geniohyoid (C1 fibers) given off as the hypoglossal nerve enters the mouth, above mylohyoid.

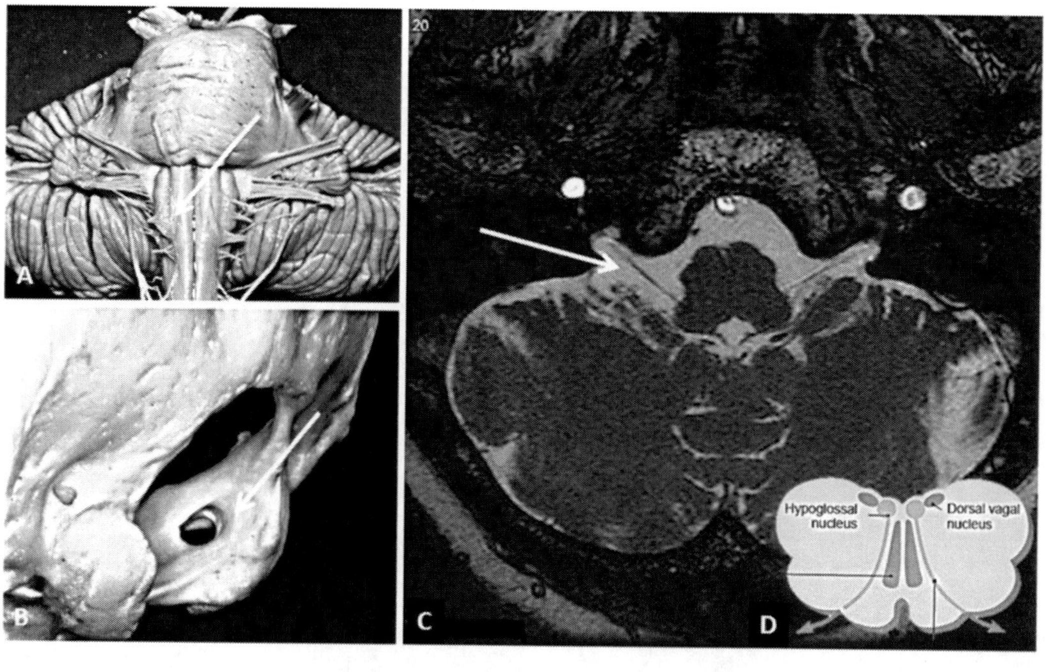

Figure 3.23. The Hypoglossal nerve (CN-XII). A, Ventral brainstem, arrow pointing towards CN-XII emerging from the pre-olivary sulcus. B, the hypoglossal canal, located at the base of the occipital condyle, between it and the jugular tubercle. C, T2 weighted MRI showing CN-XII. Taken with permission from the Rhoton collection (A, B), and from www.radiopaedia.org (C).

3.7.3.2. CN-XI -Accessory

Although all motor components to sternocleidomastoid and trapezius arise from the cervical spinal cord, for consistency it is regarded as a cranial nerve of the medulla. CN-XI fibers are mainly uncrossed. The cranial part of CN-XI (i.e., the accessory portion) is the smaller of the two. Its fibers arise from the cells of the nucleus ambiguus and emerge as four or five delicate rootlets from the side of the medulla oblongata, below the roots of the vagus. It runs laterally to the jugular foramen, where it interchanges fibers with the spinal portion or becomes united to it for a short distance; here it is also connected by one or two filaments with the jugular ganglion of the vagus. It then passes through the jugular foramen, separates from the spinal portion and is continued over the surface of the ganglion nodosum of the vagus. Through a pharyngeal branch it probably supplies the musculus uvulae and levator vali palatini. Some few filaments from it are continued into the trunk of the vagus below the ganglion, to be distributed with the recurrent nerve and probably also with the cardiac nerves.

The Spinal part (spinal portion) is firm in texture, and its fibers arise from the ventral horn cells in the cord between C1 and C5. The fibers emerge from the cord laterally between the anterior and posterior spinal nerve roots to form a single trunk, which ascends into the skull through the foramen magnum. It then exits the skull through the jugular foramen, through which it passes, lying in the same sheath of dura mater as the vagus, but separated from it by a fold of the arachnoid. As it exits from the jugular foramen, it runs backwards then descends obliquely behind the digastric and stylohyoid muscles to the upper part of the sternocleidomastoid; it pierces this muscle, and courses obliquely across the posterior triangle of the neck, to end in the deep surface of the trapezius muscle. In the posterior triangle it unites with the second and third cervical nerves, while beneath the trapezius it forms a plexus with the third and fourth cervical nerves, and from this plexus fibers are distributed to the muscle. Most consider the cranial part of the eleventh cranial nerve to be functionally part of the vagus nerve.

The accessory nerve is responsible for the motor innervation of the sternocleidomastoid and trapezius muscles. The sternocleidomastoid acts in elevation of the thoracic cage and shoulder girdle, or, with fixation of the limb, will act in lateral flexion of the head to the shoulder on the same side and rotate the head to direct the chin upward to the opposite side. The trapezius muscle is one of several muscles that elevate the shoulder girdle and retract the girdle dorsally. Clinically, CN-XI can be located at Erb`s point just superior to where the greater auricular nerve surfaces from the deep neck. The spinal accessory nerve can also be located readily in the lateral neck at the point where it disappears under the deep surface of the trapezius muscle, roughly two finger-breadths superior to the clavicle at the anterior margin of the trapezius muscle.

3.7.3.3. CN-X - Vagus

The vagus (CN-X) is located in an intermediate position between the midline and lateral aspect of the medulla, exiting through the post-olivary sulcus. CN-X exits the cranial cavity through the pars vascularis part of the jugular foramen to enter the carotid space. Within the jugular fossa lie the superior (jugular) sensory ganglion of the vagus nerve and the inferior (nodose) ganglion, which lies approximately 1cm distally. The vagus nerve descends vertically through the neck within the carotid sheath, where it lies posteriorly between the internal / common carotid artery and internal jugular vein. Refer to figures 3.24-3.27. Since the thorax is not symmetrical, the course of the left and right vagus nerves is not identical.

The left vagus nerve crosses anterior to the left subclavian artery as it enters the thorax. Its course takes it lateral to the aorta arch as it descends posterior to the hilum of the left lung and towards the esophageal hiatus, which it passes through to enter the abdominal cavity. The right vagus nerve also passes anterior to the right subclavian artery before diving into the fat surrounding the innominate vessels. It reaches the right paratracheal region before descending, like the left, posterior to the lung hilum and then medially to the esophageal hiatus, which it passes through to enter the abdominal cavity. Around the esophageal hiatus the left and right vagus nerves meet and join to form the esophageal plexus, from which an anterior and posterior vagal trunk (also called gastric nerves) form and descend into the abdomen. The trunks are not composed of equal fibers from the left and right as the anterior trunk is mainly composed of fibers from the left.

Branches (from proximal to distal):

a) From the superior ganglion - small meningeal nerve, auricular nerve (Arnold's nerve), small communicating branches.
b) From the inferior ganglion - pharyngeal nerve to the pharyngeal plexus, carotid body branches, superior laryngeal nerve - divides into internal and external laryngeal
c) From the vagus nerve - recurrent laryngeal nerve, superior and inferior cardiac nerves, anterior and posterior bronchial nerves, esophageal plexus (gastric nerves), coeliac plexus - from the right vagus, hepatic plexus - from the left vagus.

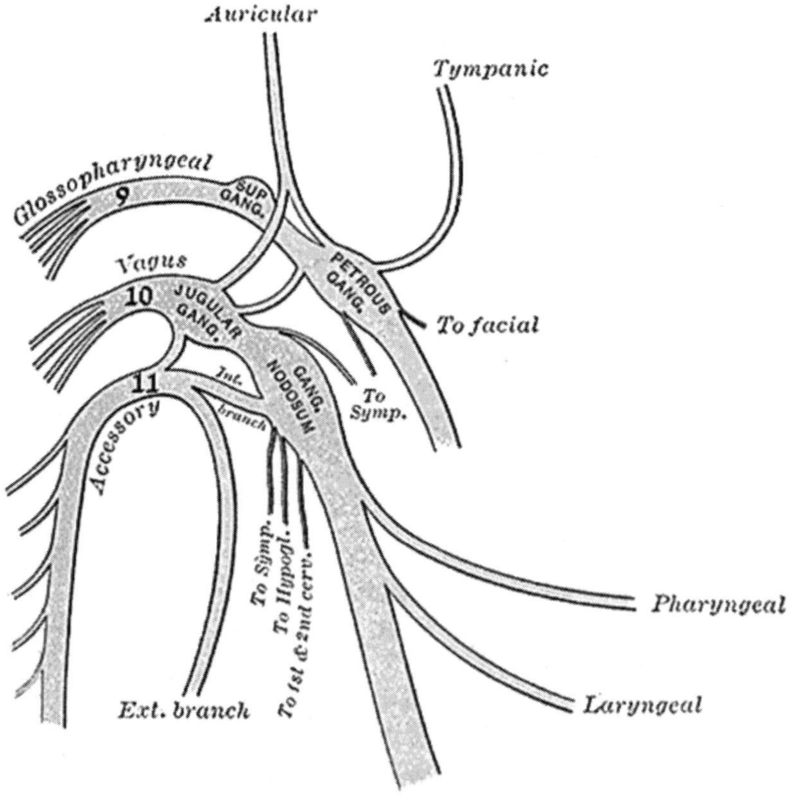

Figure 3.24. Vagus nerve illustration. Gray's anatomy images related to the vagus nerve. Images are in the Public Domain.

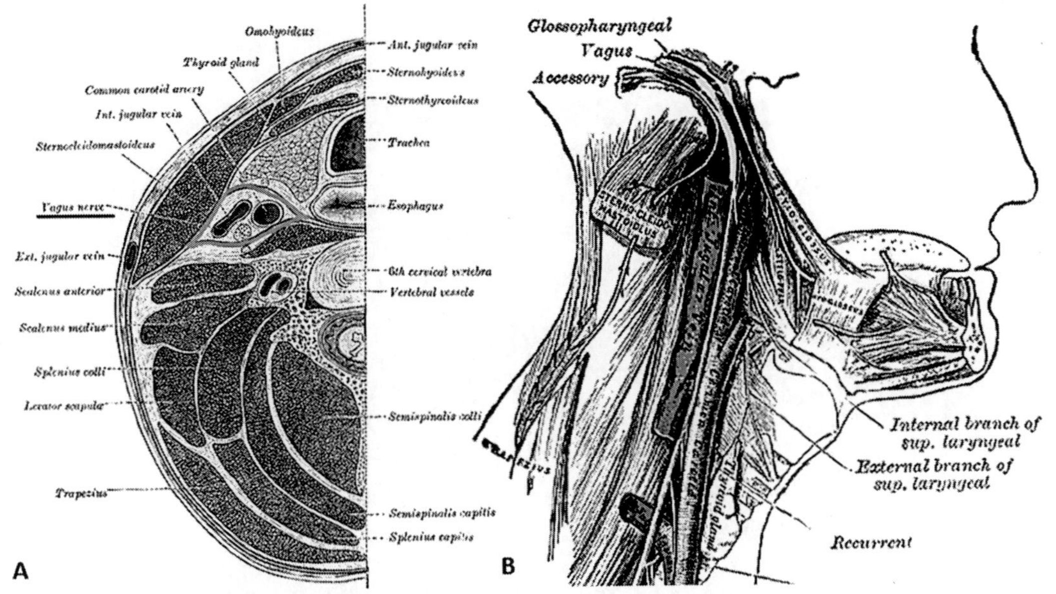

Figure 3.25. The Vagus nerve, peripheral course. A, cross section through the carotid sheath. B, neck dissection showing the peripheral branches. Refer to text. Gray's anatomy images related to the vagus nerve. Images are in the Public Domain.

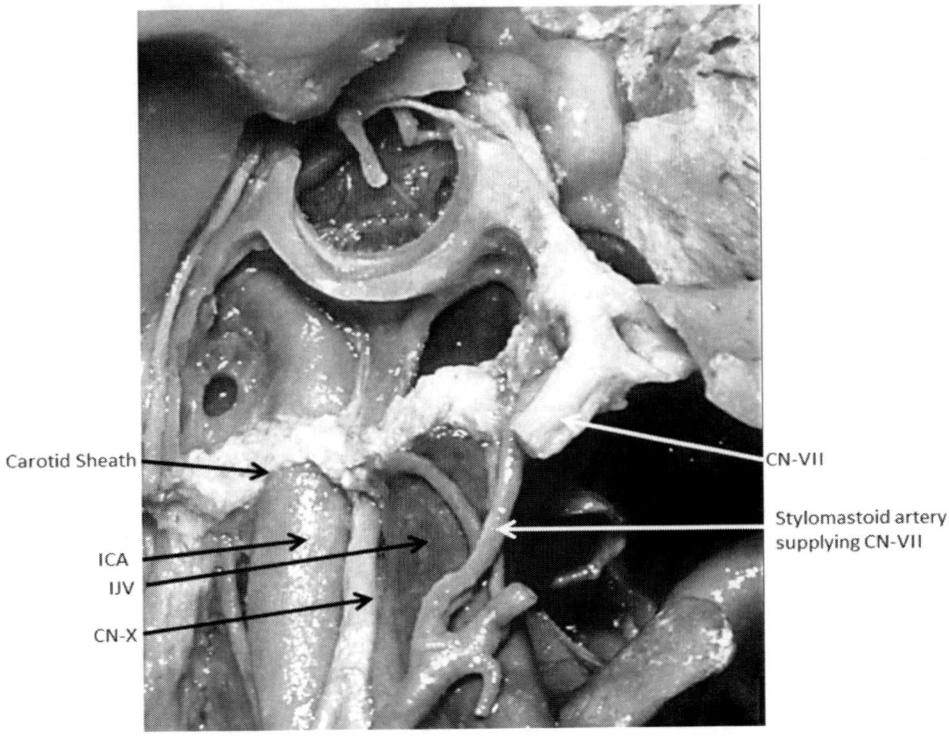

Figure 3.26. Deep neck dissection showing the content of the carotid sheath and related structures. Taken with permission from the Rhoton Collection.

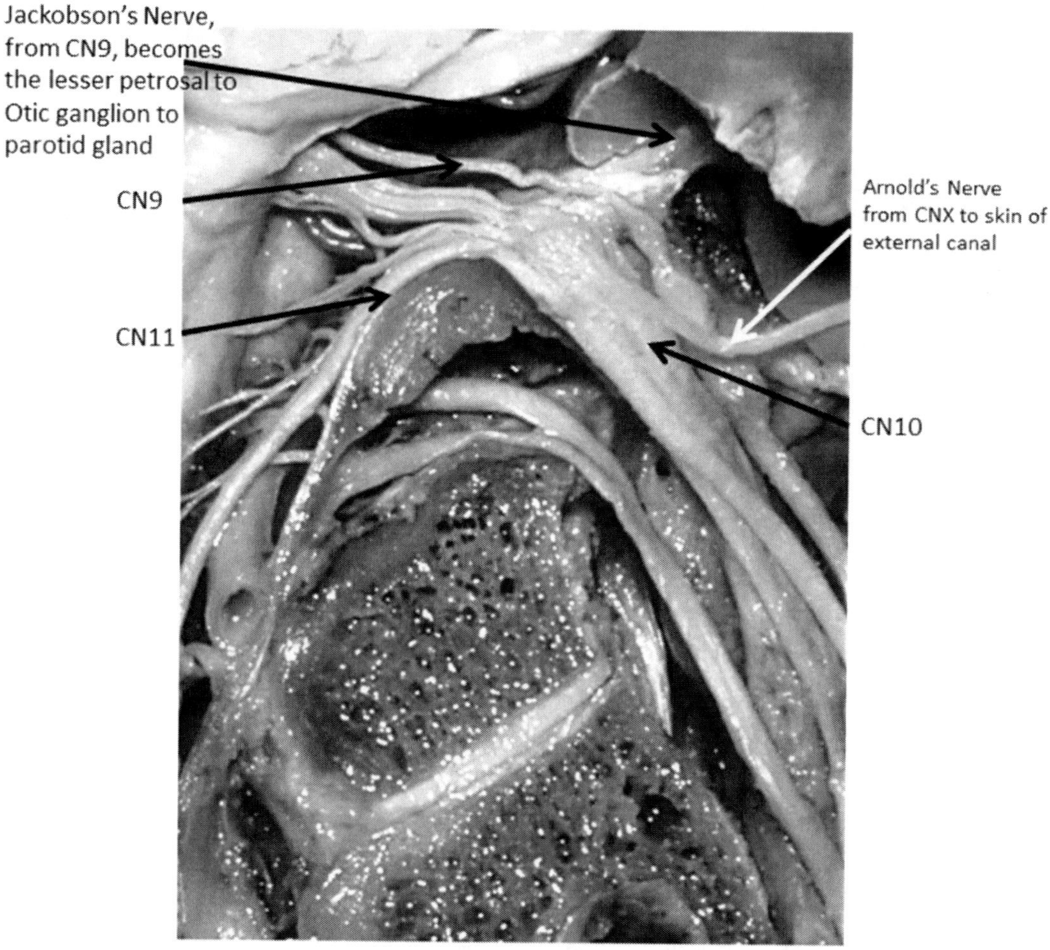

Figure 3.27. Deep neck, mastoid and temporal bone dissection showing the CN-IX-XI complex during its course through the Jugular foramen. Taken with permission from the Rhoton Collection.

3.7.3.4. CN-IX -Glossopharyngeal

The glossopharyngeal nerve (CN-IX) exits the medulla at the post-olivary sulcus, rostral to CN-X. The sensory ganglion cells lie in the superior and inferior ganglia of the nerve. The central processes pass to the nucleus of the tractus solitarius, conveying taste sensation, and to the nucleus of the spinal tract of the CN-V nerve conveying somatic sensation. The motor nucleus lies in the upper part of the nucleus ambiguous which receives bilateral supranuclear innervation from the corticobulbar fibers. This nucleus supplies the stylopharyngeus muscle. The autonomic parasympathetic fibers arise in the inferior salivary nucleus. These fibers are carried in the lesser petrosal nerve via the tympanic branch to the otic ganglion. The post ganglionic fibers are distributed to the parotid gland via the auriculotemporal nerve.

From the medulla oblongata, the glossopharyngeal nerve passes laterally across the flocculus, and leaves the skull through the central part of the jugular foramen, in a separate sheath of the dura mater, lateral to and in front of the vagus and accessory nerves. It descends in front of the internal carotid artery and beneath the styloid process and the muscles connected with it, to the lower border of the stylopharyngeus. It then curves forward, forming an arch on the side of the neck and lying upon the stylopharyngeus and middle pharyngeal constrictor muscle. From there it passes under cover of the hyoglossus muscle, and is finally distributed to the palatine tonsil, the mucous membrane of the fauces and base of the tongue, and the mucous glands of the mouth.

In passing through the jugular foramen, the nerve presents two ganglia, the superior (jugular) and the inferior (petrous). The superior ganglion is situated in the upper part of the groove in which the nerve is lodged during its passage through the jugular foramen; it is very small, and is usually regarded as a detached portion of the petrous ganglion. The inferior (petrous) ganglion is larger and is situated in a depression in the lower border of the petrous portion of the temporal bone.

The glossopharyngeal nerve functions in receiving general sensory fibers from the tonsils, the pharynx, the middle ear and the posterior 1/3 of the tongue. CN-IX receives special sensory fibers (taste) from the posterior one-third of the tongue, as well as receives visceral sensory fibers from the carotid bodies. CN-IX supplies parasympathetic fibers to the parotid gland via the otic ganglion, and it supplies motor fibers to the stylopharyngeus muscle, the only motor component of this cranial nerve. Refer to figures 3.27-3.30.

Branches:

a) **The tympanic nerve** (nerve of Jacobson) - exits the jugular foramen and passes by the inferior glossopharyngeal ganglion. It then re-enters the skull through the inferior tympanic canaliculus and reaches the tympanic cavity where it forms the tympanic plexus in the middle ear cavity. It then travels from this plexus through a canal and out into the middle cranial fossa adjacent to the exit of the greater petrosal nerve. It is here the nerve becomes the lesser petrosal nerve. The lesser petrosal nerve exits the cranium via the foramen ovale and synapses in the otic ganglion.

b) Muscular branch to the stylopharyngeus muscle.

c) Carotid branches - descend along the trunk of the internal carotid artery as far as its origin, communicating with the pharyngeal branch of the vagus, and with branches of the sympathetic nerves.

d) Pharyngeal branches - together with the pharyngeal branches of the vagus and sympathetic nerves, they form the pharyngeal plexus.

e) Tonsillar branches - supply the palatine tonsil.

f) Lingual branches to supply the vallate papillae and the mucous membrane covering the base of the tongue, follicular glands of the posterior part of the tongue, and communicates with the lingual nerve.

g) **N.B. Sinus nerve "Hering's nerve"** -The branch of the glossopharyngeal nerve to the carotid sinus is the nerve that runs downwards anterior to the internal carotid artery communicate with the vagus and sympathetic then divides in the angle of bifurcation of the common carotid artery to supply the carotid body and carotid sinus. It carries impulses from the baroreceptors in the carotid sinus (to help maintain a more consistent blood pressure) and from chemoreceptors in the carotid body.

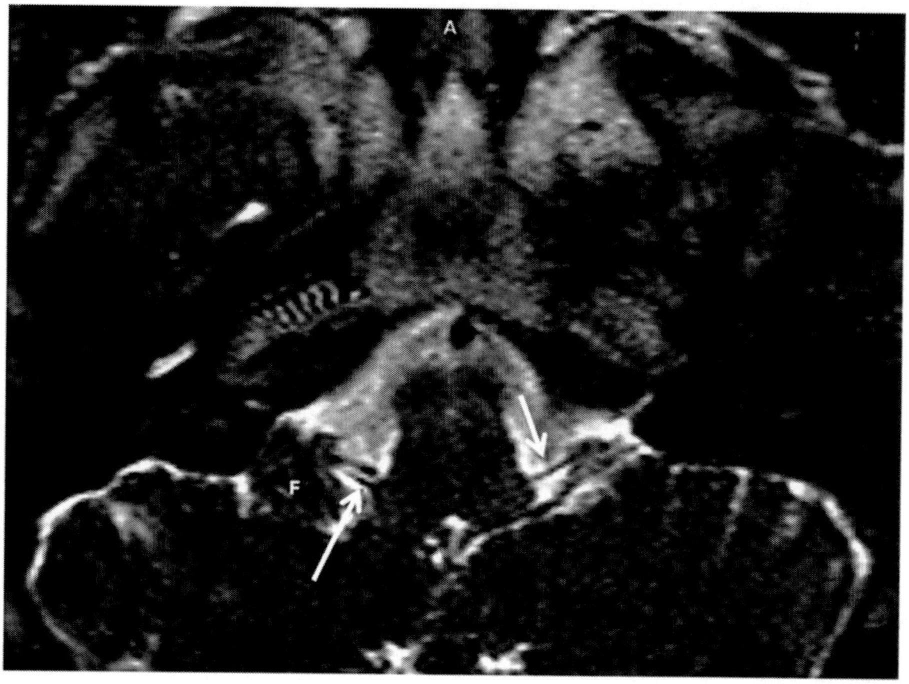

Figure 3.28. The Glossopharyngeal (CN-IX) nerve. T2-Weighted images. Taken with permission from www.radiopaedia.org.

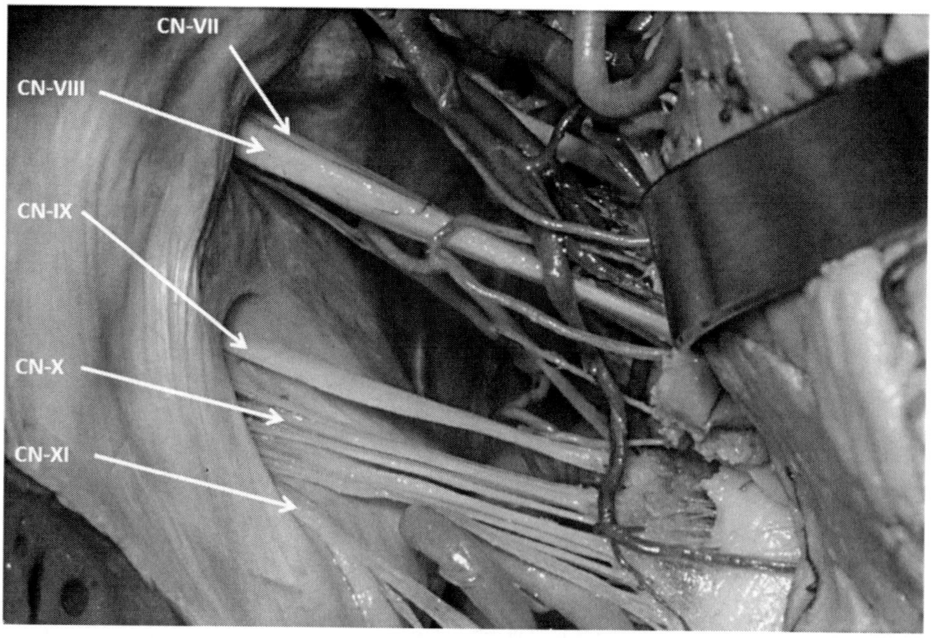

Figure 3.29. An operative view showing the entrance to the jugular foramen. CN-IX-XI can be shown, as well as CN-VII-VIII on entering the internal acoustic meatus. Taken with permission from the Rhoton collection.

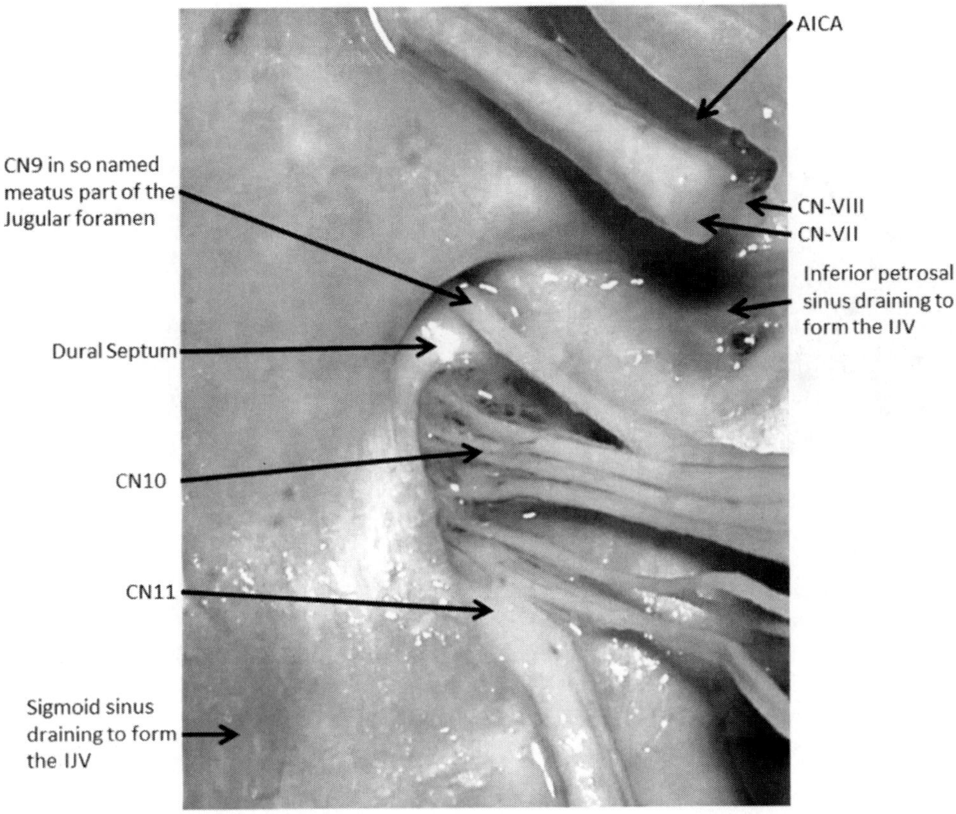

Figure 3.30. An operative view showing the entrance to the jugular foramen. CN-IX-XI can be shown, as well as CN-VII-VIII on entering the internal acoustic meatus. The segmentation of the jugular foramen is better shown here, as well as the interior petrosal and sigmoid venous sinuses forming the IJV at this location. Taken with permission from the Rhoton Collection.

3.7.4. Cranial Nerves of Pons-Medulla junction

3.7.4.1. CN-VIII - Vestibulocochlear

The vestibulocochlear (CN-VIII) nerve is the eighth cranial nerve and has two roles: It innervates the cochlea for hearing and it innervates the vestibule for acceleration sense. CN-VIII emerges between the pons and the medulla lateral to the facial nerve and nervus intermedius, passing laterally through the cerebellopontine angle to the internal acoustic meatus / canal (IAM / IAC) with the aforementioned two other nerves. In the IAM the nerve splits into 4 bundles: the cochlear nerve, superior and inferior division of the vestibular nerve and nerve from the posterior semicircular canal, separated from each other by the falciform crest and Bill's bar (see figure 3.31). The cochlear nerve relays with the first order sensory cells in the spiral ganglion, which is in the base of the spiral lamina (refer to chapter 12 for audition).

The vestibular nerve relays in the vestibular ganglion (aka ganglion of Scarpa). From here three bundles emerge: the superior division, the inferior division and the nerve from the posterior semicircular canal. The superior division of the vestibular nerve carries sensory fibers from the hair cells of the anterior and lateral semicircular canals and utricle. It is located in the postero-superior quadrant. The inferior division carries sensory fibers from the saccule. It is located in the postero-inferior quadrant, along with the nerve from the posterior semicircular canal, also in the postero-inferior quadrant passes through the foramen singulare. Refer to figures 3.31-3.32.

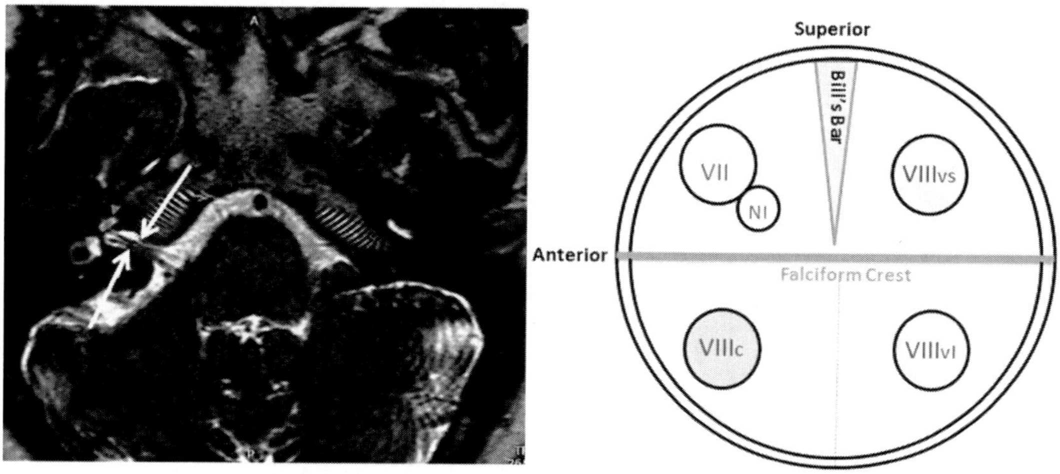

Figure 3.31. CN-VIII. A, T2 weight MRI. B, A diagram of relationship of nerves in the internal acoustic meatus. VII = facial nerve NI = nervus intermedius VIIIc = cochlear nerve VIIIvs = superior division of vestibular nerve VIIIvi = inferior division of vestibular nerve. Refer to text.

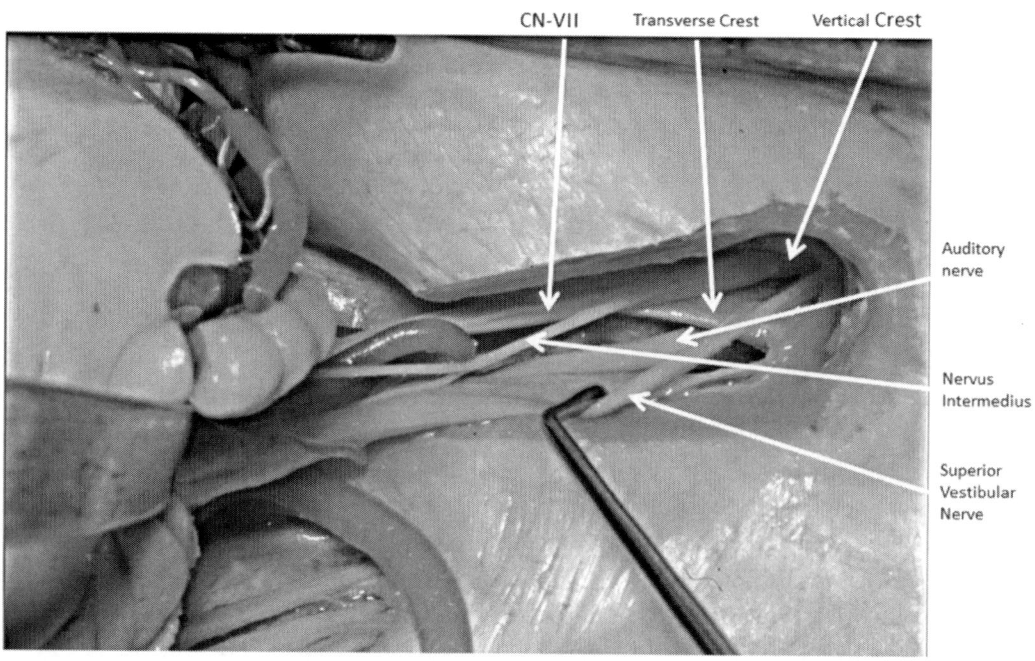

Figure 3.32. The internal Acoustic Meatus. The meatal segment of the facial nerve is seen within the internal auditory canal, which has been drilled from a retrosigmoid approach. The facial nerve is located anterior and superior within the canal. The transverse crest separates it from the auditory nerve inferiorly. The vertical crest separates it from the superior vestibular nerve posteriorly. The nervus intermedius is also seen. Taken with permission from the Rhoton collection.

3.7.4.2. CN-VII – The Facial Nerve

Three brainstem nuclei contribute to the facial nerve: one GSE, one GVE, and one GVA. The facial nerve nucleus is in the pons. Its motor fibers loop posteriorly over the abducens nerve nucleus, to form the facial colliculus on the floor of fourth ventricle. The superior salivary nucleus, next to the facial nucleus supplies GVE parasympathetic fibers. The nucleus tractus solitarius, supplies taste fibers that eventually end up in the chorda tympani. The facial nerve has six named segments: the intracranial (cisternal) segment, the meatal segment (internal auditory canal, whose length is about 8mm having no branches), the labyrinthine segment (from IAM to the geniculate ganglion, measuring 3-4mm having 3 branches (from geniculate ganglion), the tympanic segment (from geniculate ganglion to the pyramidal eminence measuring 8-11mm with no branches), the mastoid segment (from pyramidal eminence to stylomastoid foramen measuring 8-14mm having 3 branches) and the extratemporal segment (from stylomastoid foramen to division into major branches, measuring 5-20mm and having 9 branches). Refer to table 3.2 for the segments of the facial nerve. Refer to figures 3.32-3.35.

Table 3.2. Facial Nerve (CN-VII) Segments

Segment	Comments	Branches
Intracranial (cisternal)	As the nerve emerges immediately beneath the pons, lateral to the abducens nerve and medial to the vestibulocochlear nerve, it is joined by the nervus intermedius, which has emerged lateral to the main trunk. Together the two travel through the cerebellopontine angle to the internal acoustic meatus.	
Meatal segment.	Having been joined by the nervus intermedius, these nerves are located in the anterior superior quadrant, above the falciform crest and anterior to Bill's bar.	
Labyrinthine segment	As the facial nerve and nervus intermedius pass through the anterior superior quadrant of the internal acoustic meatus it enters the Fallopian canal, passing anterolaterally between and superior to the cochlea (anterior) and vestibule (posterior), and then runs back posteriorly at the geniculate ganglion (where the nervus intermedius joins the facial nerve and where fibers for taste synapse)	greater superficial petrosal nerve lesser petrosal nerve external petrosal nerve
Tympanic segment	As the nerve passes posteriorly from the geniculate ganglion it becomes the tympanic segment (8-11 mm in length) and is immediately beneath the lateral semicircular canal in the medial wall of the middle ear cavity. The bone of the Fallopian canal is often dehiscent in the area of the oval window in 25-55% of postmortem specimens, having mucosa in direct contact with the nerve. The nerve passes posterior to the cochleariform process, tensor tympani and oval window. Just distal to the pyramidal eminence the nerve makes a second turn (second genu) passing vertically downwards as the mastoid segment.	

Table 3.2. (Continued)

Segment	Comments	Branches
Mastoid segment	The mastoid segment, measuring 8-14mm in length, extends from the second genu to the stylomastoid foramen, through what is confusingly referred to as the Fallopian canal. The Chorda tympani is a terminal branch carrying both vasomotor fibers to the submandibular gland and sublingual gland and taste to the anterior two thirds of the tongue	Nerve to the stapedius Chorda tympani Nerve from the auricular branch of the vagus nerve (CN X) - pain fibers to the posterior part of the external acoustic meatus hitchhike from the jugular foramen
Extratemporal segment	As the nerve exits the stylomastoid foramen, it gives off a sensory branch that supplies part of the external acoustic meatus and tympanic membrane. It then passes between the posterior belly of the digastric muscle and the stylohyoid muscle and enters the parotid gland. Lying between the deep and superficial lobes of the gland the nerve divides into two main branches at the pes anserinus (Latin: duck foot) - a superior temporofacial and inferior cervicofacial branches. The temporal branch runs with the superficial musculoaponeurotic system (SMAS) over the zygomatic arch.	Branch to external acoustic meatus and tympanic membrane From the anterior border of the gland, five branches emerge; temporal, zygomatic, buccal, mandibular (marginal) and cervical.

The functions of the facial nerve include taste, parasympathetic and motor functions. Taste fibers to the anterior two thirds of the tongue originate in the nucleus of the tractus solitarius (NTS), travel in the nervus intermedius (preganglionic) where they join the facial nerve at the geniculate ganglion and synapse. Postganglionic fibers travel with the facial nerve and are given off as the chorda tympani, which eventually joins the lingual nerve (branch of the trigeminal nerve (CN V)).

Parasympathetic Preganglionic fibers originate in the superior salivary nucleus and join the facial nerve at the geniculate ganglion having traveled with the nervus intermedius. These fibers do not synapse in the ganglion, but rather pass through to be distributed between the greater superficial petrosal nerve (GSPN) anastomosing in the pterygopalatine ganglion. Next these travel to supply the lacrimal gland.

The lesser petrosal nerve anastomoses in the otic ganglion and supplies the parotid gland (along with fibers from the inferior salivary nucleus which arrive via the glossopharyngeal nerve to supply to the tympanic plexus). The chorda tympani anastomoses in the submandibular ganglion and supplies the submandibular gland and sublingual gland.

The facial nerve receives its arterial supply from three main sources:

a) The labyrinthine - a branch of the AICA, which supplies the meatal segment. It is supplemented by direct twigs in the cisternal position, directly from the AICA.
b) The superficial petrosal artery - a branch of the middle meningeal artery which passes retrogradely along the greater superficial petrosal nerve.

c) The stylomastoid artery - a branch of the occipital artery, which passes retrogradely into the stylomastoid foramen.

The labyrinthine segment of the facial nerve is the most vulnerable to ischemia as the connections between the labyrinthine artery and superficial petrosal artery are very tenuous, with each artery essentially being end arteries.

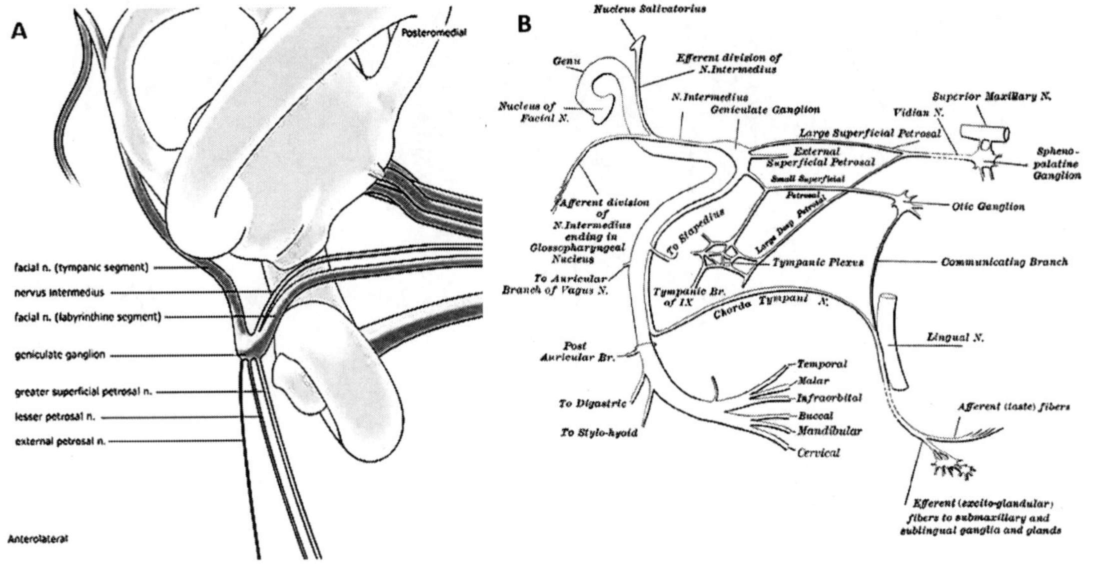

Figure 3.33. The Facial Nerve Connections. A, A simplified form, with cochlea and vestibule for orientation. Taken with permission from www.radiopaedia.org. B, Detailed. Gray's anatomy images related to the vagus nerve. Images are in the Public Domain.

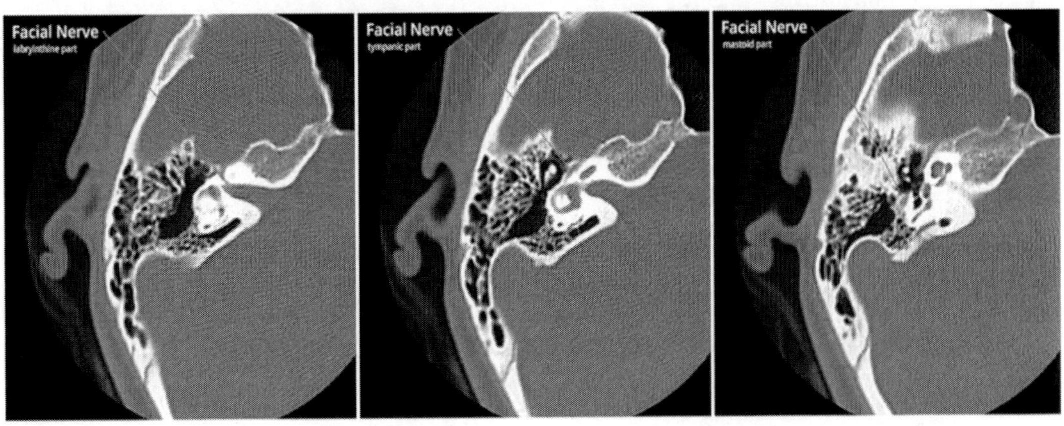

Figure 3.34. The segments of the facial nerve, as seen on CT. taken with permission from www.radiopaedia.org.

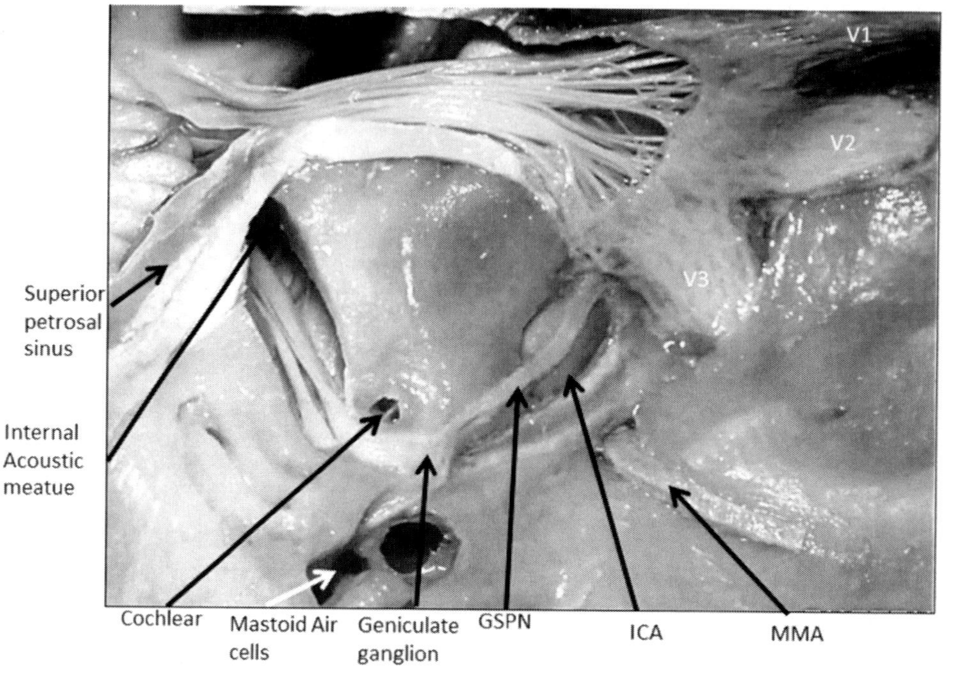

Figure 3.35a+b. Stepwise dissection through the internal acoustic meatus, cochlea and vestibule from the middle cranial fossa floor. A, bony dissection of the right internal acoustic meatus from the middle cranial fossa view showing the CN-VII, CN-VIII at the IAM, the geniculate ganglion and GSPN, the cochlear nerve. The superior petrosal sinus, the internal carotid artery (ICA), and middle meningeal artery (MMA), the trigeminal nerve are also shown. Taken with permission from the Rhoton Collection.

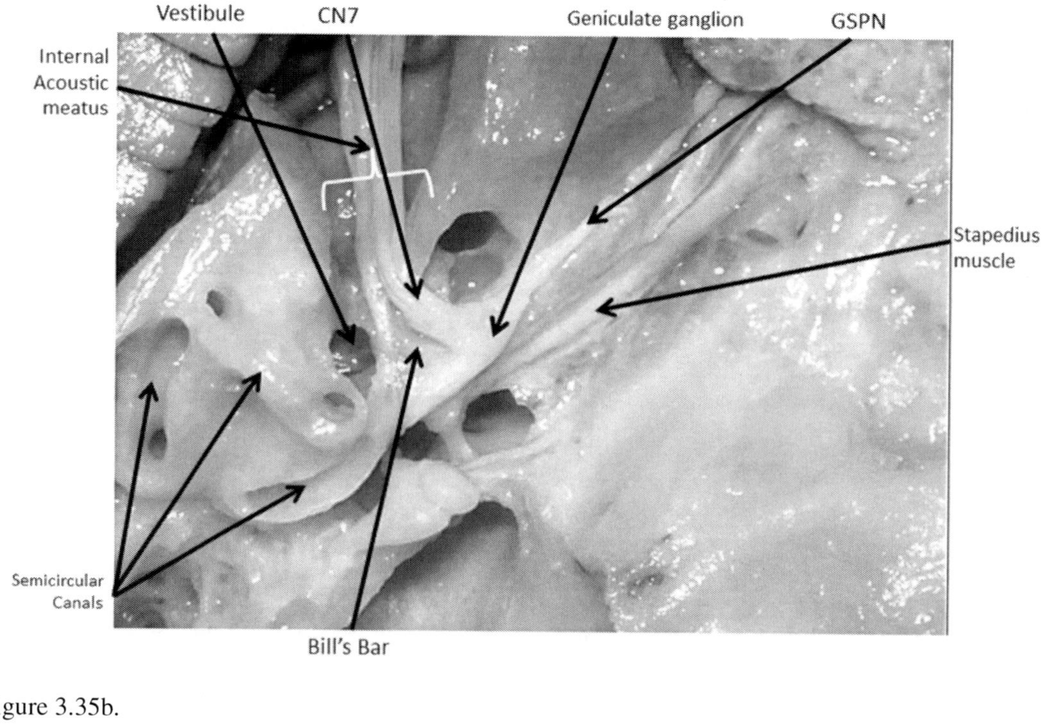

Figure 3.35b.

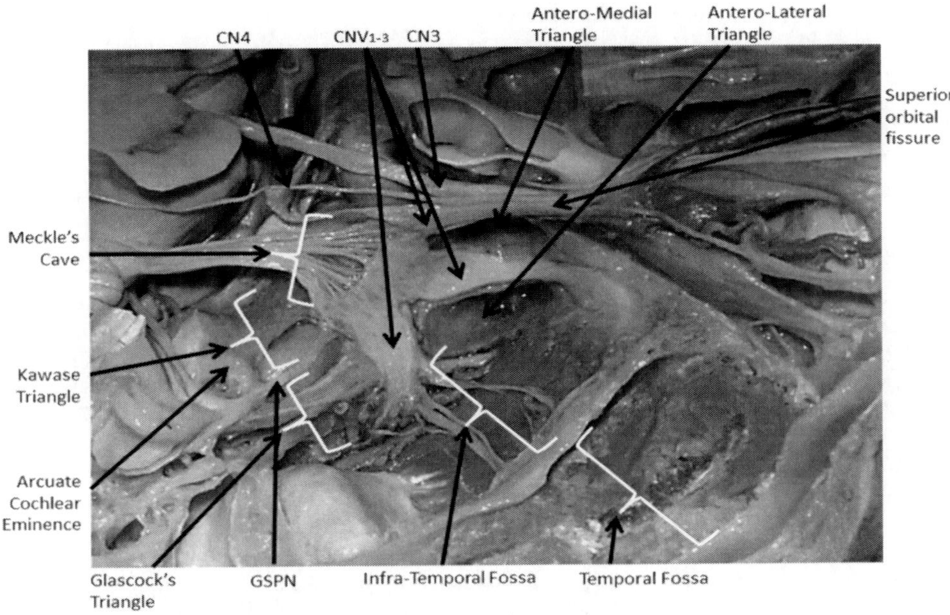

Figure 3.35c. Dissection of the right internal acoustic meatus and the right middle cranial fossa from a middle cranial fossa view. The different middle fossa zones are shown (refer to text, chapter 10). The temporal fossa, infra-temporal fossa access regions is shown. The middle fossa triangles are shown (Anteromedial and anterolateral, **Meckle**'s cave, **Kawase**'s triangle, **Glascock**'s triangle) etc. Taken with permission from the Rhoton Collection.

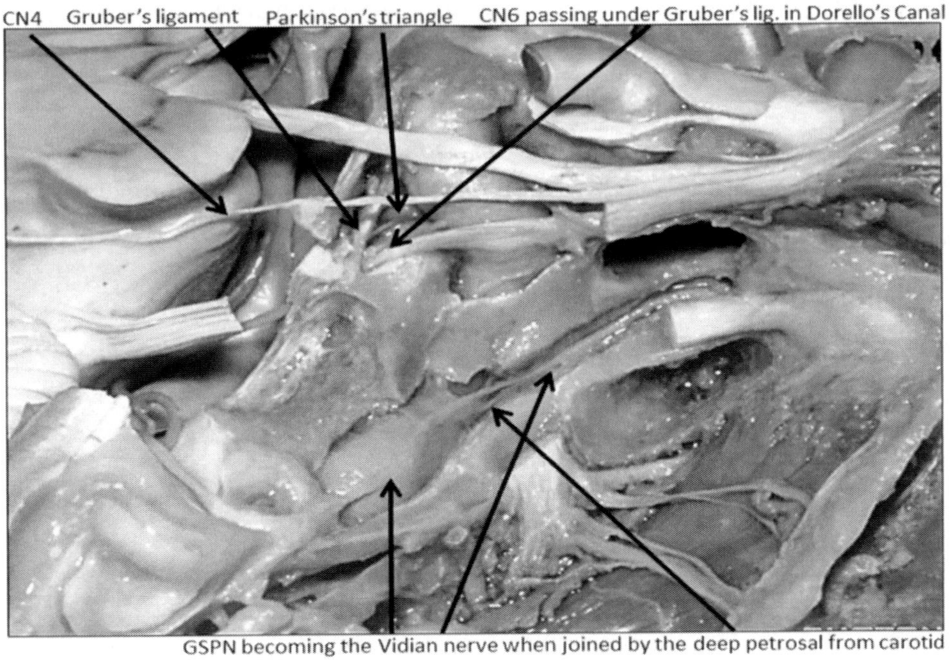

Figure 3.35d. Dissection of the right internal acoustic meatus and the right middle cranial fossa from a middle cranial fossa view. The different middle fossa zones are shown (refer to text, chapter 10). The **Parkinson**'s triangle, **Gruber**'s ligament, **Dorello**'s canal. The formation of the vidian nerve from the GSPN and the deep petrosal nerve is shown. Taken with permission from the Rhoton Collection.

3.7.4.3. CN-VI - The Abducens Nerve

The abducens nerve is the sixth cranial nerve. Its course from nucleus located in the dorsal pons, to its innervation of the lateral rectus muscle can be divided into four parts: The nucleus and intra-parenchymal portion, the cisternal portion, the cavernous sinus portion and the orbital portion. Refer to table 3.3 and figures 3.35d, 3.36, 3.37.

Table 3.3. Abducens Nerve (CN-VI) Segments

Nucleus and intra-parenchymal portion	The abducens nucleus is a small nucleus situated at the upper part of the rhomboid fossa beneath the colliculus facialis within the pons, at the floor of the rhomboid fossa, Lateral to the Medial sulcus. Its axons course through the tegmental and basilar Pons. Interneurons in the nucleus, send their axons to the contralateral medial longitudinal fasciculus (MLF), ascending to the oculomotor (CN-II)I nucleus, and forming excitatory synapses on it (discussed later).
Cisternal portion	It is the most medial of the nerves emerging from immediately below the pons (facial nerve and vestibulocochlear nerve lateral to it) at the pontomedullary junction into the prepontine cistern. It courses anteriorly toward the clivus where it runs superiorly along the clivus enclosed within fibrous sheath called Dorello's canal and pierces the dura inferior to the posterior clinoid process, passing under Gruber's ligament (refer to figure 3.35d). Then it courses over the medial petrous apex toward the cavernous sinus. It is its oblique course and relatively fixed anchor in Dorello's canal which makes it prone to stretching when raised ICP from a space occupying lesion causes transtentorial herniation (a sixth nerve palsy is the classic lateralizing sign of an extradural hematoma).
Cavernous sinus portion	Within the cavernous sinus the abducens nerve is located inferolateral to the internal carotid artery medial to the lateral wall of the sinus (refer to figure 3.36).
Orbital portion	Having entered the orbit through the superior orbital fissure within the tendinous ring it supplies the lateral rectus (refer to figure 3.37).

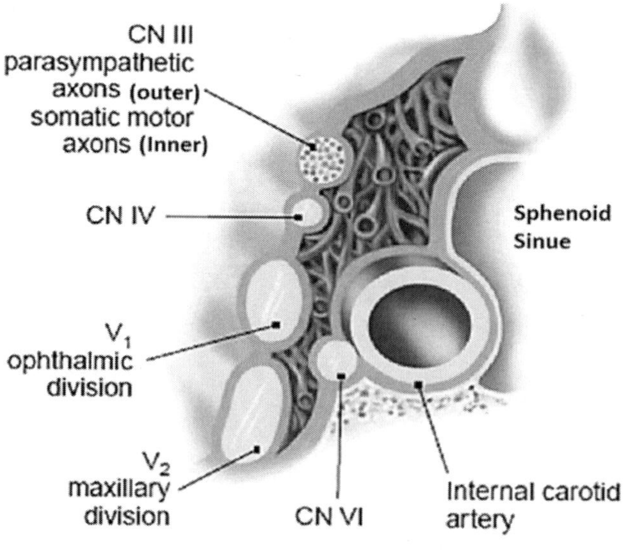

Figure 3.36. The left cavernous sinus in coronal section. Note that all blood vessels and cranial nerves are within its walls, formed by dura. The lateral wall is occupied from superior to inferior by cranial nerves CN-III, CN-IV, CN-V_1, CN-V_2. The medial wall is occupied from superior to inferior by the internal carotid artery and CN-VI. Taken with permission from www.radiopaedia.org.

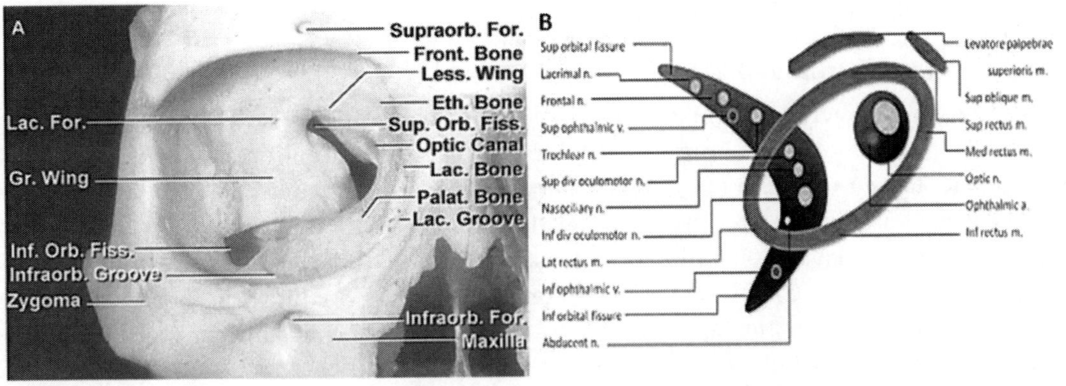

Figure 3.37. The superior orbital fissure. A, Anterior view of the right orbit. The walls of the orbit are formed by seven bones. They are the frontal, zygomatic, sphenoid, lacrimal, ethmoid, and palatine bones, and the maxilla. The superior orbital fissure is bounded above by the lesser wing of the sphenoid bone, below by the greater wing, and medially by the sphenoid body. The inferior orbital fissure is bounded posteriorly by the greater sphenoid wing and anteriorly by the maxilla. Taken with permission from the Rhoton Collection. B, Diagram of the superior orbital fissure. Taken with permission from www.radiopaedia.org.

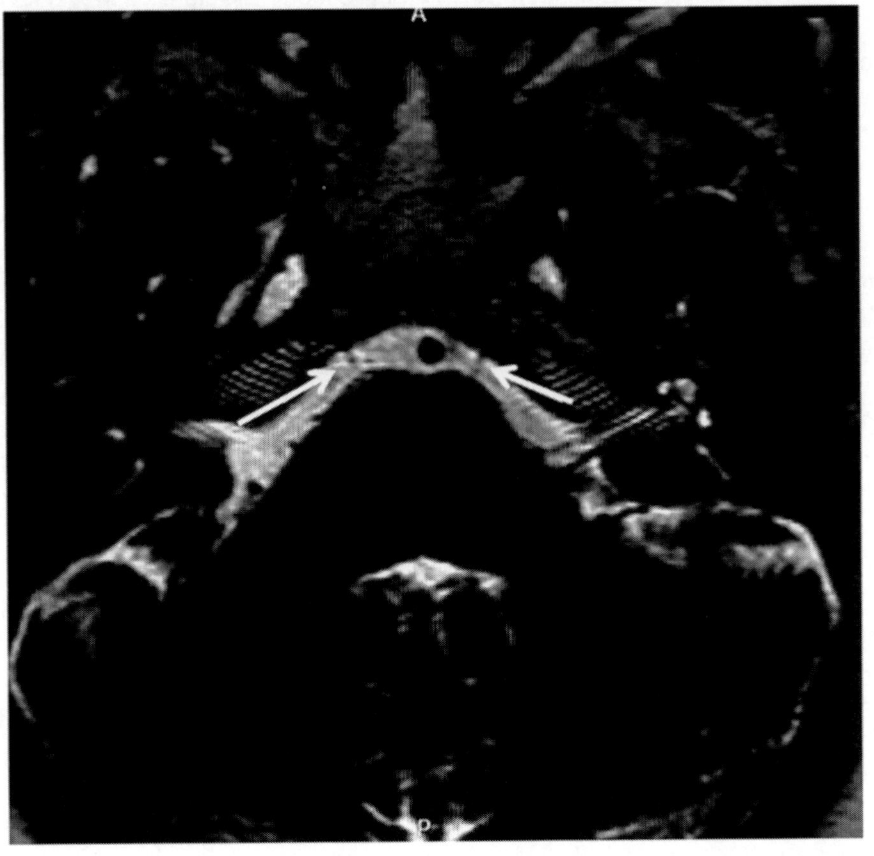

Figure 3.38. CN-VI – T2-weight MRI. Taken with permission from www.radiopaedia.org.

3.7.5. Cranial Nerves of the Pons

3.7.5.1. CN-V – The Trigeminal Nerve

The trigeminal nerve is a mixed nerve, having a sensory component (GSA, sensation of touch, pain, temperature and proprioception in the face) and motor (SVE, to the muscles of mastication, tensor tympani muscle). It is both large and complicated and has multiple brainstem nuclei (sensory and motor) as well as many interconnections with other cranial nerves. It swaps parasympathetic fibers and taste fibers willy-nilly, and divides into dozens of terminal branches. The CN-V nuclear complex runs from the midbrain to the upper cervical spinal cord consisting of 3 nuclei. The CN-V Mesencephalic nucleus mediates proprioception from the face; the CN-V chief sensory mediates vibration and light touch from the face (and hence is analogous to the function of the dorsal columns system from the body). The CN-V Spinal trigeminal nucleus mediates pain and temperature sensation from the face (and hence analogous to anterolateral system from the body). It is the rostral extension of the dorsal horn. The Spinal trigeminal tract is thus analogues to Lissauer's tract.

The CN-V fibers are arranges somatotopically, with mandibular division located dorsally and the ophthalmic division located ventrally. Superimposed in this fiber layering is the concentric "onion rings" arrangement, in which perioral areas are more rostral in the nucleus. The CN-V motor nucleus is located in upper middle pons, near the nerve's exit point from the pons. Its motor root runs inferomedial to the ganglion, along the floor of Meckel's cave, than joins the CN-V^3 division (the mandibular nerve). The motor branch innervates the muscles of mastication, tensor tympani, tensor vali palatine, mylohyoid, and the anterior belly of the digastric muscle.

The trigeminal lemniscus (analogous to the medial lemniscus for the dorsal columns system) crosses to the opposite side to ascend with the medial lemniscus to the VPM nucleus of thalamus (while medial lemniscus goes to VPL). A second smaller pathway, the dorsal trigeminal tract arises from the chief trigeminal sensory nucleus to reach the ipsilateral VPM nucleus of thalamus without crossing.

The trigeminal nerve exits at the mid ventrolateral pons into the prepontine cistern and passes anteriorly to Meckel's cave (a doubling of the dural later upon crossing the petrous ridge into the middle cranial fossa) where its fibers rely forming the Gasserian ganglion. It then divides into three main branches. CN-V1, the ophthalmic division passes at the lateral wall of the cavernous sinus inferior to trochlear nerve and then through the superior orbital fissure where it divides into the frontal, lacrimal, and nasociliary nerves. The frontal nerve divides into the supraorbital and supratrochlear nerves. Nasociliary nerve branches include a communicating branch to the ciliary ganglion, short and long ciliary nerves, the posterior and anterior ethmoidal nerves (the latter divides into internal and external nasal branches), and the infratrochlear nerve.

CN-V2, the maxillary division, passes in the lateral wall of cavernous sinus and then through the foramen rotundum to exit skull. Then it crosses the pterygopalatine fossa and enters the orbit through the inferior orbital fissure and the infraorbital canal. It emerges through the infraorbital foramen to become the infraorbital nerve. Hence orbital blow out fracture is associated with loss of sensation over the maxilla. CN-V3, the mandibular division, passes through the foramen ovale and gives motor supply to the muscles of mastication. The trigeminal nerve provides sensation for touch and pain in nasal sinuses, inside the nose, mouth, and the anterior two thirds of the tongue. Supratentorial dura pain sensation is also innervated by the trigeminal nerve (in the posterior fossa pain is mediated via the CN-X and the upper cervical roots). Refer to figures 3.35a and c, 3.36, 3.37, 3.39, 3.40.

Trigeminal neuralgia, AKA tic douloureux is a pain syndrome having recurrent episodes of brief severe lancinating pain lasting seconds to minutes, mostly in the distribution of the maxillary and mandibular branches. Usually begins after age 35, unilateral, sharply demarcated within its division. Pain episodes are provoked by chewing, shaving, touching specific trigger points of actions. The exact cause is unknown, although a neurovascular conflict with a vessel impinging on the CN-V cisternal segment (most commonly, ie in 80%, the superior cerebellar artery - SCA) has been linked, with its decompression resulting in immediate pain cessation. Still in other cases, no such neurovascular conflict can be shown.

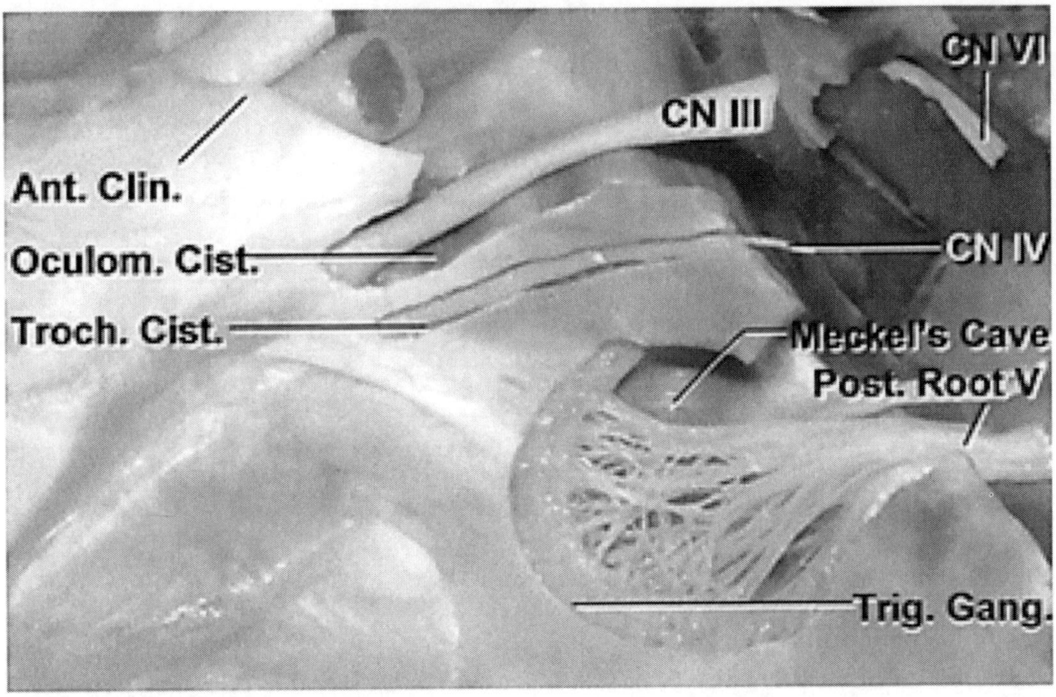

Figure 3.39. Lateral view of the left cavernous sinus. The oculomotor, trochlear, and trigeminal nerves are all enclosed in an arachnoid sac that surrounds the nerve for a short distance after they enter into the dura. The lateral wall of all three cisterns has been removed. Meckel's cave, the cistern around the posterior trigeminal root, extends forward to the middle portion of the gasserian ganglion. The oculomotor cistern extends forward in the roof of the cavernous sinus to where the nerve passes under the anterior clinoid process. The thin cistern around the trochlear nerve extends forward below the oculomotor cistern. Taken with permission from the Rhoton Collection.

3.7.6. Cranial Nerves of the Midbrain

3.7.6.1. CN-IV- The Trochlear Nerve

CN-IV is the only cranial nerve formed completely by axons that cross the midline before exiting, decussating in the most anterior part of anterior medullary velum and exiting caudal to the inferior colliculus. It is situated within the MLF. After exiting, the fibers have a long intracranial course, exiting into the superior (quadrigeminal) cistern, than coursing laterally-anteriorly through ambient cistern located on lateral midbrain. It rounds the cerebral peduncles in the ambient cistern coursing, along with the oculomotor nerve, between the superior cerebellar artery and posterior cerebral artery, and pierces the dura in-between the free and attached edge of tentorium cerebelli. Upon entering the dura, it courses rostrally within the lateral wall of the cavernous sinus (figure 3.36). It enters the orbit through the superior fissure (figure 3.37). Having entered the orbit lateral and superior to the tendinous ring it arches up and medially above superior rectus and levator palpebrea superioris to innervate the superior oblique muscle. An important source of cerebral cortical input to the CN-IV is from neurons in the frontal eye field (via the vertical gaze center of MLF). Refer to figures 3.35c and d, 3.39.

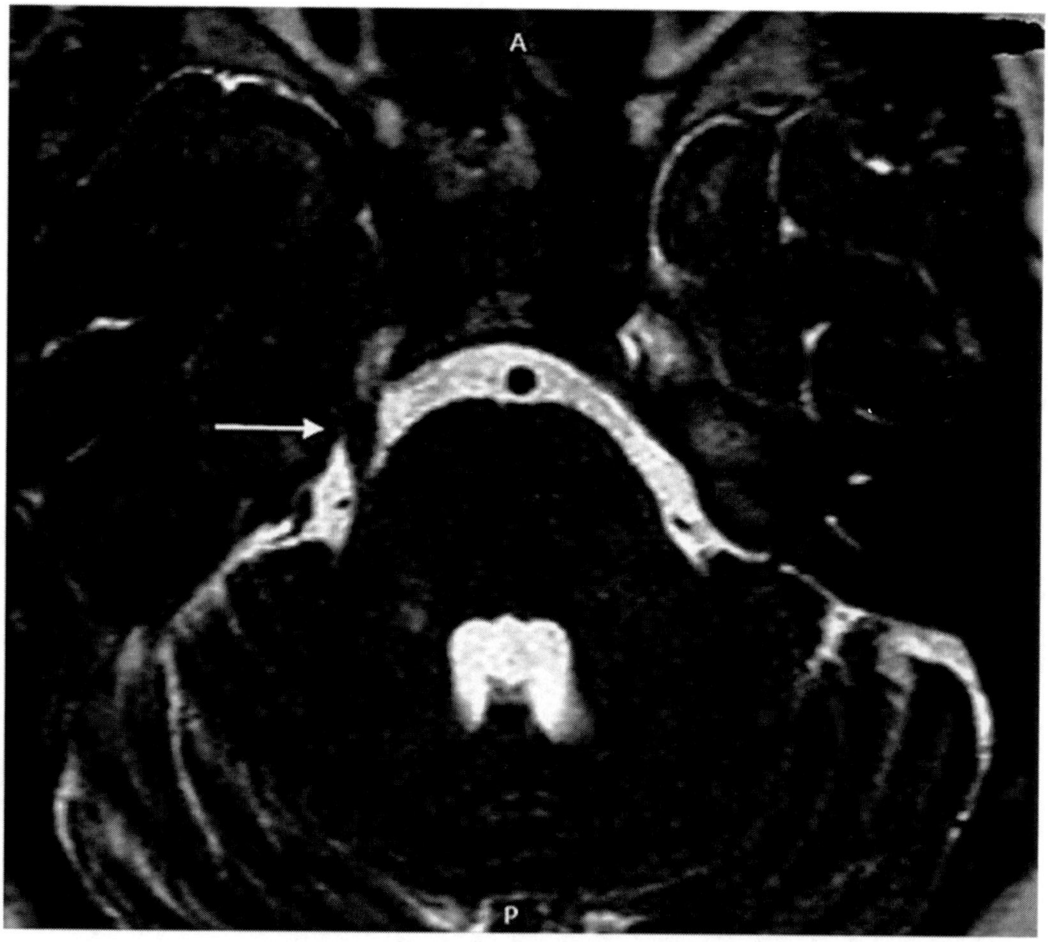

Figure 3.40. CN-V – T2-weight MRI. Taken with permission from www.radiopaedia.org.

3.7.6.1. CN-III - The Oculomotor Nerve

The oculomotor nucleus lies in the deep periaqueductal grey (PAG) matter at the level of the superior colliculus anterior to the cerebral aqueduct and posterior to the MLF. The fibers run through the tegmentum, red nucleus and medial aspect of the substantia nigra to emerge from the medial aspect of the cerebral peduncle into the interpeduncular cistern. The nerve then travel forwards, below the posterior cerebral artery (where it can be compressed by a posterior communicating artery aneurysm) and above the superior cerebellar artery, before piercing the dura mater and entering the cavernous sinus. Refer to figure 3.41.

The oculomotor nerve passes around penetrates the dura just lateral to the sella turcica, coursing within the superior aspects of the lateral wall of the cavernous sinus (figures 3.36, 3.39). The nerve than enters the orbit via the superior orbital fissure (figures 3.35c, 3.37) where it divides to a superior and inferior divisions. Within the orbit, its superior and inferior divisions, with the nasociliary nerve (a branch of the ophthalmic nerve) between them and the abducens nerve (CN VI) below all three pass through the tendinous ring (refer to figure 3.42). The superior division, the smaller of the two, runs above the optic nerve and gives branches to superior rectus and levator palpebrae which it supplies with motor fibers. Additionally it also supplies the later with sympathetic fibers which it picked up from the internal carotid artery. The inferior division supplies the inferior rectus muscle, medial rectus muscle (this branch passes below the optic nerve), and the inferior oblique muscles. It also gives off the parasympathetic root to the ciliary ganglion. Refer to figure 3.43. smooth muscles require GVE innervation through the ciliary ganglion (sphincter papillae, ciliary muscles).

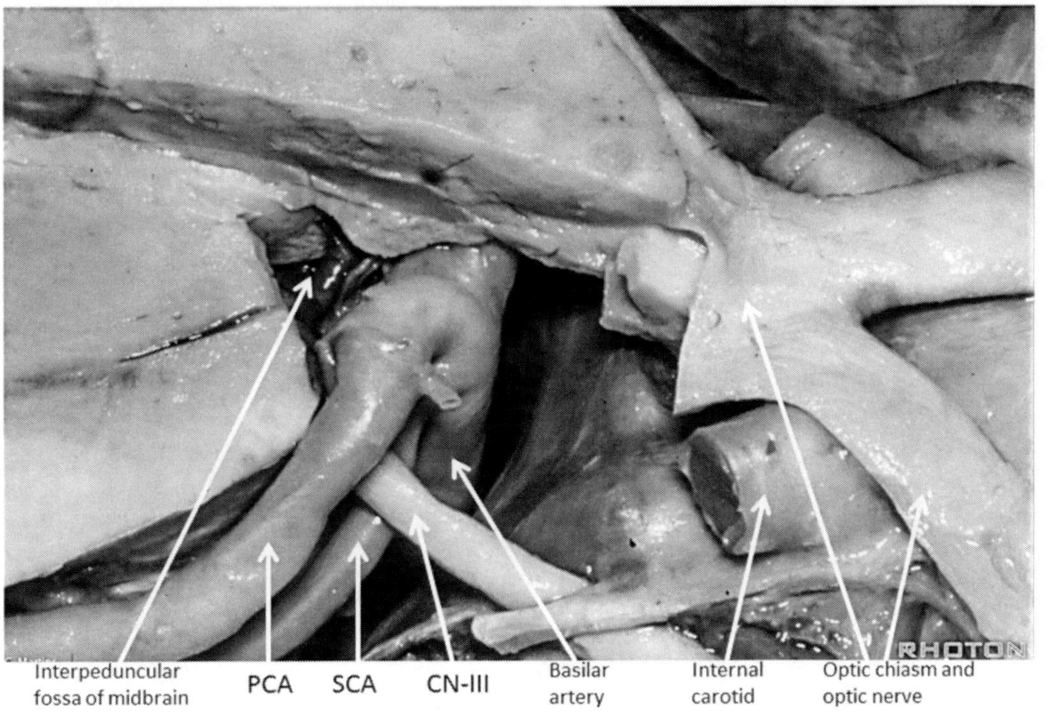

Figure 3.41. A lateral view on the brainstem at midbrain level showing the exit point of the oculomotor nerve at the interpeduncular cistern, between the trunks of the superior cerebellar artery (SCA) and the posterior cerebral artery (PCA). It is in this location that a PCA or a posterior communicating artery aneurysm can cause a peripheral CN-III palsy. Taken with permission from the Rhoton Collection.

Oculomotor palsy, a clinical finding of great importance, due to the CN-III close proximity both to the different vascular structures discussed previously as well as the medial aspects of the temporal lobe, i.e., the uncus (discussed later in the chapter on herniation syndromes) manifests with the eyeball coming to a "down and out" position. Paralysis of levator palpebrae superior causes a mild closure of the eye (ptosis). The pupil is dilated and unresponsive to light.

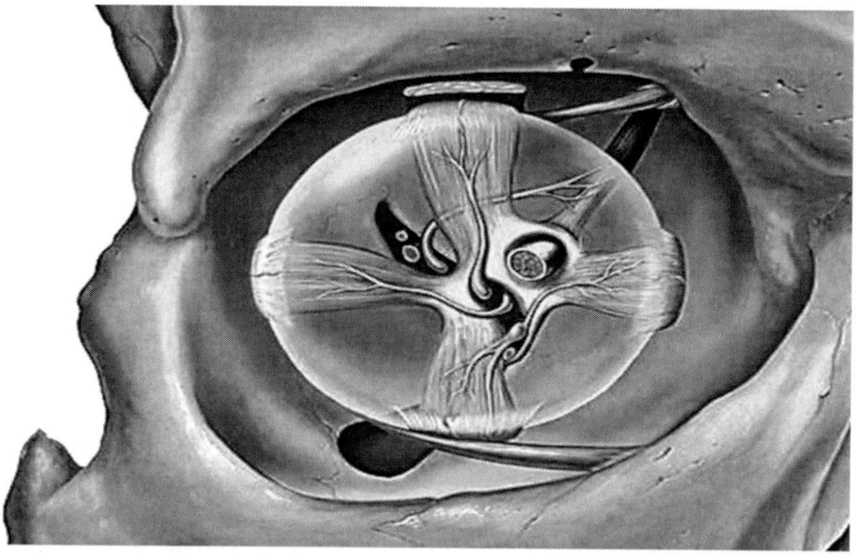

Figure 3.42. Anterior view of the orbit anterior view of the orbit. Note the tendinous ring onto which converge the extraocular muscles. Taken with permission from www.radiopaedia.org.

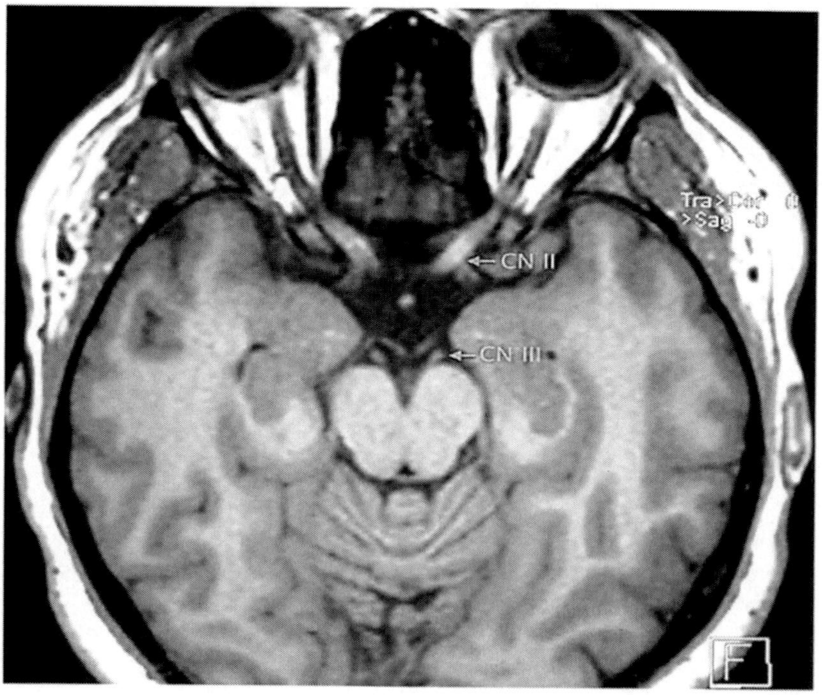

Figure 3.43. Axial T1 weight MRI showing the labeled CN-III at its origin from the interpeduncular fossa and CN-II. Taken with permission from www.radiopaedia.org.

3.7.7. Eye Movements and Pupillary Control

3.7.7.1. Extraocular Muscles, Nerves

Six extraocular muscles, originating in a common tendinous ring at the orbital apex control the eyeball movements. These insert into the sclera (figure 3.42). In addition to horizontal and vertical movements, torsional movements, in which the eye is rotated about its axis are facilitated via the oblique muscles. The superior oblique muscle, via the trochlea (pulley like loop), produces intorsion. The inferior oblique muscle produces extorsion. Depending on eye position, the rectus muscles can also produce torsional movements, and the oblique muscles can take important role in contributing to vertical eye movements.

CN-III, IV, VI pass through the cavernous sinus, entering the orbit through the superior orbital fissure (figure 3.37). CN-III Supplies all extraocular muscles except lateral rectus and superior oblique, CN-IV innervates the superior oblique muscle and CN-VI innervates the lateral rectus muscle. Refer to chapter 11 for an overview of the visual system.

3.7.7.2. The Pupil and Other Ocular Autonomic Pathways

3.7.7.2.1. Parasympathetic Control

Light activates retinal ganglionic cells, projecting to both optic tracts via chiasm. Nerve fibers in the extra-geniculate pathway (discussed later) continue in the brachium of superior colliculus past the lateral geniculate nucleus (LGN, nucleus of thalamus) to the pretectal nuclei where they synapse. Upon synapsing, these fibers continue bilaterally to the Edinger-Westphal nucleus (the Visceromotor nucleus of CN-III), in part through the posterior Commissure (discussed in later chapters). The preganglionic fibers then reach the ciliary ganglion via CN-III, located in the orbit. Postganglionic fibers continue as the short ciliary nerve to the pupillary constrictor muscle, causing miosis. A bilateral pupillary response (the accommodation response) may also occur through a different circuit: visual signals relayed to visual cortex, cortical activation of the pretectal nuclei, than as described previously, via the Edinger-Westphal nucleus.

Contraction of the ciliary muscle of the lens is also parasympathetic nervous system mediated, by the same pathway essentially. The ciliary muscle acts as a sphincter, thus upon contraction causes relaxation of the suspensory ligament of the lens, causing the lens to become more convex.

3.7.7.2.2. Sympathetic Control

The sympathetic control of the pupil begins with a descending pathway from the hypothalamus that travels in the lateral brainstem and cervical spinal cord (similar to the spinothalamic tract), to reach the first and second thoracic levels of the spinal cord, to the intermediolateral cell column of the upper thoracic spinal cord (the lateral gray matter horn, sympathetic center). From there, the preganglionic sympathetic information exits the spinal cord via the ventral roots of spinal nerves T1+T2. These nerves reach the paravertebral sympathetic chain, reaching up to superior cervical ganglion (the so named stellate ganglion) where they synapse. Postganglionic fibers re-enter the skull via the carotid plexus located on the internal carotid artery, entering through the carotid canal. These nerves accompany the ophthalmic artery (the first intracranial terminal branch of the internal carotid artery) through the optic canal into the orbit. Within the orbit these nerves innervate the pupillary dilatory muscle (dilator pupillae, a much weaker muscle), as well as the superior tarsal muscle (Muller's). This innervation explains why in Horner's syndrome (Sympathetic information block to the face and orbit, caused by many causes), the clinical manifestation includes both ptosis, miosis and unhydrosis (lack of sweating).

3.7.7.3. Supranuclear Control of Eye Movements

The medial and lateral rectus muscles, mediating horizontal movements of the eyeball, are controlled by CN-III, VI cranial nerves. The nuclei of these cranial nerves are interconnected via the MLF (a white matter bundle that connects the nuclei of cranial nerves CN-III, IV, VI, and VIII bilaterally). The CN-VI nuclear complex does more than just control abduction of the ipsilateral eye. Rather it is the horizontal gaze center, controlling horizontal movements of both eyes in the direction ipsilateral to the side of nucleus. The paramedian pontine reticular formation (PPRF), located in the pontine tegmentum near CN-VI nucleus, is an additional important horizontal gaze center. It provides input from the cortex and other pathways.

Vertical and vergence eye movements are mediated via the superior and inferior rectus muscles as well as the oblique muscles. Centers controlling these vertical movements are located in the midbrain reticular formation and pretectal area. The ventral midbrain portion mediates downgaze coordination, whereas the dorsal region located in vicinity of the posterior commissure, mediates upward gaze coordination. The exact anatomical location for centers coordinating vergence is not absolutely defined. These are probably located in midbrain reticular formation.

3.8. Brainstem Vascular Supply

3.8.1. Overview

The vertebrobasilar arterial system gives rise to multiple branches that provide the blood supply to the brainstem and cerebellum, as well as to most of the thalamus, inferomedial occipital and temporal lobes. The vertebral artery (VA) arises from the subclavian artery. The VA ascends posterior to the internal carotid artery in the transverse foramina of the cervical vertebrae. It gives off numerous small and spinal branches. It finally combines with the contralateral vertebral artery to form the basilar artery (refer to chapter 9). The vertebrobasilar arterial system has several named branches which is required knowledge as well as many small branches. When discussing the blood supply to the brainstem per-se, these are the posterior inferior cerebellar artery (PICA), the anterior inferior cerebellar artery (AICA) and the superior cerebellar artery (SCA). The posterior cerebral arteries (PCA), supply mainly the cerebral cortex, hemispheral deep structures and diencephalic structures, and no substantial portion of the posterior fossa of brainstem structures. The PCA's arise from the tip of the basilar artery; CN-III passes between SCA and PCA. The PCA's are discussed in chapter 9. Refer to figure 3.44 for a schematic representation of these arteries.

Each of the three neurovascular complexes in the posterior fossa includes one of the Three cerebellar arteries, one of the three parts of the brainstem, one of the three cerebellar peduncles, one of the three cerebellar surfaces, one of the three fissures between the brainstem and the cerebellum, and one of the three groups of cranial nerves. The upper complex is related to the SCA, the middle complex is related to the AICA, and the lower complex is related to the PICA. The upper complex includes the SCA, midbrain, superior cerebellar peduncle, cerebellomesencephalic fissure, tentorial cerebellar surface, and the oculomotor, trochlear, and trigeminal nerves. The middle complex includes the PICA, pons, middle cerebellar peduncle, cerebellopontine fissure, petrosal surface, and the abducens, facial, and vestibulocochlear nerves. The lower complex includes the PICA, medulla, inferior cerebellar peduncle, cerebellomedullary fissure, suboccipital surface, and the glossopharyngeal, vagus, accessory, and hypoglossal nerves. Refer to figures 3.44-3.47.

The PICA is the first branch, arising at the level of the medulla. PICA origin is variable, with the majority arising from the VA, but 18-20% arises extracranially inferior to foramen magnum, and 10% arise from the basilar rather than vertebral artery. In 2% PICA are bilaterally absent. PICA has a variable territory depending on the size of the AICA. Typically it may supply the posteroinferior cerebellar hemispheres (up to the great horizontal fissure), the cerebellar tonsils (85% of the time), biventral lobule (80%), nucleus gracilis (85%), superior semilunar lobule (50%), inferior portion of the vermis and the lower part of the medulla (50%). Refer to table 3.4 for a description of the different PICA segments. PICA branches include small perforating medullary branches coming from the anterior and lateral segments, and the tonsillohemispheric and inferior vermian branches coming from the supratonsillar segment.

The AICA, in 99% of cases, arises from the basilar artery, but where along the vessel is variable. 75% arise from its lower third, 16% from its middle third and 9% from the vertebrobasilar junction. The amount of tissue supplied by the AICA is variable (depending on the PICA - AICA dominance) but usually includes the middle cerebellar peduncle, inferolateral portion of the pons, the flocculus and the anteroinferior surface of the cerebellum. Branches include the internal auditory branch that passes into the IAM, the lateral branch that passes around the flocculus and into the hemispheric fissure and the medial branch that supplies the biventral lobule.

The SCA arises from the distal basilar artery, just below the PCA and typically supplies the whole superior surface of the cerebellar hemispheres down to the great horizontal fissure, the superior vermis, the dentate nucleus, most of the cerebellar white matter and parts of the midbrain.

Although, unlike the AICA and PICA the SCA is rarely absent, it is frequently duplicated. Unilateral duplication is seen in 28%, bilateral duplication is seen in 8% and triplication can be seen in 2%. The upper branch, when multiple, may arise from the PCA and usually supplies the vermis, whereas the lower branch supplies the hemisphere. Branches include perforating branches to the pons, midbrain and inferior colliculus, the lateral (marginal) branch, hemispheric branches, supplying the dentate nucleus, superior vermis medial quadrigeminal lobule and the superior semilunar lobule and a superior vermian branch.

Table 4.4. Brainstem Arterial Segments

PICA	Anterior medullary	From PICA origin around the inferior aspect of the medullary olive
	Lateral medullary	Curves forming the 'caudal loop' which is located anteroinferior to the tip of the cerebellar tonsil, but does NOT relate to the tonsillar position.
		The apex of the loop is above foramen magnum (FM) in 60% of cases, at the level of FM in 10% and below in 30%. Its relationship to the vertebral artery is also variable, 84% lateral and 16% medial
	Posterior medullary	Ascends posterior to the medulla behind CN IX and CN X and along the posterior medullary velum.
	Supra-tonsillar	The junction between the posterior medullary segment and the supratonsillar segment is upwardly convex and is the site of origin of small choroidal branches: it is known as the "choroid point". This point has a constant relationship with the 4th ventricle and was used prior to cross-sectional imaging to asses for shift in its position.
AICA	Anterior pontine	Each segment may be composed of one or more trunks, depending on the level of bifurcation of the main trunk. Refer to figure 3.45
	Lateral pontomedullary	
	Flocculonodular	
	Cortical	
SCA	Prepontine	Anterior pontomesencephalic
	Ambient	Lateral pontomesencephalic
	Quadrigeminal	Cerebellomesencephalic
	Cortical	

Smaller branches, like the paramedian branches, usually respect the midline, with individual branches supply either the right or left paramedian regions. These branches extend variable distances from the ventral surface, with the longest branches reaching all the way to the ventricle. Additional smaller branches include the Short and long circumferential arteries. Refer to table 4.5 for a summary of vascular territories.

Table 4.5. Vascular Territories in the Brainstem

Medulla	Medial	Paramedian branches of anterior spinal artery caudally, Paramedian branches of vertebral artery Rostrally.
	Lateral	Penetrating branches of vertebral artery, PICA.
Pons	Medial	Paramedian branches of basilar artery.
	Lateral	Circumferential branches Of the basilar artery.
		AICA in more caudal Pons.
		Inner ear is supplied by the labyrinthine artery, arising from AICA.
	Rostral	Pontine artery, a short circumferential artery.
	SDL*	SCA
Midbrain		Artery from top of basilar and proximal PCA.
	Medial	Paramedian branches from top of basilar enter interpeduncular fossa to supply medial midbrain and thalamus.
		The artery Of Percheron supplies bilateral medial midbrain and thalamus.

*Superior Dorsolateral.

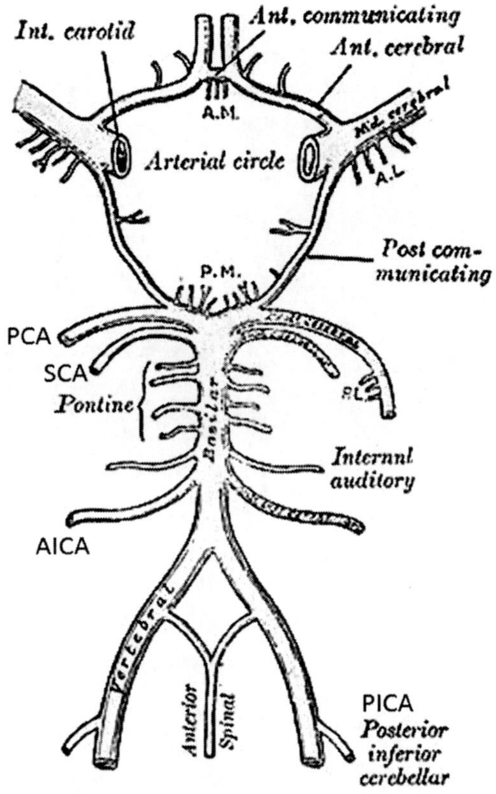

Figure 3.44. Arterial circulation at the base of the brain. Original diagram from Gray's anatomy, now out of copyright.

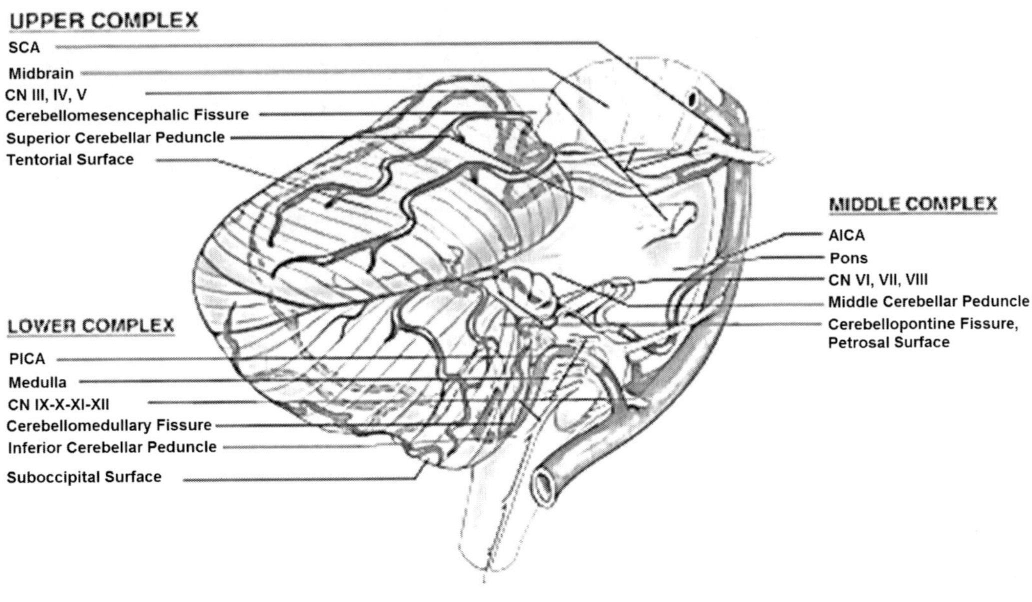

Figure 3.45. Vascular territories of the brainstem and cerebellum. A.I.C.A., anteroinferior cerebellar artery; CN, cranial nerve; Fiss., fissure; Ped., peduncle; P.I.C.A., posteroinferior cerebellar artery. Taken with permission from the Rhoton Collection.

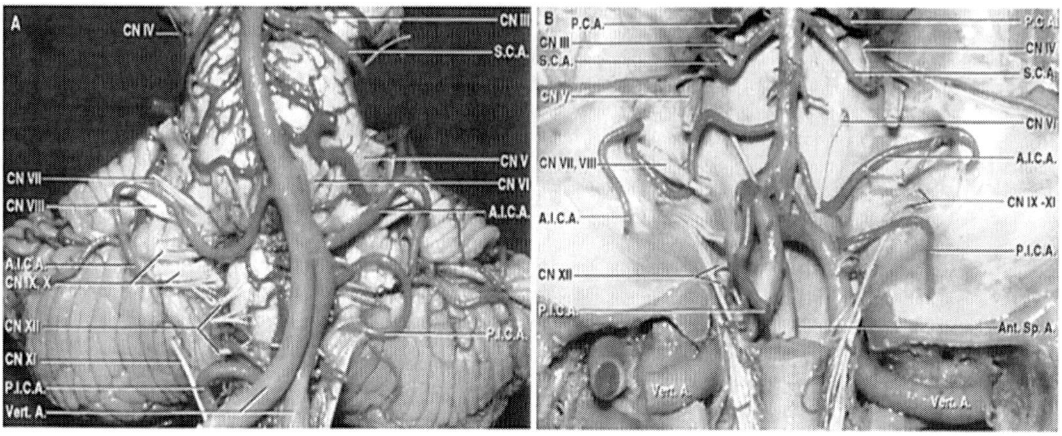

Figure 3.46. A, anterior view of the brainstem and cerebellar arteries. B, posterior view of the cranial base with the cranial nerves and arteries preserved. A., artery; A.I.C.A., anteroinferior cerebellar artery; Ant., anterior; CN, cranial nerve; P.C.A., posterior cerebral artery; P.I.C.A., posteroinferior cerebellar artery; S.C.A., superior cerebellar artery; Sp., spinal; Vert., vertebral. Taken with permission from the Rhoton Collection.

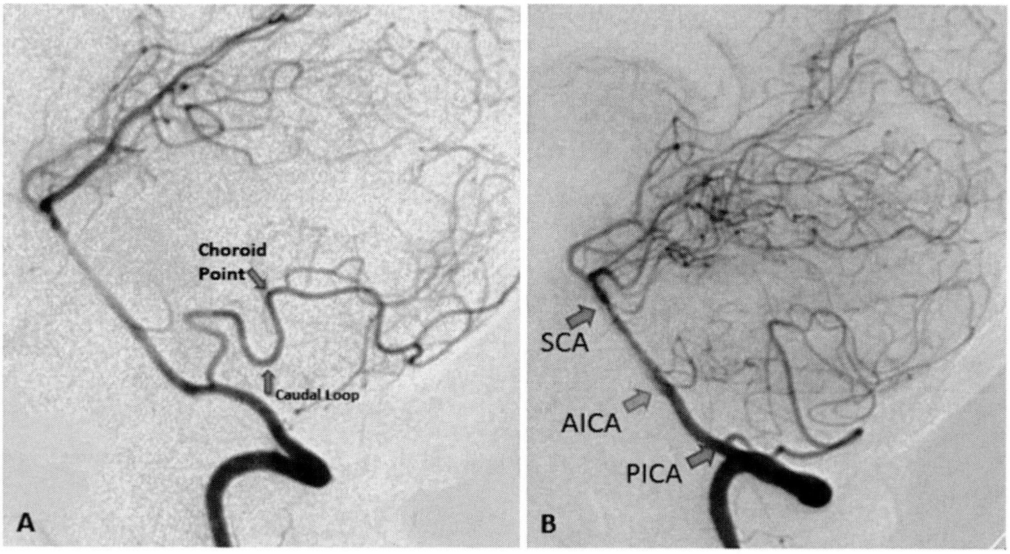

Figure 3.47. Vertebrobasilar angiogram, lateral view. A, the Choroid and caudal points of PICA. B, the three major vessels supplying the posterior fossa and brainstem are depicted. Taken with permission from www.radiopaedia.org.

3.8.2. General Features of Posterior Circulation Disease

Atherosclerosis and other etiologies may result in preferential vertebrobasilar system insufficiency clinical presentation, owing to the lower flow and relative lack of laminar flow in this system. Generally speaking, signs of brainstem ischemia may include crossed signs (i.e., face and body affected on different sides with the face being ipsilateral to the lesion site and the body contralateral, due to the location of decussation). Cranial nerves abnormalities, especially eye movement abnormalities are very important localizing signs. Pupillary abnormalities, nystagmus are additional hints to a vestibular or pontine location. Vertebral positional insufficiency may manifest with Bow-Hunter syndrome (head position dependent loss of consciousness).

Midbrain dysfunction may manifest with CN-III palsy, pupil dilation, ataxia, decorticate posturing and impaired consciousness, all owing to the anatomy discussed previously. Pontine dysfunction may manifest with a bilateral Babinski sign (UMN pyramidal dysfunction sign), weakness, perioral numbness, "salt and pepper" (pins and needles) facial tingling, bilateral upper / lower visual loss and irregular respirations, ocular bobbing or shivering (due to the location of these centers in the pons). Medullary dysfunction may manifest with vertigo, ataxia, nystagmus, nausea or vomiting.

3.8.2.1. Posturing Reflexes

These reflexes are seen in patients with damage to the descending UMN pathways. The presence of either implies a severe brain injury. Decortication posture occurs in response to a painful stimulus, manifesting with the flexion of upper limb musculature and parallel extension of lower extremities musculature. Primate instincts, hanging from tree branches are thought to be the etymology. This occurs when the brainstem is transected above the level of the red nucleus. Decerebration posture occurs in in response to a painful stimulus, manifesting with the extension of all limbs. This occurs when the brainstem is transected below the level of the red nucleus, showing a slightly worse outcome. Refer to figure 3.48. These reflexes depend on brainstem function, their presence suggests damage to descending pathways, with some brainstem function left intact.

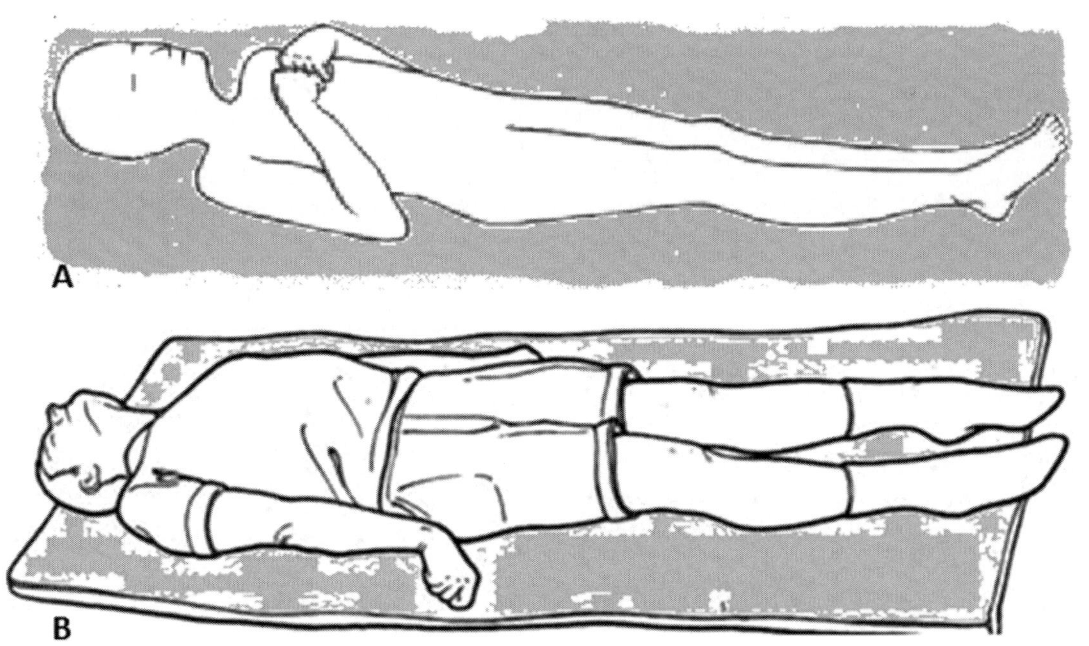

Figure 3.48. Pathological Posturing reflexes. A, Decorticate posturing, with elbows, wrists and fingers flexed, and legs extended and rotated inward. B, Decerebrate rigidity or abnormal extensor posturing.

3.8.3. Specific Clinical Vascular Syndromes of the Brainstem

Refer to table 4.6 for a short summary of clinical vascular syndromes of the brainstem.

Table 4.6. Brainstem Stroke Syndromes Overview

Syndrome	Anatomical location	Clinical manifestation
Anton	Bilateral occipital lobe stroked Bilateral PCA or Top of Basilar syndrome	Visual deficit without recognition of blindness (visual agnosia)
Claude	Dorsal midbrain Syndrome Ipsilateral CN-III palsy with contralateral ataxia	
Dejerine	Medial medullary Syndrome. Basilar artery, vertebral artery, anterior spinal artery.	Contralateral spastic weakness (pyramidal) sparing face, Loss of vibration / position sense (medial lemniscus), Ipsilateral tongue weakness
Foville's	Inferior medial pontine syndrome. Basilar artery perforators	Contralateral weakness (Corticospinal), Facial weakness (CN-VII nucleus), Lateral gaze deficit (CN-VI nucleus)
Locked-in	Basilar artery	Paralysis of all movements except vertical gaze and eyelid opening (Supranuclear ocular motor pathways preserved). Sensation and conscious preserved
Marie-Foix	AICA occlusion	Ipsilateral ataxia, nausea, vertigo, decreased hearing, Contralateral hemiparesis
Milard-Gubler	Basilar artery perforators, Base of Pons syndrome	Contralateral weakness (Corticospinal), diplopia, strabismus, ipsilateral facial weakness
Raymond	Perforators of basilar artery	Lateral gaze deficit (CN-VI), Weakness (pyramidal tract)
Top of the Basilar	Generally embolic or post-angio stent complication, Sudden onset of altered mental status, ophthalmoplegia, papillary and visual field abnormalities	
Wallenberg	Vertebral artery occlusion / dissection, PICA occlusion.	Facial pain and sensory loss (CN-V nucleus), Ataxia (Restiform body), Nystagmus, nausea, vomiting, vertigo Dysphagia, hoarseness, Dysarthria Ipsilateral Horner's syndrome, Contralateral loss of pain and temperature (spinothalamic) Hiccups (reticulophrenic)
Weber	PCA midbrain perforators leading to ventral midbrain infarct	Contralateral weakness (Corticospinal) Lateral gaze deficit & ipsilateral pupillary dilatation (CN-3), Contralateral corticobulbar dysfunction

Chapter 4

The Diencephalon and the Third Ventricle

4.1. Abstract

The diencephalon holds more of a conceptual challenge than a detailed structure to memorize for the medical student. A clear three dimensional view of the third ventricle and surrounding structures eludes many students and with it, a lack of understanding of these structures. Realizing this, the chapter is built in a layer-like fashion, beginning with relevant embryological key points; next the organization of the diencephalon is presented, followed by a short description of its different components. Great care was taken to focus only on those clinically important details, forming an overview for a future clinician. Emphasis was put on highlighting important pitfalls, and omitting data having no clinical relevance. The dorsal thalamus, hypothalamus, pituitary gland, ventral thalamus and epithalamus are described. Each of these components is presented grossly first and then the key microstructural and connections are presented. The internal capsule (not a part of the diencephalon) is discussed in this chapter for the ease of understanding the three dimensional anatomy. The chapter closes with a synopsis of the third ventricle using dissections to show the different key features.

4.2. Overview

The diencephalon is a portion of the forebrain, situated between the telencephalon and brainstem. It is the main processing center for information destined to reach the cortex from all ascending sensory pathways (except olfaction), and many other subcortical cell groups. Its two halves contain symmetrically distributed cell groups, separated by the space of the third ventricle. The diencephalon is composed of different components: The dorsal thalamus (true thalamus), the hypothalamus and related pituitary gland, the ventral thalamus (i.e., the subthalamic nucleus) and the Epithalamus. Each of these structures will be discussed in this chapter with its relevant clinical and anatomical key points. Refer to figure 4.1.

The dorsal thalamus is the largest of the diencephalic components, consisting of pools of neurons projecting to all areas of the cerebral cortex. Thalamic nuclei receive a wide range of sensory information, ranging from somatosensory, visual, or auditory inputs. These thalamic nuclei than actively modify the information, processing it to different degrees and transmit it to the correct areas of the cerebral cortex as well as to subcortical regions. Other thalamic nuclei receive input from subcortical motor areas, modify it and then project it to those parts of the cortex influencing the successful execution of the motor act. A few thalamic nuclei receive a more diffuse input, process it and send it in a diffuse way to other cortical areas, modulating conscious sensations. Thus the thalamus functions in both the motor, sensory and diffuse realms of neurological processing.

The hypothalamus, forming the lower part of the walls and the floor of the third ventricles has many nuclear subdivisions. It is connected to the forebrain, brainstem and spinal cord. The hypothalamus is involved in control of VM (GVE) functions. It is the central processing and integration of the neuroendocrine control of homeostasis. It directly "controls" and secretes hormones via the pituitary gland, connected to its lower aspect via a stalk. The ventral thalamus, also termed as the subthalamic nucleus (linked in function to the basal ganglia) is the only diencephalic component not bordering on the third ventricle. It is involved in advanced motor processing, being part of the so called motor circuitry. It is a target for deep brain stimulation surgery in treating disorders such as Parkinson's disease and essential tremor. The Epithalamus, composed to the pineal gland and related centers is located at the dorsal aspects of the third ventricle and is functionally related to the limbic system.

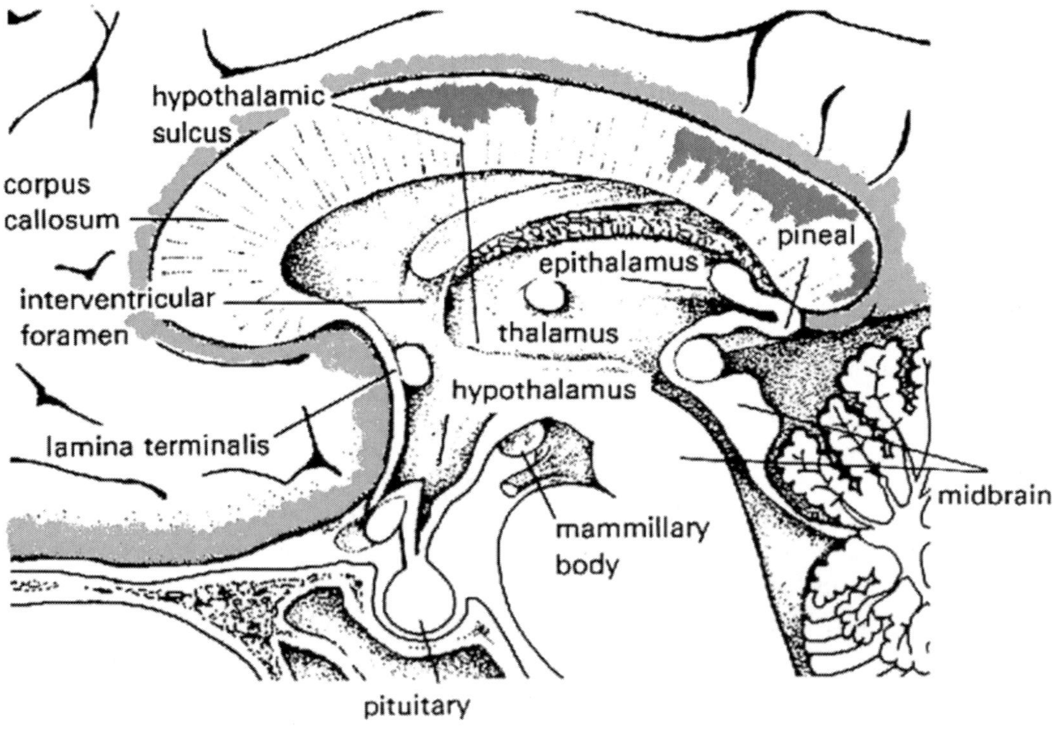

Figure 4.1. Midsagittal illustration of the diencephalon and related structures. Taken with permission from www.radiopaedia.org.

4.3. Neuro-Embryology of the Diencephalon

4.3.1. Roof Plate, Epiphysis and the Choroid

The diencephalon, which develops from the median portion of the prosencephalon, is thought to consist of a roof plate and two alar plates but to lack a floor or basal plates. Interestingly, sonic hedgehog genes, a ventral midline marker, are expressed in the floor of the diencephalon, suggesting that a floor plate does exist. The roof plate of the diencephalon consists of a single layer of ependymal cells covered by vascular mesenchyme. Together these layers give rise to the choroid plexus of the third ventricle. The most caudal part of the roof plate develops into the pineal body, or epiphysis. This body initially appears as an epithelial thickening in the midline, but by the seventh week it begins to invaginate. Eventually it becomes a solid organ on the roof of the mesencephalon that serves as a channel through which light and darkness affect endocrine and behavioral rhythms. In the adult, calcium is frequently deposited in the epiphysis and then serves as a landmark on radiographs of the skull. A portion of the roof will give rise to the habenular (a thickening in which the habenular nucleus will develop). Refer to figure 4.2.

The choroid plexus develops anteriorly to the habenular region, formed by the roof plate and adjacent pia. In the developed brain is remains suspended from the roof. It is continuous through the interventricular foramina (of Monro) with that of the lateral ventricle.

Elsewhere, specialized patches of ependyma lying on the midline form unpaired structures. These are termed as the circumventricular organs, having fenestrated capillaries, no blood brain barrier, able to sample and blood as well as releasing metabolites and neuropeptides into the CSF.

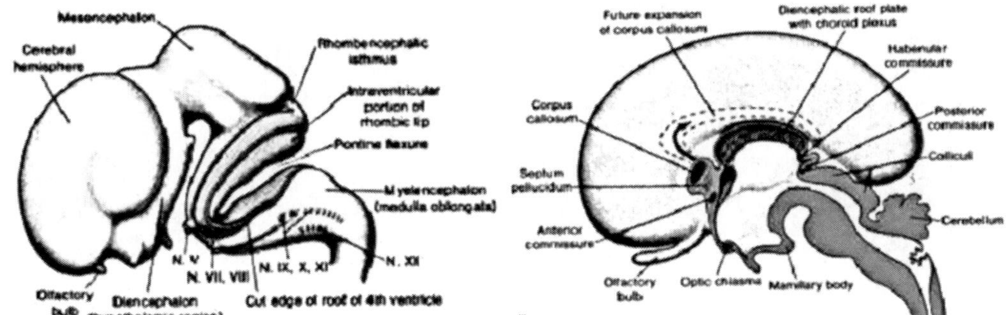

Figure 4.2. Medial surface of the right half of the brain in a 4-month embryo showing the various commissures. Broken line represents the future site of the corpus callosum. The hippocampal commissure is not indicated. Taken from Gray's anatomy, out of copyright and in the public domain.

4.3.2. Alar, Plate, Thalamus and Hypothalamus

The alar plates form the lateral walls of the diencephalon. The hypothalamic sulcus is a shallow groove, found in the wall of the third ventricle, extending rostrally from the aqueduct to the ventricle edge of the interventricular foramen of Monro (see figure 4.1). It divides the alar plate into dorsal and ventral regions, the thalamus and hypothalamus respectively. The dorsal thalamus, on sides of the third ventricle increases rapidly in size, projecting into the lumen of the diencephalon and partially fuses across the space, forming the Massa Intermedia (Interthalamic adhesion). The hypothalamus, forming the lower portion of the alar plate, differentiates into a number of nuclear areas that regulate the visceral functions, including sleep, digestion, body temperature and emotional behavior. One of these groups, the mammillary body, forms a distinct protuberance on the ventral surface of the hypothalamus on each side of the midline. Refer to figure 4.3.

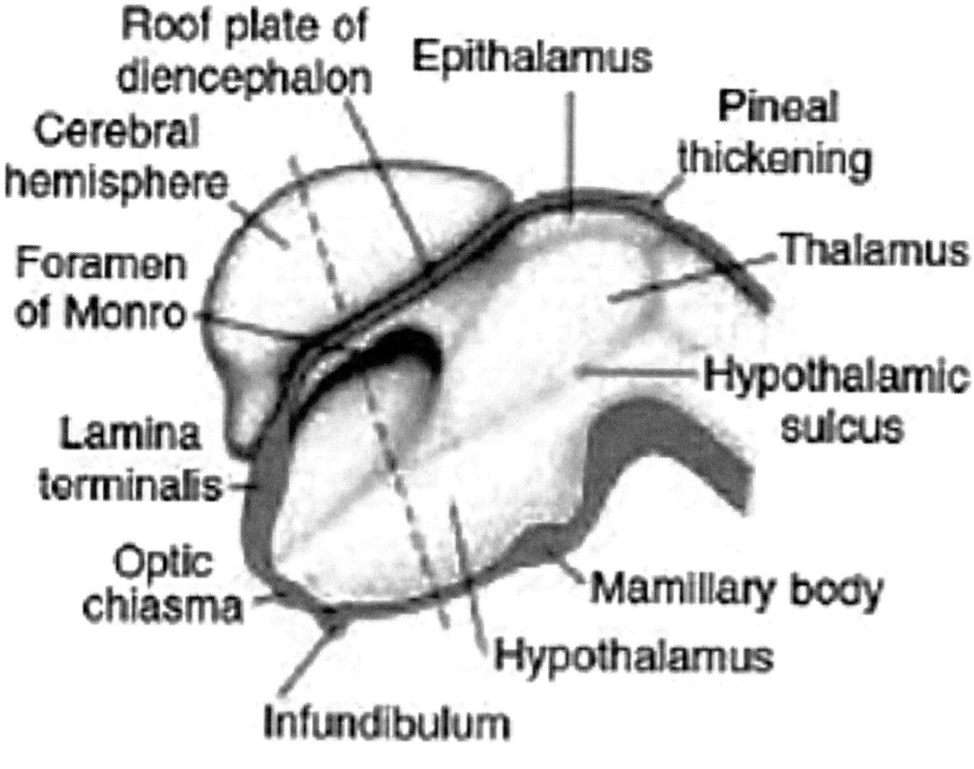

Figure 4.3. Medial surface of the right half of the prosencephalon in a 7 weeks embryo.

4.3.3. The Pituitary (Hypophysis) Gland

The pituitary gland develops from two completely different parts: An ectodermal out pocketing of the stomodeum immediately in front of the buccopharyngeal membrane (the primitive oral cavity), known as Rathke's pouch, and a downward extension of the diencephalon, the infundibulum. Rathke's pouch appears at 3 weeks old embryonic age, as an evagination of the oral cavity. By the end of the second month it loses its connection with the oral cavity and is then in close contact with the infundibulum. With further development, cells in the anterior wall of Rathke's pouch proliferate to form the anterior lobe of the pituitary (the so named adeno-hypophysis). A small extension of this lobe, the pars tuberalis, grows along the stalk of the infundibulum and eventually surrounds it. The posterior wall of Rathke's pouch develops into the pars Intermedia of the hypophysis, having little significance in humans. The infundibulum forms the posterior lobe (neurohypophysis).

4.4. Basic Organization of the Diencephalon

Refer to table 4.1 for a bullet presentation of the basic organization of the diencephalon and key points.

Table 4.1. Basic Organization of the Diencephalon

Diencephalon-Midbrain junction	Medial aspect of hemisphere	A line between posterior commissure to caudal edge of mammillary body.
	Ventral surface	A line following the caudal edge of optic tract.
Diencephalon-Telencephalon junctions	Less distinct, represented laterally by the internal capsule and rostrally by the Monro foramina, lamina terminalis, optic chiasm. Refer to figures 4.4, 4.5, 4.7, 4.11, 4.12, 4.14	
Third ventricle	Vertically oriented, between the two thalami, hypothalamic. In addition to its connection to the aqueduct and lateral ventricles, it has small recesses associated with the Optic chiasm, infundibulum, and pineal gland. Refer to figures 4.13, 4.21-4.24	
Thalamus	Dorsal to hypothalamic sulcus, extending from the Monro foramina to the level of the splenium of corpus callosum.	
Hypothalamus	Ventral to hypothalamic sulcus, bordered anteriorly by the lamina terminalis and caudally by a line extending from the mammillary body to its intersection with the hypothalamic sulcus. Refer to figures 4.14-4.15	
Ventral thalamus	The Subthalamus, does not border on the 3rd ventricle, rather has a position caudal to hypothalamus rostral to Diencephalic-Midbrain junction, lateral to the midline. Refer to figures 4.7, 4.14	
Epithalamus	Its structures are located Posteriorly & Dorsally, in close apposition to Posterior commissure. Refer to figures 4.19-4.21	
	Include the pineal gland, habenular nuclei, stria Medullaris thalami (the main affarent bundle for these nuclei).	

4.5. Dorsal Thalamus (Thalamus)

4.5.1. Overview

The Thalamus is a paired and symmetrical structure in the brain, and the main part of the diencephalon. It is the pathway through which signals are sent from cerebrum to the midbrain (brainstem) via the cerebral peduncles and vice versa. The thalamus has many functions including functioning as a translator of prethalamic inputs into readable form, it processes and relays sensory information selectively to various parts of the cerebral cortex, it regulates sleep and wakefulness, its thalamo-cortico-thalamic circuits are involved in consciousness, and he functions in arousal, mediating the level of awareness and activity. Blood supply for the thalamus comes from a number of arteries including polar and paramedian arteries, inferolateral (thalamogeniculate) arteries, and posterior (medial and lateral) choroidal arteries. These are all branches of the posterior cerebral artery. Refer to figures 4.4-4.6.

The thalamus participates in motor, sensory and limbic systems. Its outputs project to the cortex. Since very little Information reaches the cortex without passing through the thalamus, it is regarded as the gateway to or from the thalamus. The External medullary lamina is a layer of myelinated axons that cover its lateral aspect (fibers entering /leaving the subcortical white matter). Within it, nerve clusters form the thalamic reticular nucleus. At the medial surface of the thalamus, bordering the third ventricle, the external medullary lamina and reticular nucleus blend with the thalamic fasciculus and zona incerta, forming an interface. Refer to figure 4.7. The internal medullary lamina is a layer of myelinated fibers, extending into the substance of the thalamus, forming boundaries dividing the thalamus into its principal cell groups (Y-Shaped oriented rostrally). Anterior, medial, lateral, and intralaminar nuclear groups are formed (the latter are located in the portion of the internal medullary lamina separating the lateral & medial nuclear groups). The thalamic reticular nucleus is a group of midline thalamic nuclei, a diffuse population of neurons located in the external medullary lamina.

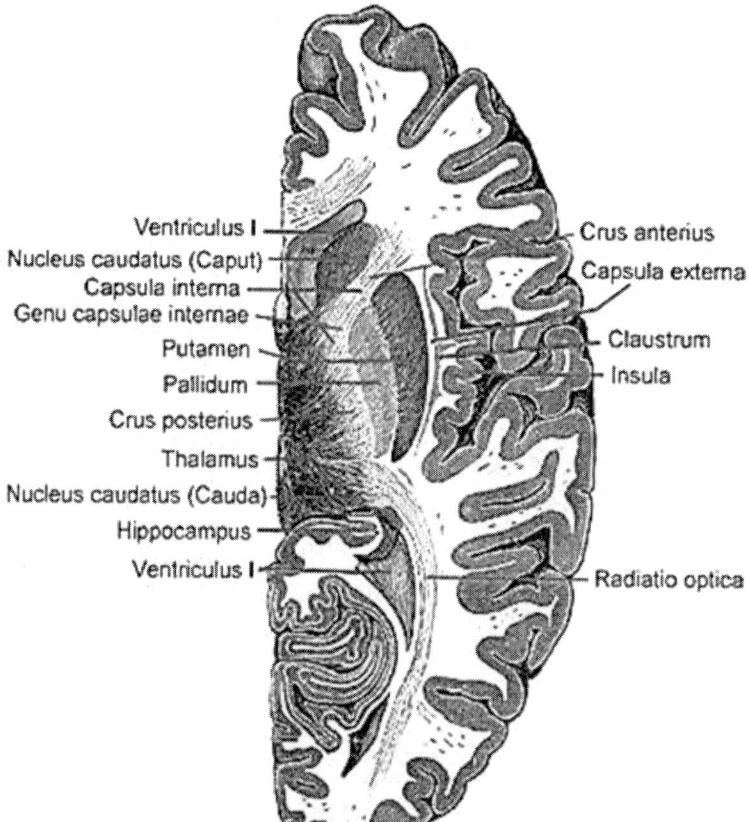

Figure 4.4. Thalamus and Basal ganglia location, axial view. Image taken from Gray's anatomy, out of copyright and in the public domain.

The medial and lateral geniculate nuclei (MGN, LGN respectively) are attached to the caudolateral portion of the thalamus (considered a part of the lateral nuclear group, but at time considered as a separate part of the diencephalon, the metathalamus). The LGN processes visual information. Visual information from retinal ganglion cells is channeled via the optic chiasms to the lateral LGN. The LGN is composed of 6 layers. Three layers (layer number 2, 3, 5) receive input from the ipsilateral eye whereas the three other layers (1, 4, 6) receive input from the contralateral eye. LGN fibers project to the primary visual cortex (located in the occipital lobe, Brodmann area 17, discussed separately) forming the optic radiation. Refer to figure 4.8. Not all visual information carrying fibers terminate in LGN; some extend to the superior colliculi via the brachium of the superior colliculus. The superior colliculus mediates gaze and head turning reflexes, as well as lens and pupil accommodation. Other fibers continue to terminate at the hypothalamus, aiding in the tuning of circadian rhythms. The visual system is discussed separately in chapter 11.

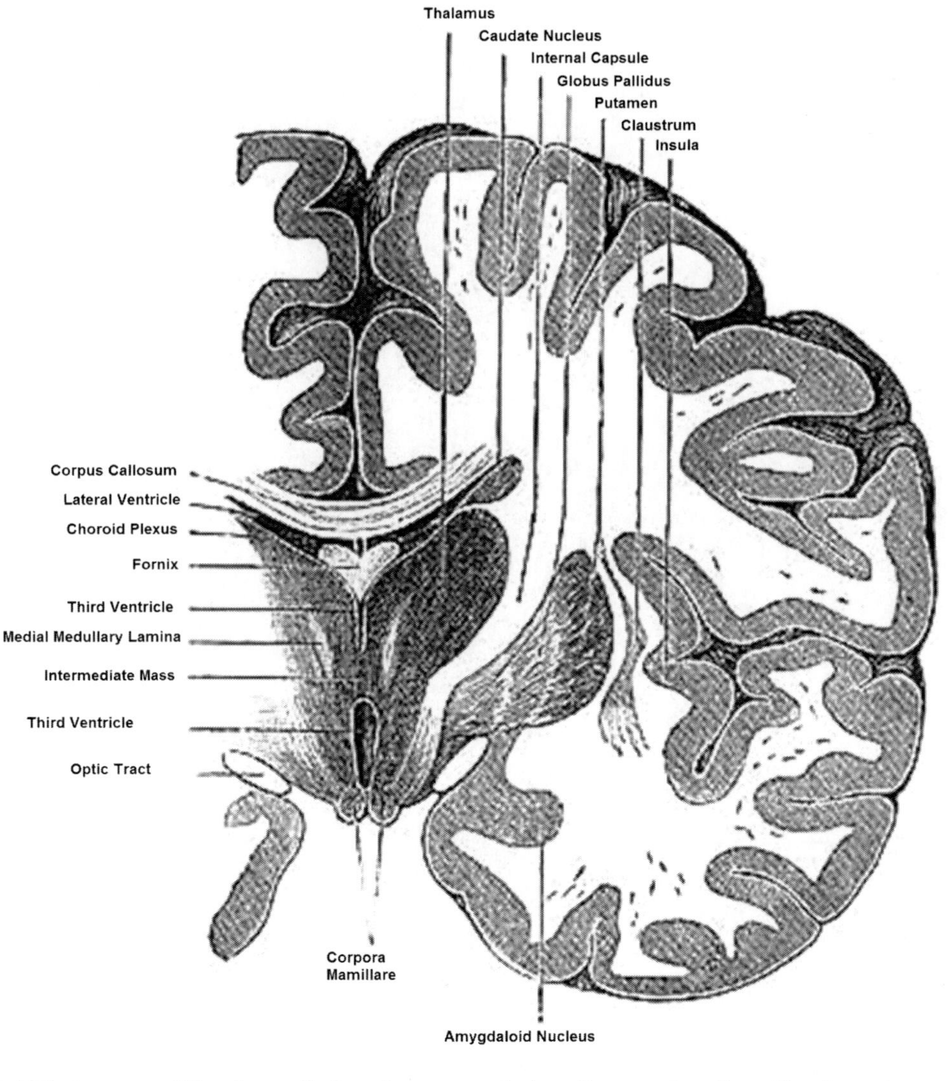

Figure 4.5.Thalamus and Basal ganglia location, coronal view. Image taken from Gray's anatomy, out of copyright and in the public domain.

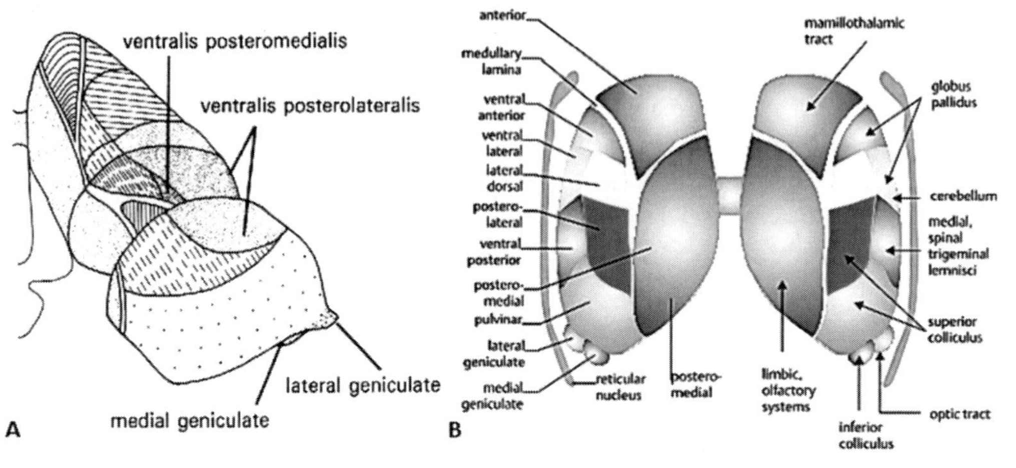

Figure 4.6. The thalamus. A, the internal architecture showing the subdivision formed by the internal medullary "Y" shaped lamina. Image taken from Gray's anatomy, out of copyright and in the public domain. B, A scheme showing the main nuclear groups and inputs of the thalamus.

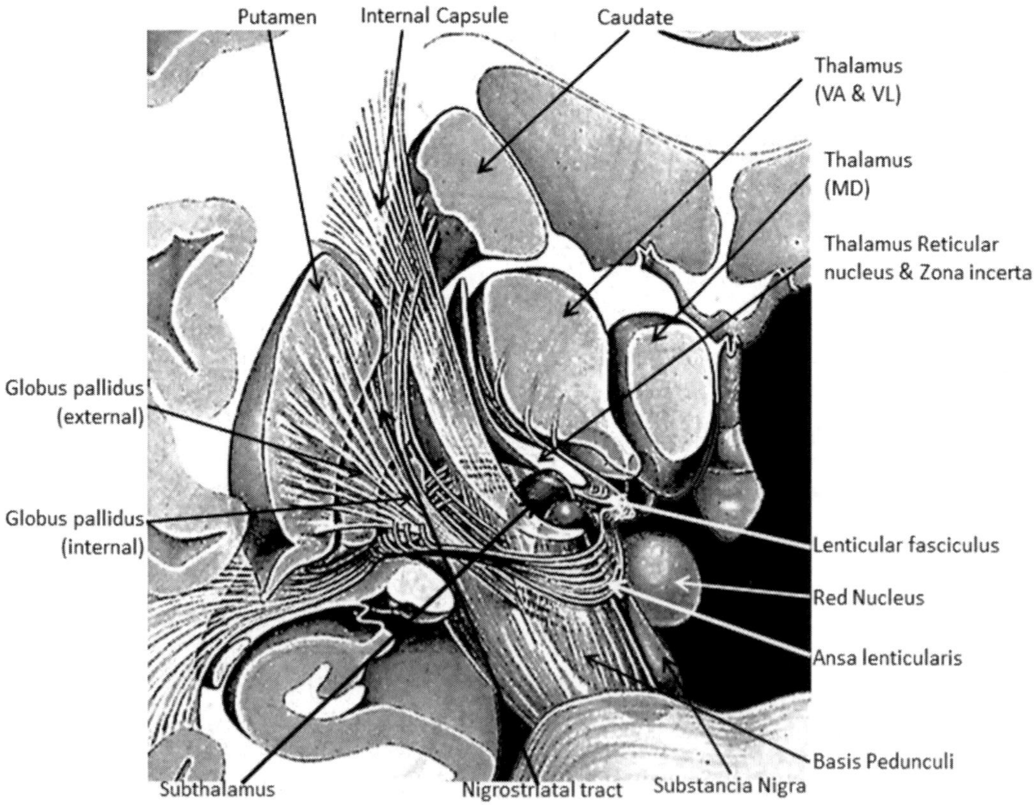

Figure 4.7. A schematic reconstruction of the efferent fiber systems leaving the lenticular nucleus connecting to the thalamus and other structures. Image adopted and modified, taken from Gray's anatomy, out of copyright and in the public domain.

Auditory information from the cochlea is channeled to the medial geniculate nucleus (MGN). The path auditory information takes to the MGN is complicated and includes the cochlea and spiral ganglion, via the auditory component of the vestibulocochlear nerve (CN-VIII) to the cochlear nuclei of the pons and medulla and via the lateral lemniscus to the inferior colliculus. From the inferior colliculus, fibers reach MGN via the brachium of the inferior colliculus.

En route from the cochlear nuclei to the inferior colliculi many fibers form synapses on various brain stem nuclei including the superior olive and trapezoid body (sound source localization), and these nuclei send secondary and tertiary fibers to inferior colliculi as well. The MGN sends fibers to the primary auditory cortex (located at the superior temporal gyrus, Brodmann areas 41, 42, discussed separately), forming the auditory radiation. The auditory system is discussed separately in chapter 12.

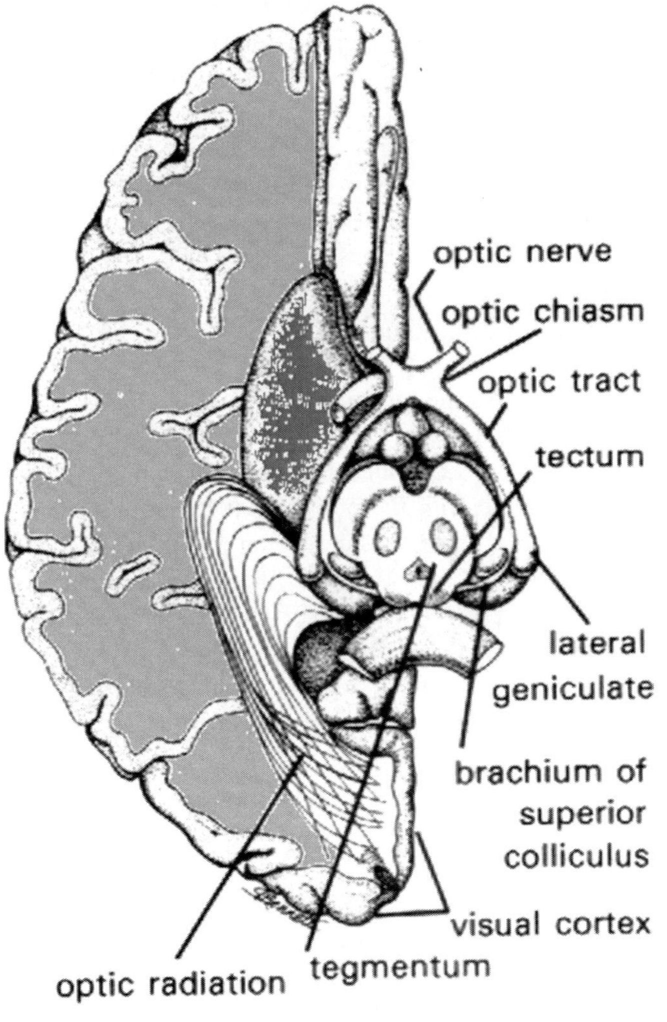

Figure 4.8. An illustration of the inferior brain surface highlighting the optic pathways and radiation. Image taken from Gray's anatomy, out of copyright and in the public domain.

4.5.2. Anterior Thalamic Nuclear Complex

The anterior thalamic nuclear complex consists of a large principal nucleus and two small nuclei. It forms a prominent wedge on the rostral aspect, caudolateral to Monro foramina, forming the so called anterior thalamic tubercle. The internal medullary lamina rostrally, partially encapsulates the anterior nucleus. Its cells receive limbic projections from the mamillary nuclei via the mammillo-thalamic tract and from the medial temporal lobe via the fornix (discussed separately). The output of the anterior thalamic nuclei is primarily directed to the cingulate gyrus, through anterior limb of internal capsule (discussed later).

4.5.3. Medial Thalamic Nuclear Complex

The dorsomedial (DM) nucleus, the most prominent and important representative of this group, has a large parvicellular (small cell group caudally), and magnocellular (large cell group rostrally) parts. The DM nucleus has also a small paralaminar part adjacent to the internal medullary lamina. Its two larger parts are linked to regions of the frontal and temporal lobes as well as to the amygdaloid complex (discussed in the chapter on the limbic system functions). Paralaminar cells receive input primarily from the frontal lobe and substancia nigra, and are involved in eye movement control.

4.5.4. Lateral Thalamic Nuclear Complex

The lateral thalamic nuclear complex is grouped into dorsal and ventral tiers. The dorsal tier includes the lateral dorsal nucleus (LD), the lateral posterior (LP) nucleus and the pulvinar. The LD nucleus has reciprocal connections with the cingulate gyrus (small). The LP nucleus has reciprocal connections with the parietal lobe. The pulvinar is the larger of this nuclear complex, having anterior, medial, lateral and inferior subdivisions. The pulvinar inferior division receives input from the superior colliculus and project to visual association cortices. Other pulvinar regions project to areas of the temporal, parietal and frontal lobes concerned with visual function and eye movement.

The ventral tier can be divided into an anterior (ventro-anterior, VA) nuclear group, a lateral (ventro-lateral, VL) nuclear group and a posterior (ventro-posterior, VP) group. The VA nuclei, together with the VL nuclear groups are important motor nuclei, composed of a large parvicellular portion and a small magnocellular part. Efferent fibers from it are diffuse. The VL nuclear group is divided into an oral (pars oralis), medial (pars medialis) and a caudal (pars caudalis) parts. Pars oralis is the largest, receiving dense projection from the globus pallidus (basal ganglia). Pars medialis has its main input arriving from the cerebellar nuclei.

The VP nuclear group is commonly divided into medial and lateral subgroups, forming the VPM and VPL nuclei respectively. The VPL is the final point of synapse for the dorsal columns-medial lemniscus tract and the spinothalamic fibers. Fibers terminate here in a somatotopic manner in a way that cervical representation is located medially, gradually moving laterally with lower body regions representation. Thus, all sensory modalities information from the body ends at the VPL. The VPM is the final point of synapse for the trigeminothalamic fibers from the spinal trigeminal nucleus and the principle trigeminal nucleus. You should recall that these tracts convey analogous sensory information, and thus the equivalent role of VPL for the body is served by the VPM for the face. Both VPM, VPL nuclei project to the primary somatosensory cortex, located at the postcentral gyrus of the parietal lobe. The ventro-postero-inferior (VPI) nucleus is a small cell group situated between VPL, VPM. VPI neurons process vestibular input mainly, projecting to the lateral postcentral gyrus. Ventral intermediate nucleus fibers are located between VL and VPL. These receive cerebellar input, projecting to the precentral gyrus.

LGN and MGN are considered a part of the lateral nuclear group. MGN receives ascending auditory input from the brachium of the inferior colliculus, and project it to the primary auditory cortex via the auditory radiation. LGN receives visual input from the retina via the optic tract and projects it to the primary visual cortex via the optic radiation. The posterior nuclear complex is located at posterior thalamus, at the level of the pulvinar and geniculate nuclei. It consists of the supra-geniculate nucleus, nucleus limitans and the posterior nucleus. It receives and sends to the cortex nociceptive cutaneous information from somatosensory pathways.

4.5.5. Intralaminar Nuclear Complex

This nuclear complex is embedded within the internal medullary lamina. It is a discontinuous group of cells. These cells project to the striatum and to other thalamic nuclei, as well as diffusely to the cortex. The centromedian (CM) nucleus projects to the striatum and to motor areas of the cortex. The parafascicular (PF) nucleus projects to the rostral lateral areas of the frontal lobe. Other nuclei receive input from ascending pain pathways, and project to sensory association cortex located at the parietal lobe.

4.5.6. Midline Nuclear Complex and the Thalamic Reticular Nucleus

The midline thalamic nuclear complex is the least understood component of the thalamus. Its paratenial nucleus is located just ventral to the rostral portion of stria medullaris thalami. Other midline nuclei are associated with the massa interthalamica. Efferents from this group reach the amygdaloid complex and the anterior cingulate cortex (role uncertain). The thalamic reticular nucleus lies within the external medullary lamina, and between it and the internal capsule. Reticular nucleus fibers project into the dorsal thalamus nuclei, but not to the cerebral cortex directly. Affarents from the cortex and thalamic nuclei, reach this nuclear complex via collaterals of thalamocortical & corticothalamic fibers. These neurons modulate (gate) the response of thalamic neurons to incoming cerebral cortical input.

4.5.7. Summary

As described previously, the thalamic nuclei can be viewed in two different ways. The nuclear complexes can be segregated into specific and non-specific categories in terms of the content of the sensory or motor information conveyed. Specific nuclei include the MGN, LGN, VPM, and VPL. In these, the input is derived from a single sensory system. All other nuclei can be regarded as non-specific in that sense. Another scheme divides the nuclear complexes into relay and association nuclei, i.e., according to the discrete versus diffuse projection of a certain nucleus. In this view, relay nuclei projecting to a single functionally uniform region include nuclei like the VL, VPL, VPM, and the geniculate nuclei. Association nuclei, projecting to association (non-motor, non-sensory) cortex include the pulvinar and the VA nuclei.

4.6. The Internal Capsule

The internal capsule is a deep subcortical structure that contains a concentration of white matter projection fibers. These fibers form the corona radiata (refer to figures, 4.4, 4.9). Anatomically, this is an important area because of the high concentration of both motor and sensory projection fibers.

Fibers forming it pass between the Diencephalon (Thalamus mostly) and cortex, as a fan-shaped mass. The internal capsule passes from the central core of the hemisphere into the brainstem. Although it consists of axons linking the thalamus and cortex, it also contains cortical efferents, projecting into the brainstem (corticorubral, corticoreticular, corticobulbar), or spinal cord (corticospinal).

The internal capsule is made up of five parts. These are the anterior limb, genu, posterior limb, retrolentiform and sublentiform parts of the internal capsule. Refer to figures 4.4, 4.9-4.12. Refer to table 4.2 for an overview of the parts of the internal capsule.

The blood supply of the internal capsule is variable but is commonly from small perforating branches of the middle cerebral artery and anterior cerebral artery. These include the lateral lenticulostriate arteries and the recurrent artery of Heubner respectively (discussed in chapter 9). In addition, the anterior choroidal artery (AChA) from the internal carotid artery supplies the posterior limb of the internal capsule.

Table 4.2. The Internal Capsule

Anterior limb	Lies between the head of the caudate nucleus medially and the lentiform nucleus laterally.	
	Contains the anterior thalamic radiation and frontopontine fibers.	
Genu	Lies medial to the apex of the lentiform nucleus, reaching almost the ventricular surface at the level of Monro foramina (figure 4.10-4.11).	
	Contains corticonuclear fibers (i.e., corticobulbar fibers)	
Posterior limb	Lies between the thalamus medially and the lentiform nucleus laterally	
	Content	Corticospinal fibers lying in anterior 2/3 of posterior limb
		The middle thalamic radiation which contains somatosensory fibers from the ventral posterior thalamic nucleus.
Retrolentiform part	Lies behind the lentiform nucleus. Contains the geniculo-calcarine or optic radiation	
Sublentiform part	Lies below the lentiform nucleus. Contains the auditory radiation fibers.	

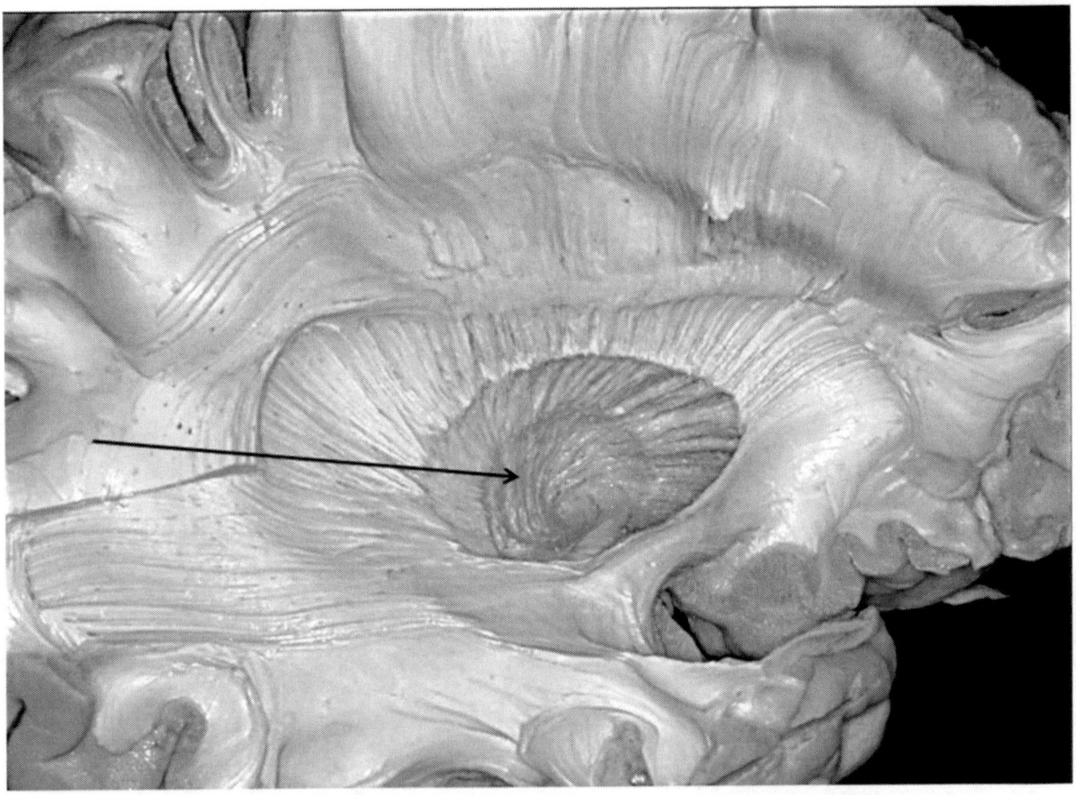

Figure 4.9. The Internal capsule, shown in a right hemispheral white matter dissection, with the right lentiform nucleus removed. Taken with permission from the Rhoton Collection.

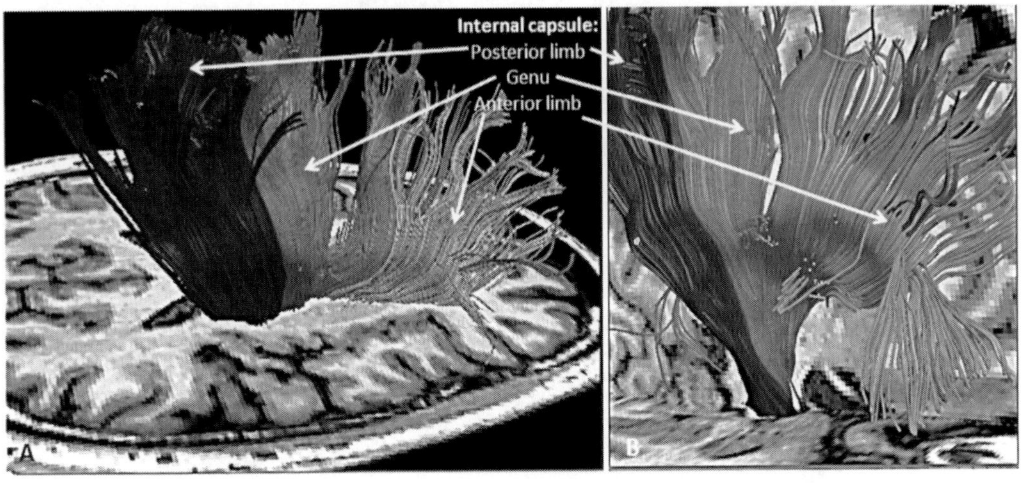

Figure 4.10. Diffusion Tensor Imaging (DTI) MRI showing the reconstruction of the different segments of the internal capsule in axial (A) and coronal (B) views. Taken with permission from the Rhoton Collection.

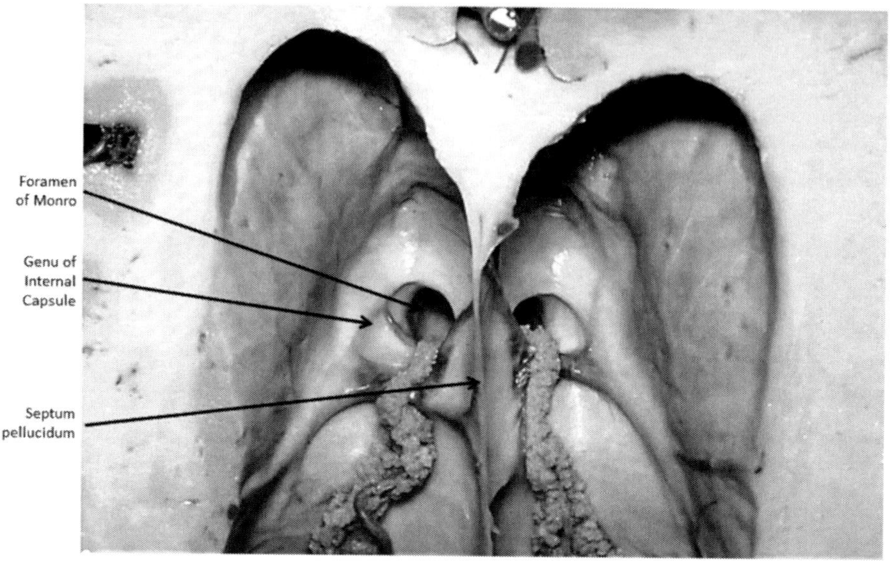

Figure 4.11. A view into the lateral ventricle and the foramen of Monro. The genu of the internal capsule and its proximity to the foramen of Monro is shown. Taken with permission from the Rhoton Collection.

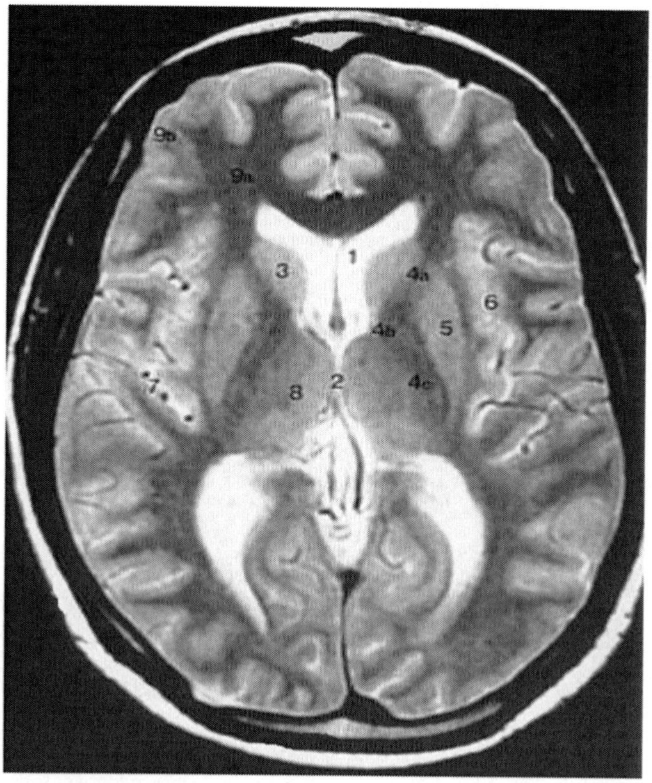

Figure 4.12. T2-weighted MRI at the level of the internal capsule. 1-Lateral ventricle, 2-Third ventricle, 3-Caudate nucleus, 4a-Anterior limb of internal capsule, 4b-Genu of internal capsule, 4c-Posterior limb of internal capsule, 5-Lentiform nucleus, 6-Insula, 7-Insular artery, 8-Thalamus, 9aWhite matter, 9bGray matter. Taken with permission from www.radiopaedia.org.

4.7. The Hypothalamus

4.7.1. Overview

The hypothalamus is involved mainly in autonomic (VM-visceromotor and VS-viscerosensory) functions as well as endocrine activities. It is the central nervous system center for neuroendocrine coordination and control, the primary autonomic center. As such, it controls the homeostasis and different bodily functions by coordinating a neural (ANS - autonomic nervous system, sympathetic and parasympathetic) and an endocrine (via the pituitary) tools to broadcast its decisions. Together with related limbic structures, the hypothalamus receives sensory information and regulates the motor systems that modify the internal environment via four mechanisms. First, it is the principal modulator of ANS. Second, it is a VS transducer having neurons with specialized receptors capable of responding to changes in the temperture, osmolarity of blood, hormonal levels. Third, it regulates the activity of the anterior pituitary through the production of inhibitory and releasing hormones and lastly, it has its own endocrine function, by producing and releasing oxytocin and antiduiretic hormone into the circulation, via the posterior pituitary. Refer to figures 4.1, 4.13 - 4.14

4.7.2. Hypothalamic Boundaries

The discussion on the borders of the hypothalamus overlaps that of the third ventricle, and should be viewed together. The anterior hypothalamic border is formed by the lamina terminalis, a thin membrane, extending ventrally from the anterior commissure to the rostral edge of the optic chiasm. It is a remnant of the telencephalic brain vesicle. The lamina terminalis separates the hypothalamus from the anterior septal nuclei. The dorsal border of the hypothalamus is defined by the hypothalamic sulcus (discussed previously, a shallow groove separating it from the dorsal thalamus). The lateral-anterior border of hypothalamus is formed by the substancia innominate (discussed later), whereas the lateral-posterior border is formed by the medial edge of the posterior limb of internal capsule. The medial border is formed by the inferior portion of the third ventricle. Posteriorly, there is no sharp border, merging into the midbrain tegmentum and the PAG.

4.7.3. Hypothalamic Zones

The hypothalamus is divided into three zones. The lateral zone extends the full rostro-caudal length of the hypothalamus, and is separated from the medial zone by a line drown through the fornix in the sagittal plane. Diffused cluster of neurons, intermingled with longitudinally oriented axon bundles (forming the Medial Forebrain bundle) occupy this zone. No nuclei are present in this zone, although the supraoptic nucleus is partially here. The lateral zone cells are involved in cardiovascular function, food and water intake regulation etc. (i.e., the hunger and satiety centers, as well the thirst center).

The medial hypothalamic zone is divided from rostral to caudal to three regions. These are the chiasmatic, tuberal and mamillary regions. The chiasmatic region has five nuclei: the preoptic nucleus (mediating hormone release and body temperture regulation), the supraoptic nucleus (mediating hormone release), the paraventricular nucleus (mediating hormone release regulation), the anterior (cardiovascular function) and the suprachiasmatic (circadian rhythms) nucleus. The tuberal region contains the dorsomedial nucleus, the ventromedial nucleus (the food intake or satiety center) and the arcuate nucleus, which delivers hormones to the portal vein, En route to the adenohypophysis. The mammillary region contains the posterior nucleus (mediating elevation of blood pressure, shivering) and the mammillary nucleus, which consists of a large medial and a small lateral nuclei.

The third zone, the periventricular zone, includes the nerves that border the ependymal surfaces of the third ventricle. Refer to figure 4.15

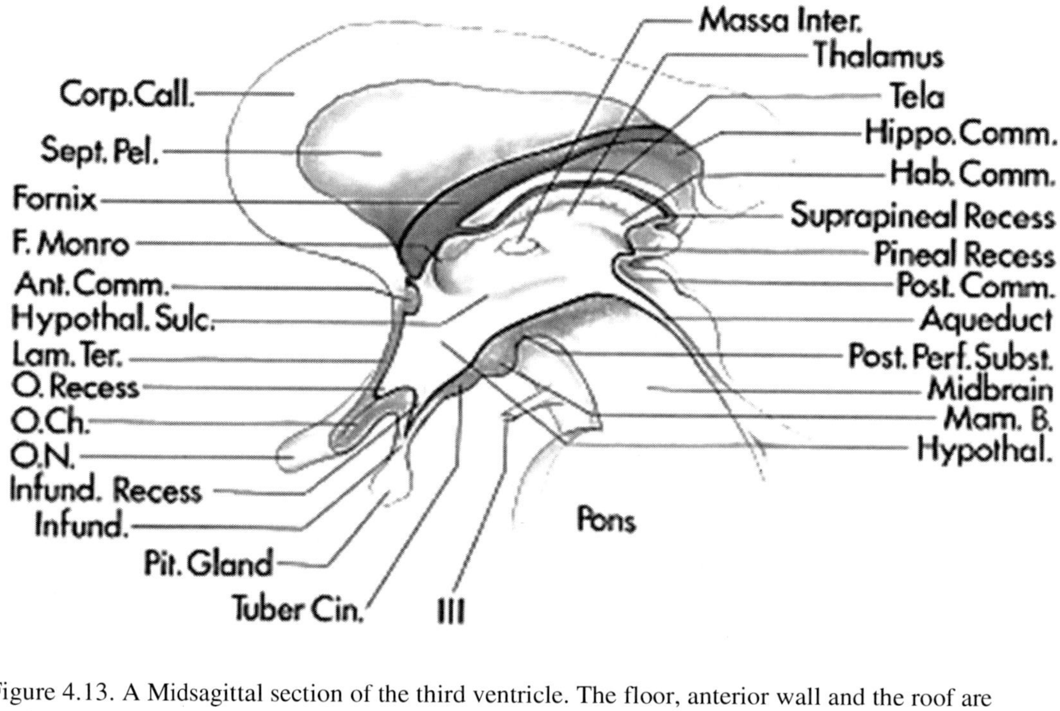

Figure 4.13. A Midsagittal section of the third ventricle. The floor, anterior wall and the roof are marked. The hippocampal commissure, corpus callosum, and septum pellucidum are above the roof. The posterior wall extends from the suprapineal recess to the aqueduct and includes the habenular commissure, pineal gland, pineal recess, and posterior commissure. The hypothalamic sulcus forms a groove between the thalamic and hypothalamic surfaces of the third ventricle. Ant., anterior; B., body; Call., callosum; Ch., chiasm; Cin., cinereum; Comm., commissure; Corp., corpus; For., foramen; Hab., habenular; Hippo., hippocampal; Hypothal., hypothalamic, hypothalamus; Infund., infundibular, infundibulum; Inter., intermedia; Lam., lamina; Mam., mamillary; N., nerve; O., optic; Pel., pellucidum; Perf., perforated; Pit., pituitary; Post., posterior; Sept., septum; Subst., substance; Sulc., sulcus; Ter., terminalis. Taken with permission from the Rhoton Collection.

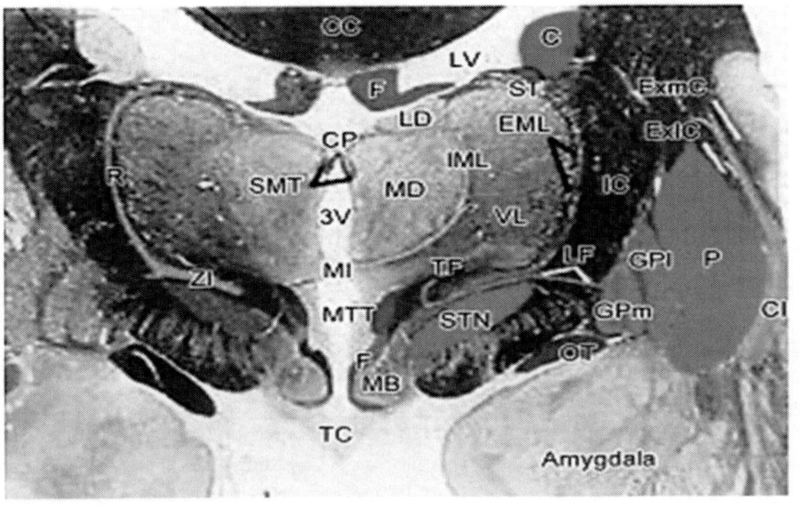

Figure 4.14. The Internal anatomy of the diencephalon and basal ganglia, at lenticular fasciculus. Corpus Callosum (CC), Lateral Ventricle (LV), Fornix (F, both dorsally and ventrally), Body of Caudate (C), Stria Terminalis (ST), Stria Medullaris Thalami (SMT, thin band of white matter on medial surface of MD), Choroid Plexus forming roof of third ventricle (3V), Mediodorsal Nucleus (MD), Lateral Dorsal Nucleus (LD), Internal Medullary Lamina (IML), Ventral Lateral Nucleus (VL), External Medullary Lamina (EML), Reticular Nucleus (R) and Zona Incerta (ZI), Subthalamic Nucleus (STN), Internal Capsule (IC), Extreme Capsule (ExmC), Claustrum (Cl), External Capsule (ExlC), Putamen (P), Globus Pallidus (GPm, GPl), Optic Tract (OT), Amygdala, Lenticular Fasciculus (LF), Thalamic Fasciculus, (TF, contains pallido-thalamic and cerebello-thalamic fibers) Mammillothalamic Tract (MTT). Tuber cinereum (TC, contains median eminence of hypothalamo-hypophyseal portal system). Taken with permission from www.radiopaedia.org.

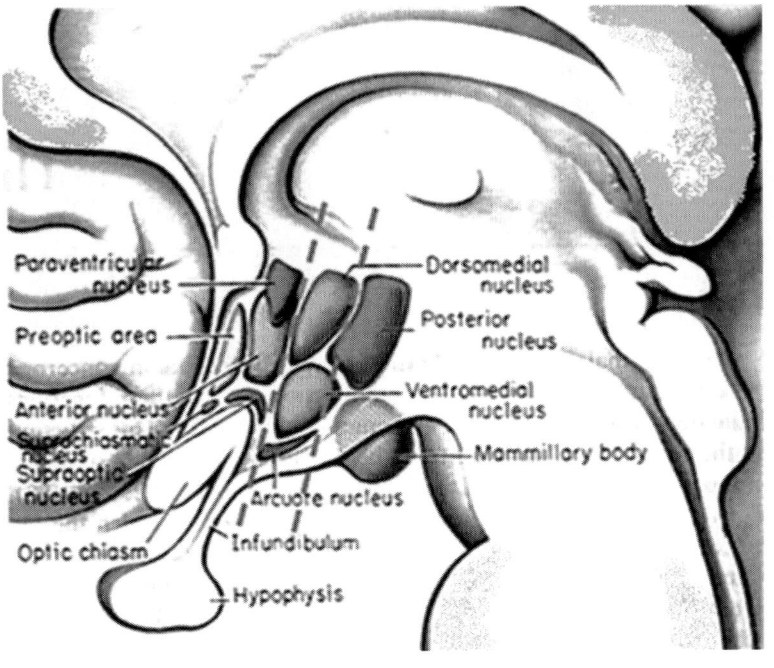

Figure 4.15. The hypothalamic zones. Refer to the text. Image taken from Gray's anatomy, now out of copyright and in the public domain.

4.7.4. Hypothalamic Functional Centers

The segregation of the different hypothalamic nuclei into functional centers and groups makes more physiological sense, albeit less anatomical one. Refer to table 4.3 for a summary of this simplified view.

Table 4.3. Hypothalamic Functional Centers

Nucleus	Function	
Anterior	Heat loss	Sweating and vasodilation centers
Posterior	Heat conservation	Vasoconstriction, shivering centers, metabolic rate increases, cessation of sweating
Supraoptic & paraventricular	Water balance	Secretion of vasopressin/ADH, secretion of oxytocin (birth process, lactation), thirst (regions near supraoptic nuclei), appetite dependent metabolism rates
Median eminence & arcuate	Secretion of hormone releasing and inhibiting factors, appetite (arcuate nucleus)	
Preoptic area (four nuclei)	Regulation of gonadotrophic hormones, reduction in heart rate and blood pressure, regulation of body temperature	
Ventromedial	Satiety center	
Dorsomedial	Gastrointestinal stimulation	
Lateral	Hunger (and thirst) center	
Suprachiasmatic	The "biological clock"	

4.7.5. Hypothalamus Blood Supply

The description of the pituitary blood supply and venous drainage is given later in the chapter. All branches supplying the hypothalamus arise from the circle of Willis. The anterior medial group is supplied by branches of the anterior communicating artery and the anterior cerebral artery (ACA, first segment). These branches serve the preoptic, supraoptic and septal nuclei. The postero-medial group is supplied by branches of the Posterior communicating artery and the posterior cerebral artery (PCA, first segment). These branches serve the nuclei of the tuberal and mamillary regions. The hypophyseal arteries, divided into a superior and inferior groups of arteries are small branches all arising from the internal carotid artery, but from different segments. The inferior branches arise from the cavernous (C4) segment of the internal carotid artery, whereas the superior branches arise from its intradural (C6) segment. Refer to chapter 9 for a discussion on the carotid arterial system.

4.7.6. Hypothalamic Affarent Fibers Systems

The fornix is the largest single input to the hypothalamus. The fibers of the fornix largely originate in the hippocampus. The fornix arises from neurons in the subiculum and hippocampus (both of the hippocampal Formation). When approaching the anterior commissure, the fornix is divided to a precommissural bundle (from hippocampus mainly), and a larger postcommissural bundle (mainly from subiculum). The fornix is discussed in greater details in chapter 7. The Amygdalofugal bundle fibers exit the amygdala, course through the substancia innominata to enter the hypothalamus and thalamus. This bundle is composed of two systems: the stria terminalis (originating from the medial portion of the amygdala, terminating in the septal nuclei and preoptic area) and the ventral amygdalofugal pathway, arising from the basolateral amygdaloid complex, passing under the lentiform nucleus through the substancia innominata into the hypothalamus (refer to figure 4.7). The medial forebrain bundle, passes bidirectional through the lateral hypothalamic region. It consists of ascending axons originating from all throughout the neuroaxis, terminating in the hypothalamus, and others that exit the hypothalamus to reach forebrain and brainstem. It is a diffuse structure, containing mainly fibers coursing through the Lateral hypothalamic zone.

Other affarent fiber systems to the hypothalamus include the mamillary peduncle (arising from the medial portion of midbrain reticular formation), the thalamohypothalamic tract (arising from the DM-nucleus of thalamus), the corticohypothalamic tract (being the only direct neocortical projection originating from the prefrontal cortex) and the retinohypothalamic tract, arising from the suprachiasmatic nucleus (receiving from the retina). These fibers arise as direct axons from the optic chiasm, or as collaterals of the retinogeniculate fibers.

4.7.7. Hypothalamic Efferent Fibers Systems

Hypothalamic efferent fibers systems include both ascending fibers (to forebrain) and descending fibers. Among the ascending fibers system, a few are to be mentioned. The mamillary fasciculus originates from the medial mamillary nucleus, passing dorsally and then bifurcates into the mammillothalamic tract (projecting to anterior nucleus of thalamus, important in the circuit of Papez, discussed in the limbic system) and the mammillotegmental tract (projecting to tegmental nuclei of midbrain).

Important descending tracts, projecting to brainstem and spinal targets include the hypothalamospinal tract (arising from the paraventricular nucleus, descending through the PAG, and reticular formation of midbrain and rostral Pons to terminate on neurons of the intermedio-lateral Cell column), the hypothalamomedullary tract (similar path, terminating in nucleus solitaries and dorsal Vagal nucleus), the dorsal longitudinal fasciculus (arising from medial zone nuclei) and the mammillotegmental tract (arising from the medial mamillary nucleus).

4.8. The Pituitary Gland

4.8.1. Overview and Gross Anatomy

As discussed in the neuro-embryology chapter (4.3.3), the anterior pituitary lobe (e.g., the adenohypophysis) is derived from Rathke's pouch. Its posterior wall forms the intermediate lobe of the pituitary gland, having a less prominent function in humans. The posterior pituitary lobe (e.g., the neurohypophysis) develops as an evagination of the floor of the developing third ventricle. Hypothalamic cell bodies are located within the hypothalamus, secreting neurohypophysis hormones in the posterior pituitary gland.

The pituitary fossa, the housing of the pituitary gland, is located in the sella turcica of the sphenoid bone. As discussed in chapter 1, the sella turcica forms the pituitary fossa with its floor formed by the sphenoid sinus. The pituitary is surrounded by dura, both below it, as the lining of the sella Turcica as well as above it. The diaphragma sella is the dural coverings over the superior portion of the pituitary fossa. The pituitary stalk communicates with the main cranial cavity through a hole in the diaphragma sella. Figure 4.16 presents the dural coverings of the skull base and the diaphragma sella. Bordering the pituitary fossa are important neurovasucular structures. The cavernous sinus with its cranial nerve contents, the internal carotid artery (coming to lie very close to the gland at its cavernous portion), the optic chiasm tract and nerve, the third ventricle etc. Refer to figures 4.17-4.18 for the pituitary gland and its relationships in sagittal and coronal dissections.

As shown in figure 4.17, the intercavernous carotid produces prominences in the lateral wall of the sphenoid sinus below and anterior to the gland. Intercavernous sinuses courses along the anterior and posterior margins of the diaphragm. The basilar sinus, located on the back of the dorsum, is the largest connection across the midline between the posterior edges of the paired cavernous sinuses. The inferior hypophyseal artery arises from the posterior bend of the intercavernous carotid and is directed medially toward the posterior lobe. The cavernous sinuses are located on the lateral side of the gland and separate the gland from the intracavernous carotids. The superior hypophyseal arteries arise from the medial side of the supraclinoid carotid and pass to the chiasm and stalk. The anterior intercavernous sinus crosses the anterosuperior margin of the gland, and the inferior intracavernous sinus extends below the gland interconnecting the cavernous sinuses.

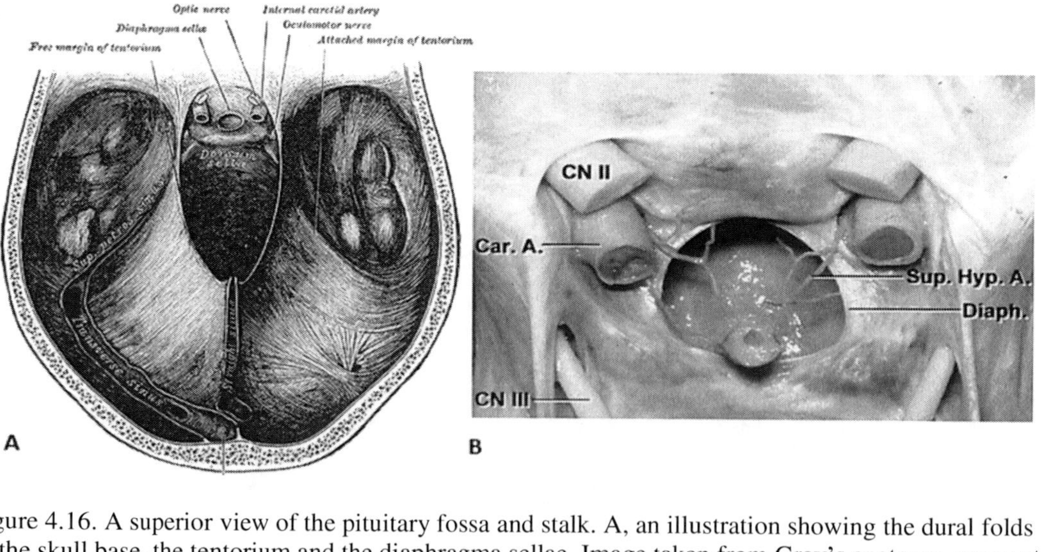

Figure 4.16. A superior view of the pituitary fossa and stalk. A, an illustration showing the dural folds of the skull base, the tentorium and the diaphragma sellae. Image taken from Gray's anatomy, now out of copyright and in the public domain. B, dissection of the sellar region showing the optic nerve (CN-II), the oculomotor (CN III) nerve entering the cavernous sinus, the internal carotid artery emerging from the cavernous sinus (car.A.), the superior hypophyseal artery (Sup.Hyp.A) and the pituitary gland exposed below a large natural opening in the diaphragm sellae. Taken with permission from the Rhoton Collection.

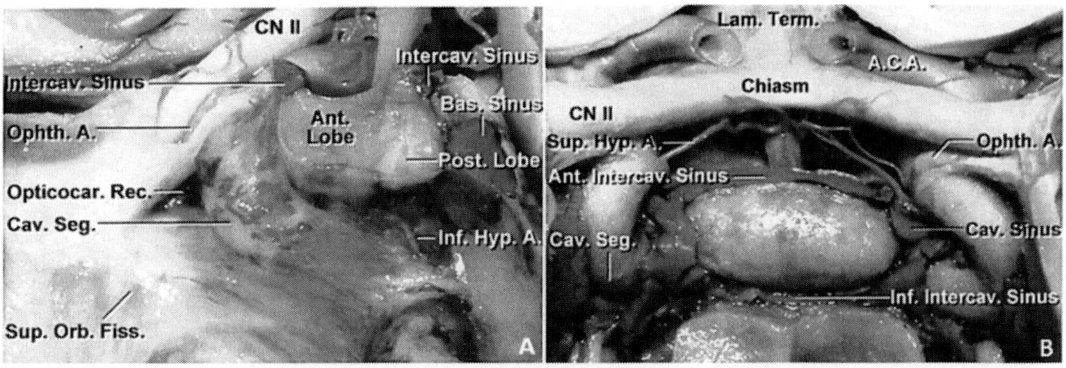

Figure 4.17. The pituitary gland and its relationships. A, A midsagittal section of the sella extending through the anterior and posterior lobes and sphenoid sinus. B, Anterior view of the pituitary gland region. Taken with permission from the Rhoton Collection.

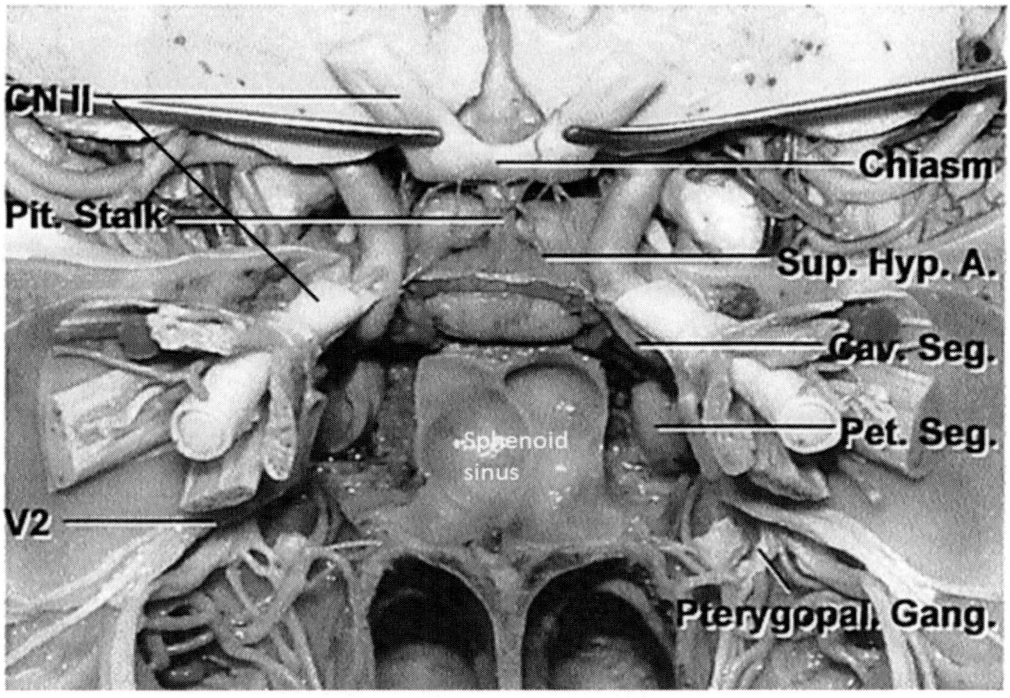

Figure 4.18. A Transnasal route to the sphenoid sinus and sella. The optic nerves have been elevated to show the suprasellar area and the relationships between the orbital apex, optic canals, nasal cavity, pterygopalatine fossa, and the petrous and intracavernous segments of the internal carotid artery. The superior hypophyseal arteries pass to the lower margin of the optic chiasm and the pituitary stalk. A., artery; Car., carotid; Cav., cavernous; CN, cranial nerve; Gang., ganglion; Hyp., hypophyseal. Taken with permission from the Rhoton Collection.

4.8.2. Endocrine Functions of the Pituitary and Hypothalamus

The release of hormones by the anterior pituitary glandular cells is controlled by hypothalamic neurons through the hypophyseal portal system. A portal vascular system (also present in the liver and kidneys) refers to the presence of two capillary beds in continuity. Its manifestation anatomically in the pituitary can be best described in a step-wise fashion:

1) Pituitary cells receive arterial blood from the inferior and superior hypophyseal arteries. Both are internal carotid artery branches, entering the stalk where they branch out into many sinusoids.
2) The first capillary plexus is located in the median eminence. Hypothalamic neurons are lying adjacent to the third ventricle project to the median eminence, secreting releasing hormones (RH) and inhibitory hormones (IH).
3) RH and IH are carried by the hypophyseal portal veins to the anterior pituitary. All RH and IH are peptides except the prolactin IH which is dopamine.
4) The second capillary plexus is located in the anterior pituitary gland. Hormones released in the anterior pituitary gland enter the blood stream, drained into the inferior hypophyseal vein to the inferior petrosal sinus or to the cavernous sinus (60% to the inferior petrosal).
5) Blood drains through the venous sinusoidal system to reach the internal jugular veins.

The posterior pituitary lobe has also a capillary plexus, picking up the secreted hormones (oxytocin and vasopressin) secreted in the posterior pituitary lobe by neurons terminals whose cell bodies are in the supraoptic and paraventricular nuclei. Refer to table 4.4 for a short overview of the endocrine functions of the pituitary and hypothalamus, not in the scope of this book.

Table 4.4. Endocrine Functions of the Pituitary and Hypothalamus

Anterior pituitary (Adenohypophysis)	ACTH	Adrenocorticotrophic hormone
	GH	Growth hormone
	PRL	Prolactin
	TSH	Thyroid stimulating hormone
	LH	Luteinizing hormone
	FSH	Follicle stimulating hormone
Intermediate lobe	POMC	Pro-opio-melanocortin
	MSH	melatonin stimulating hormone
Posterior lobe (Neurohypophysis)	OTC	Oxytocin
	ADH	anti-diuretic hormone, Vasopressin

4.9. Ventral thalamus – Subthalamic Nucleus

The Subthalamic nucleus (STN) is a lens shaped cell group situated rostral and dorsal to substancia nigra and ventral to the lenticular fasciculus. The cells receive input from motor areas of the cortex, and project to substancia nigra. The nuclear cells are reciprocally connected with the globus pallidus. Lesions in this region result in a characteristic condition termed as hemiballisimus. The Subthalamic nucleus has a few unique features making it an attractive target for treatment of motor circuit diseases, such as Parkinson's disease and Essential tremor. In choosing a target for a surgical procedure, it should have a tight representation of the entire body, far from major arterial and venous vessels, allowing for a small intervention to result in a homogeneous, whole body effect. That is the case with the STN. The STN itself has subdivisions, with only the dorsal aspect of which focused on motor functions. Its ventral area has limbic functions, among other. This issue is beyond the scope of this book. Refer to figures 4.7, 4.14 for the STN details.

The prerubral area, AKA the "fields H of Forel", is white matter tracts located rostral to the red nucleus and medial to the subthalamic nucleus. This bundles are traversed by fibers from the lenticular fasciculus (Forel's field H_2), entering the thalamic fasciculus. Zona incerta is located dorsal to subthalamic nucleus, separated form it by the lenticular fasciculus. It contains output neurons, projecting to many locations (cortex, superior colliculus, pretectal region, basilar pons etc).

4.10. The Epithalamus

The epithalamus term encompass the pineal gland, habenular nuclei and the stria medullaris thalami. The pineal gland is a richly vascularized connective tissue structure containing glial cells and pinealocytes, no neurons. It is a rudiment of the third eye. Pinealocytes synthesize melatonin from serotonin, via enzymes sensitive to diurnal fluctuations.

The photonic stimulus is indirect, via the retinal ganglion cells, projecting to the suprachiasmatic nucleus which influences neurons of the intermediolateral cell column in the spinal cord. These preganglionic sympathetic neurons project to the superior cervical (stellate) ganglion, which innervates the pineal gland via postganglionic fibers traveling on branches of internal carotid artery. Refer to figures 4.19 - 4.21.

The habenular nuclei are located anterior to the pineal gland, consisting of a large lateral nucleus and a small medial nucleus. Both nuclei contribute to the habenulo-interpeduncular tract (fasciculus retroflexus), terminating in the midbrain interpeduncular nucleus. The habenular commissure is a small bundle of fibers, riding on dorsal edge of posterior commissure, connecting the habenular regions of the two sides. The stria Medullaris thalami, the main epithalamic output, arches over the dorsal surface of the thalamus, near the Midline, conveying input to both Habenular nuclei. Refer to figures 4.20 - 4.21.

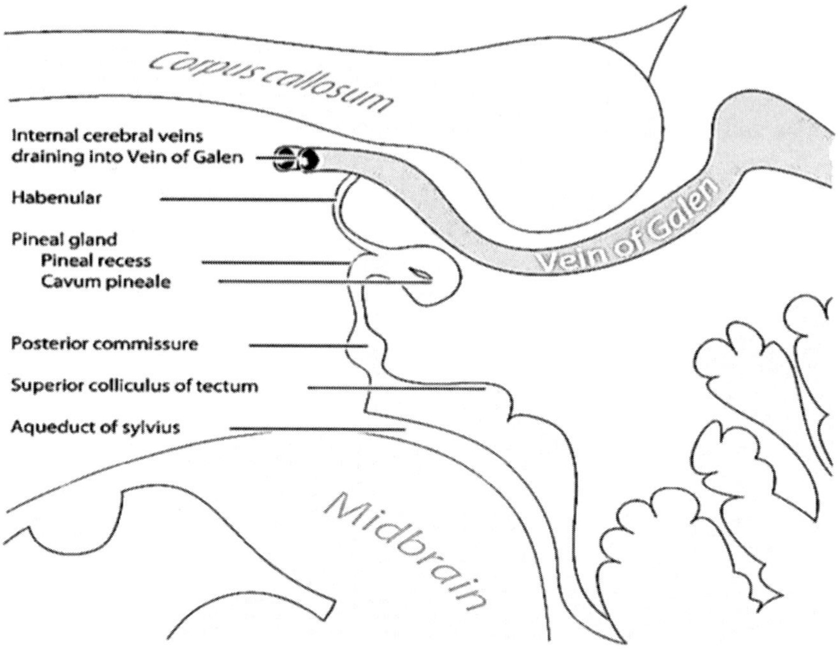

Figure 4.19. The pineal Region. Taken with permission from www.radiopaedia.org.

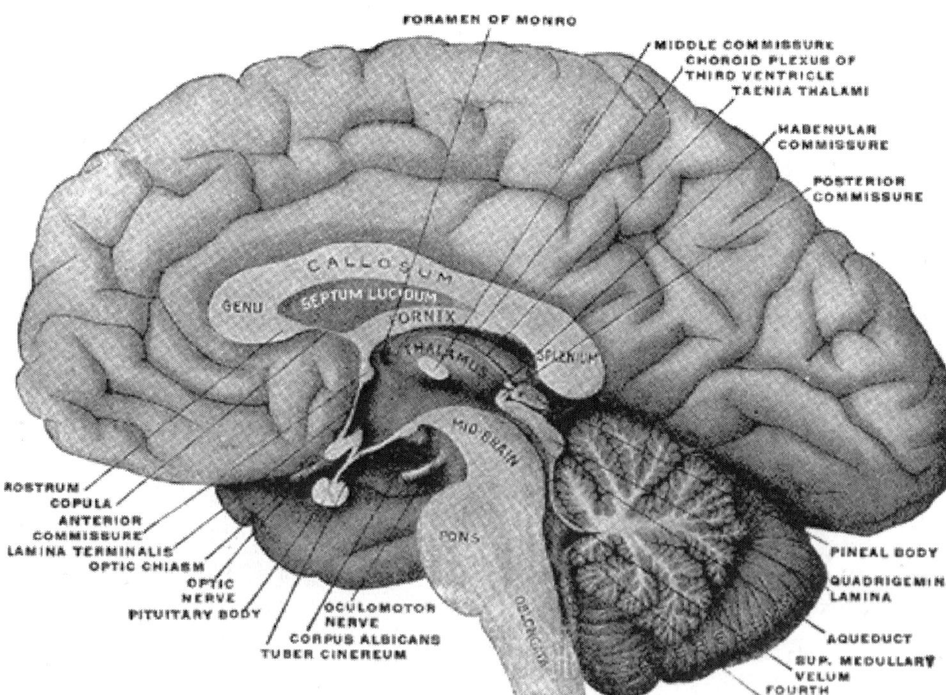

Figure 4.20. The Epithalamus. The stria medullaris thalami is bolded. Taken from Gray's anatomy (now in the public domain and out of copyright).

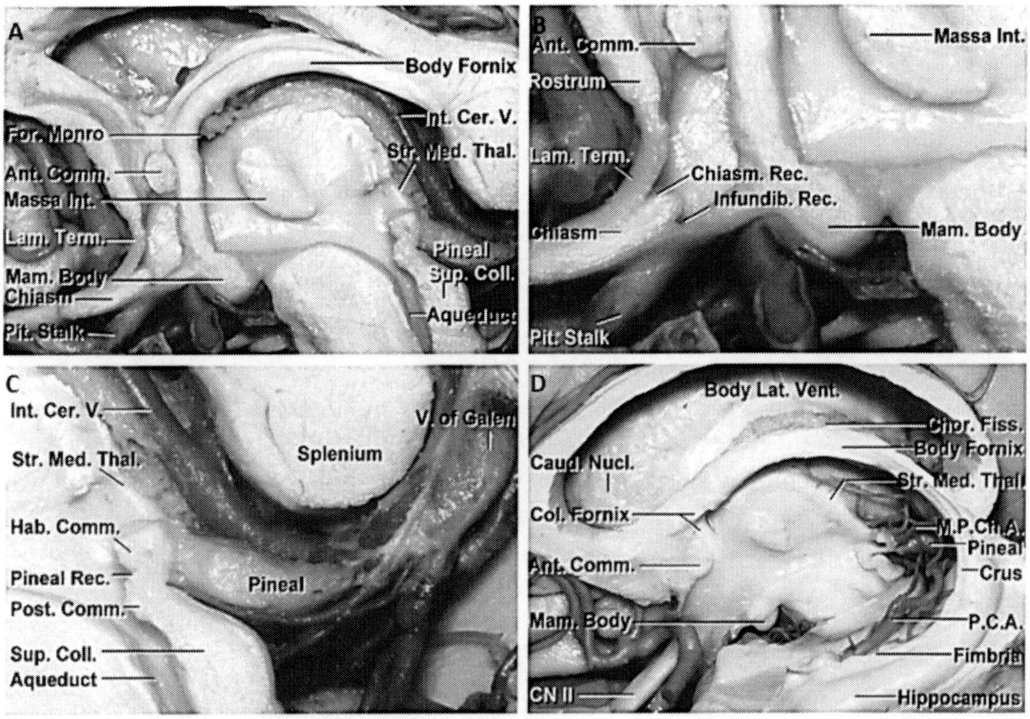

Figure 4.21. The third Ventricle. A, Overview. B, Enlarged floor. C, Enlarged view of the posterior part of the third ventricle. D, lateral view of the third ventricle with the hippocampus and fornix preserved. A., artery; A.C.A., anterior cerebral artery; Ant., anterior; Bas., basilar; Call., callosum; Car., carotid; Caud., caudate; Cer., cerebral; Chiasm., chiasmatic; Chor., choroid; CN, cranial nerve; Col., column; Coll., colliculus; Comm., commissure; Corp., corpus; For., foramen; Hab., habenular; Infund., infundibular; Int., intermedia, internal; Interpos., interpositum; Lam., lamina; Lat., lateral; Mam., mamillary; Med., medial; M.P.Ch.A., medial posterior choroidal artery; Nucl., nucleus; P.C.A., posterior cerebral artery; Pell., pellucidum; Pit., pituitary; Plex., plexus; Post., posterior; Rec., recess; Sag., sagittal; Sept., septal, septum; Str., straight; Sup., superior; Term., terminalis; Thal., thalami; V., vein; Vel., velum; Vent., ventricle. Taken with permission from the Rhoton Collection.

4.11. Synopsis of the Third Ventricle

Figures 4.21-4.22 presents the wall and spatial anatomy of the third ventricle. The anterior wall is made up of the lamina terminalis and the anterior commissure. The optic chiasm, mamillary bodies, and midbrain are in the floor. The chiasmatic recess is located above the optic chiasm and behind the lamina terminalis. The infundibular recess is located below and behind the optic chiasm. The lamina terminalis blends into the rostrum of the corpus callosum. The anterior commissure is positioned between the rostrum of the corpus callosum and the columns of the fornix. The thalamus and hypothalamus form the lateral wall of the third ventricle.

Looking at the posterior wall of the third ventricle, it is formed by the aqueduct, pineal, and habenular and posterior commissures. The pineal recess extends into the base of the pineal in the interval between the habenular and posterior commissures. The body of the fornix forms the roof of the third ventricle.

The velum interpositum, through which the internal cerebral veins course, is located between the body of the fornix and the stria medullaris thalami. The quadrigeminal cistern and pineal region are located anteromedial to the crus of the fornix, and the ambient cistern and posterior cerebral artery are located medial to the temporal horn and the fimbria. Opening the choroidal fissure adjacent to the body of the fornix exposes the third ventricle. The medial posterior choroidal arteries turn forward beside the pineal to reach the velum interpositum.

Looking at the roof of the third ventricle (figure 4.23), the choroid plexus is attached along the choroidal fissure located between the body of the fornix and the thalamus. The superior choroidal veins course along the choroid plexus. The thalamostriate veins pass through the posterior margins of the foramen of Monro. The columns of the fornix pass anterior and superior to the foramen of Monro. The body of the fornix forms the upper part of the roof of the third ventricle. The tela choroidea spans the interval below the body of the fornix and forms the upper wall of the velum interpositum in the roof of the third ventricle. The velum is positioned between an upper layer of tela attached to the lower surface of the body of the fornix and a lower layer of tela attached below the internal cerebral veins to the stria medullaris thalami.

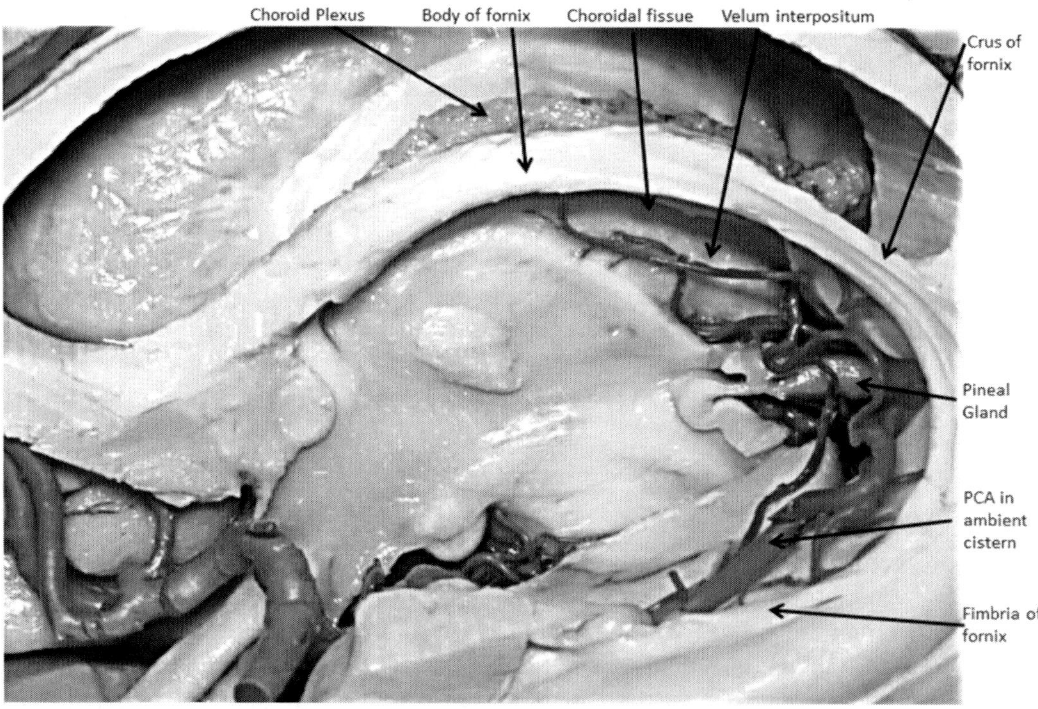

Figure 4.22. The third ventricle, highlighting the choroidal fissure and its relation to the crus of fornix and other structures. Taken with permission from the Rhoton Collection.

The internal cerebral veins and medial posterior choroidal arteries course in the velum interpositum (figure 4.23). The tela is a thin, arachnoid-like membrane, through which the internal cerebral veins and the medial posterior choroidal arteries can be seen. The anterior septal veins pass above the foramen of Monro. The anterior septal veins course along the septum and join the internal cerebral veins near the foramen of Monro. Opening the tela, we can see the massa intermedia, mamillary bodies, and posterior commissure within the ventricle. The aqueduct is positioned below the posterior and habenular commissures. The pineal recess extends posteriorly between the habenular and posterior commissures into the base of the pineal.

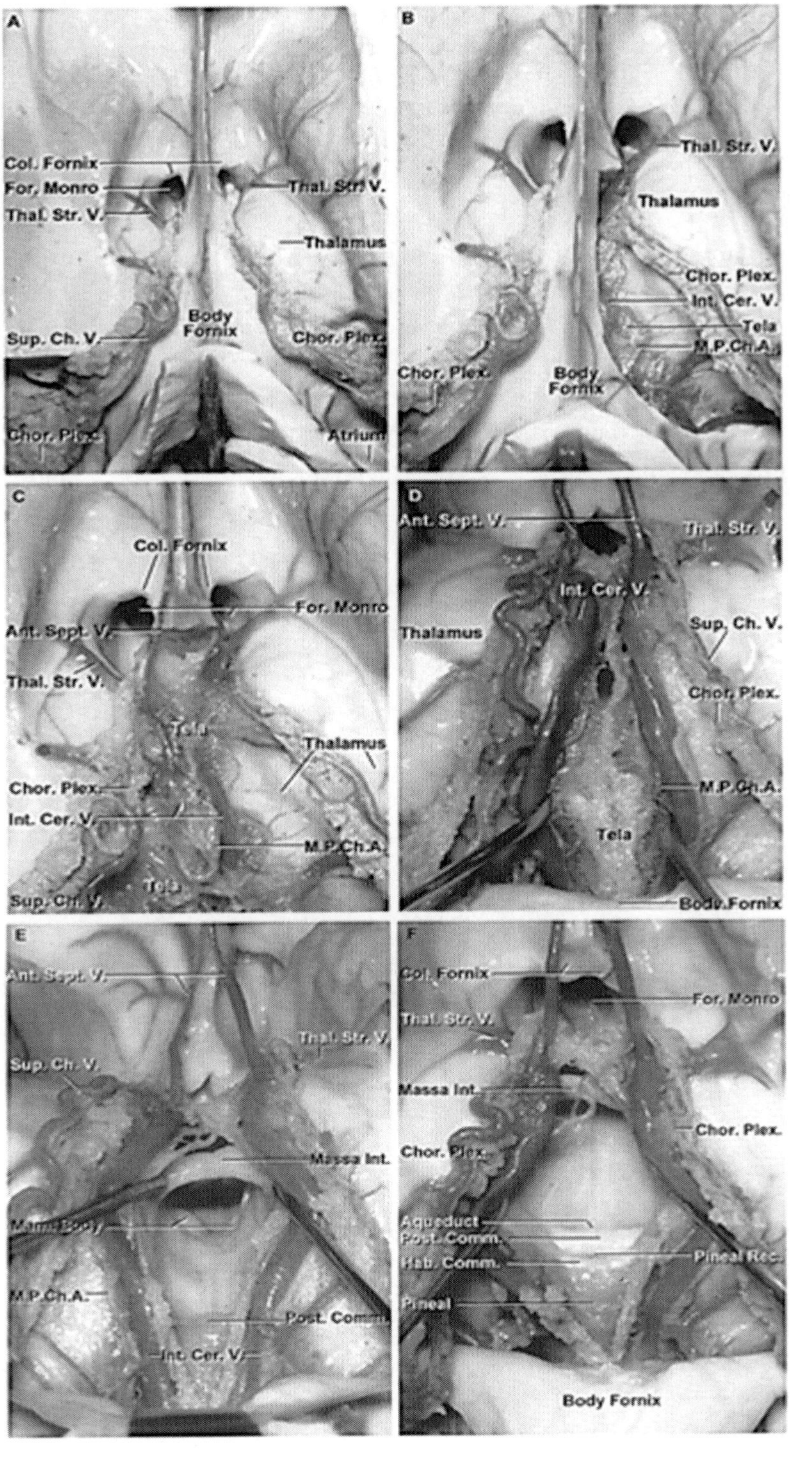

Figure 4.23. The Roof of the third ventricle. Superior views. A, the upper part of the hemispheres has been removed to expose the frontal horn and body of the lateral ventricle. B, the right lateral edge of the fornix has been removed to expose the upper layer of tela choroidea. C, the body of the fornix has been folded backward. The upper layer of tela that rests against the lower surface of the body of the fornix has been preserved. D, the upper layer of tela has been removed to expose the internal cerebral veins and medial posterior choroidal arteries. The internal cerebral veins have been retracted laterally. E, the tela has been opened to expose the massa intermedia, mamillary bodies, and posterior commissure. F, the exposure has been directed to the posterior part of the third ventricle. Ant., anterior; Cer., cerebral; Ch., choroidal; Chor., choroid; Col., column; Comm., commissure; For., foramen; Hab., habenular; Int., intermedia, internal; Mam., mamillary; M.P.Ch.A., medial posterior choroidal artery; Plex., plexus; Post., posterior; Rec., recess; Sept., septal; Sup., superior; Thal.Str., thalamostriate; V., vein. Taken with permission from the Rhoton Collection.

Looking at the floor of the third ventricle (figure 4.24), it is located medial to the uncus and anterior perforated substance and above the midbrain. From anterior to posterior, the floor includes the lower margin of the optic chiasm, the pituitary stalk surrounded by the tuber cinereum, mamillary bodies, and the midbrain. The interpeduncular fossa is located below the posterior part of the floor. The anterior part of the optic tract extends along the lateral margin of the floor, but further posteriorly, the tracts deviate laterally away from the floor to pass around the upper margin of the cerebral peduncle.

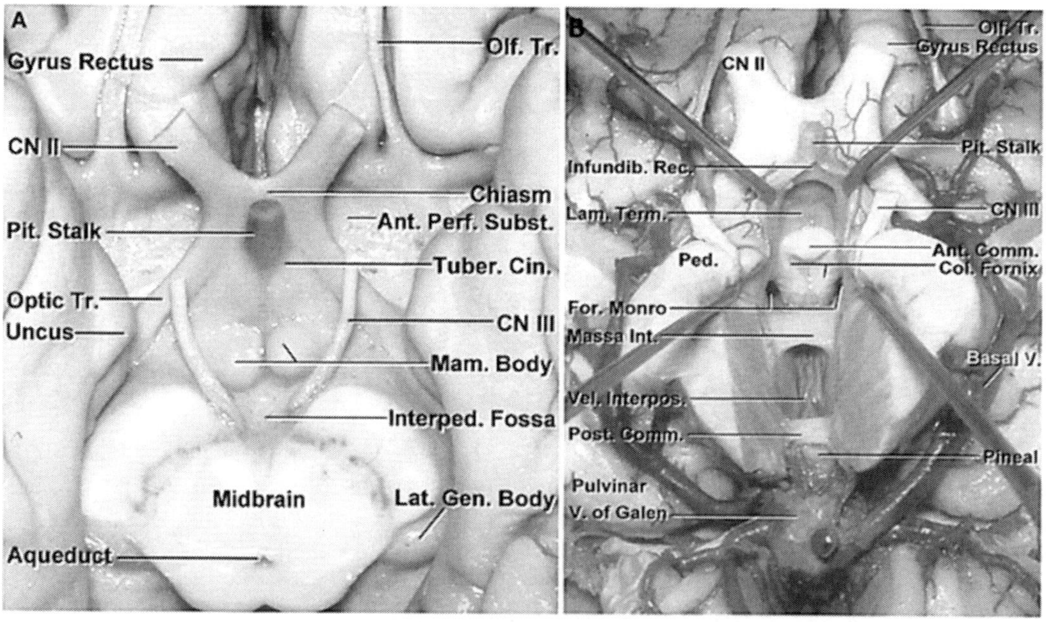

Figure 4.24. A, the floor of the third ventricle. B, inferior view with the floor of the third ventricle removed to expose the roof. The pituitary stalk has been reflected forward to expose the ventricular side of the infundibular recess and lamina terminalis. Taken with permission from the Rhoton Collection.

The lamina terminalis (figure 4.24b) slopes upward from the upper edge of the chiasm to the area in front of the anterior commissure where it blends into the rostrum of the corpus callosum. The columns of the fornix cross above and anterior to the foramen of Monro and descend toward the mamillary bodies. The massa intermedia crosses the midportion of the third ventricle. The velum interpositum, in which the internal cerebral veins and medial posterior choroidal arteries course, is positioned between the thalami in the roof of the third ventricle. The posterior commissure is exposed below the pineal gland. The vein of Galen, into which the basal veins empty, is located just behind the third ventricle.

Chapter 5

The Basal Ganglia

5.1. Abstract

The basal ganglia form a cluster of gray matter nuclei in the depth of the cerebral hemispheres. The key anatomical features related to these structures, are mostly in detailing the white matter pathways and tracts and the interconnections these share with surrounding structures and with the cerebral cortex. Their importance is immense for motor, sensory as well as learning and limbic functions. Much of current research on motor diseases like the parkinsonism spectrum, tremor, dystonia etc. is focused on unraveling the details of these connections. For our purpose, a systematic review, describing the relevant embryological key points.

This is followed by a short overview of the gross anatomical features and a short description of the key tracts needed as a basic working knowledge for the aspiring medical student. Major connections of the basal ganglia are discussed, separated into afferent, efferent and intrinsic subchapters as well as a focused view on the direct and indirect pathways.

The chapter ends with a short description of blood supply to the basal ganglia and related structures with its very common devastating clinical manifestation.

5.2. Neuro-Embryology of the Basal Ganglia

The corpus striatum received its descriptive name due to the face that in cross-section, this region has a striated appearance. Its cells appear in the floor of the developing lateral ventricle at the time when primordial cell groups in the wall of the 3rd ventricle give rise to diencephalic structures (refer to chapter 4).

During development it is bisected by axons to and from the cerebral cortex, forming the internal capsule (refer to chapter 4). The internal capsule divides it into the medial caudate nucleus and the lateral putamen nucleus. Diencephalic cells migrate across the internal capsule to assume a position medially to putamen. These cells give rise to the globus pallidus (GP). Putamen and GP are termed together as the lenticular nucleus.

The site where the hemisphere wall is attached to the roof of the diencephalon remains thin, forming the future choroid plexus (protruding into the lateral ventricle, forming the choroidal fissure).

Above the fissure, the wall of the hemisphere is gradually thickened, forming the hippocampus (refer to chapter 7). With development and proliferation, the hemispheres bulge over the lateral diencephalon, mesencephalon and the cephalic metencephalon. Corpus striatum later expands and divides into the caudate nucleus located dorsomedially and the lentiform nucleus located ventrolaterally. This division is caused by nerve fibers passing down from the hemisphere cortex, breaking this nuclear mass (i.e., the internal capsule fibers). Refer to figure 5.1.

With further development, the medial aspect of the hemisphere wall and lateral wall of diencephalon fuse, bringing caudate nucleus and thalamus close to each other. Continuous growth results in formation of the frontal, temporal, parietal and occipital lobes. The area between the frontal and temporal lobes becomes depressed, known as insula (at birth almost completely covered by adjacent lobes).

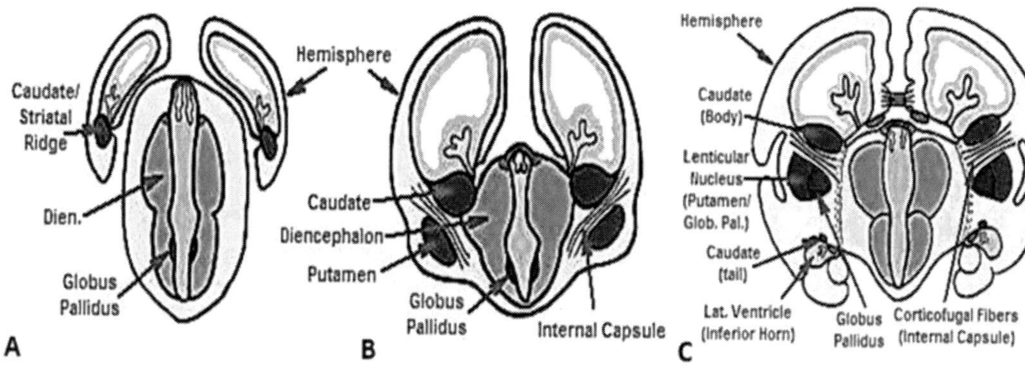

Figure 5.1. A-C, Stepwise Development of the basal ganglia.

5.3. Overview of the Basal Ganglia

The basal ganglia comprise a distributed set of brain structures in the telencephalon, diencephalon, and mesencephalon. The forebrain originated structures include the caudate nucleus, the putamen, the nucleus accumbens (or ventral striatum) and the globus pallidus. Together, these structures are named the corpus striatum. The basal ganglia definition focuses on the functional characteristics of these nuclei, and in this respect, they consist of the caudate and lenticular nuclei (together forming the dorsal basal ganglia), nucleus accumbens and parts of the adjacent olfactory tubercle (forming the ventral striatum), and substancia innominata (the ventral pallidum).

Substancia nigra and the subthalamic nucleus are not considered part of the basal ganglia, but have important structural and functional relationship with the caudate and lenticular nuclei. The basal ganglia function primarily in the motor sphere. Refer to figures 5.2-5.4.

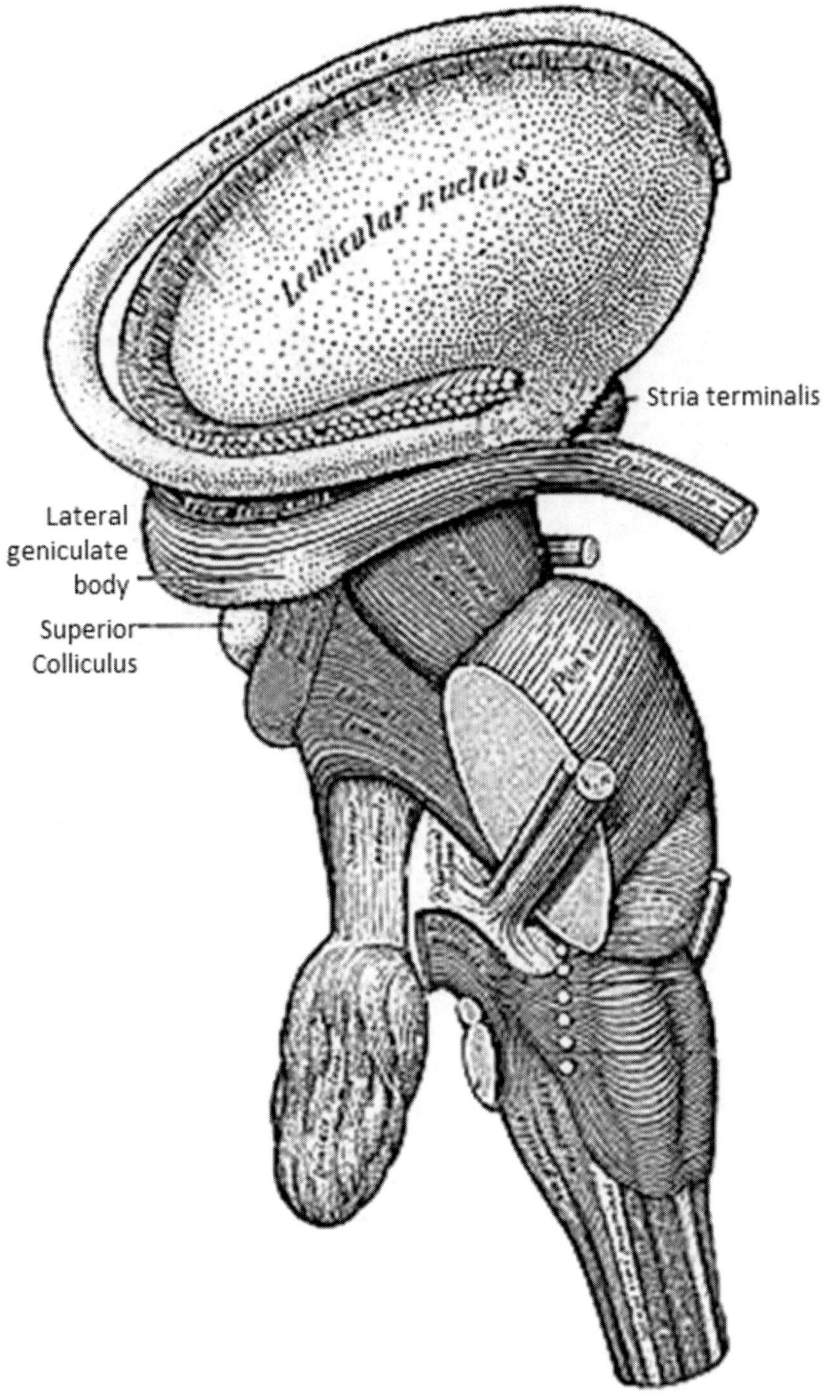

Figure 5.2. The basal ganglia and diencephalon showing the continuous and intimate connection. Taken from Gray's anatomy (out of copyright and in the public domain).

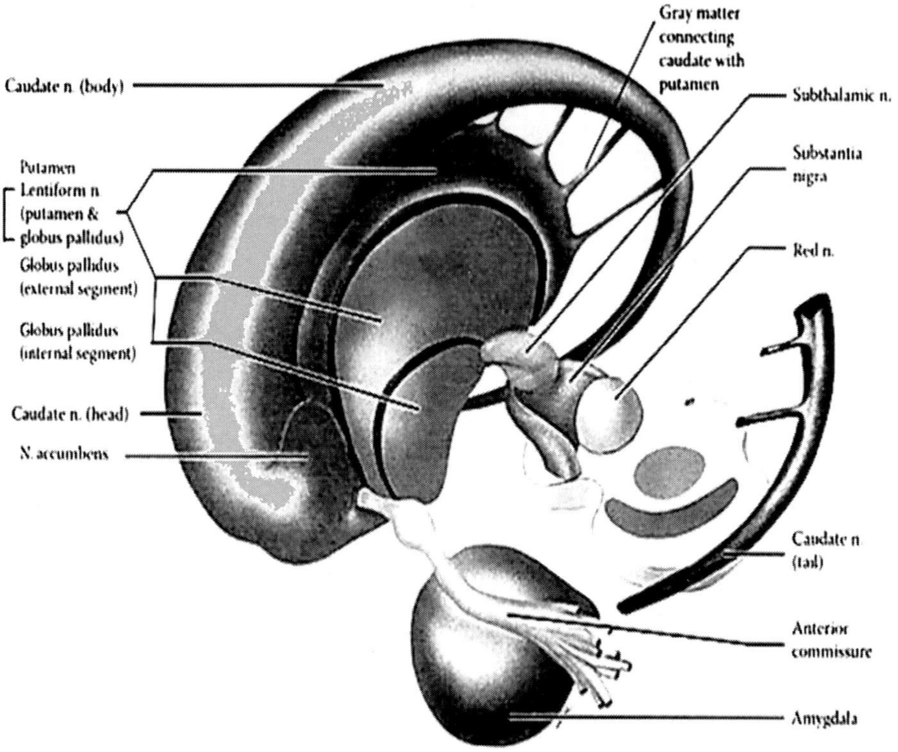

Figure 5.3 The basal ganglia complex in three dimensions. Note the continuous relationship between the caudate nucleus, nucleus accumbens and the putamen. Taken from Gray's anatomy (out of copyright and in the public domain).

5.3.1. The Caudate and Lenticular Nuclei

Together, these structures form the corpus striatum, which is segregated into the neostriatum (a term encompassing the caudate nucleus and putamen) and the paleostriatum (referring to the globus pallidum). The globus pallidum and putamen form the lenticular nucleus.

The caudate nucleus is a C-shaped structure that is closely associated with the lateral wall of the lateral ventricle. It is largest at its anterior pole (the head), and its size diminishes posteriorly as it follows the course of the lateral ventricle (the body) all the way to the temporal lobe (the tail), where it terminates at the amygdaloid nuclei. The head of the caudate nucleus forms a prominent bulge in the anterior horn of the lateral ventricle, and diminishes in size at about the level of the Monro foramina (but continues as the body). The body of the caudate nucleus is located in the lateral wall of the body of the lateral ventricle. At the lateral wall of the collateral trigon, it then turns ventrally and anteriorly to continue rostrally as the tail. The tail of the caudate nucleus is located in the dorsolateral wall of the temporal horn, forming part of the roof of the temporal horn of the lateral ventricles. Thus, the C-shaped form of the caudate nucleus follows the C-shape form of the lateral ventricle, begin "hugged" by the ventricles, with the head found "below" the ventricle and the tail found "above" it.

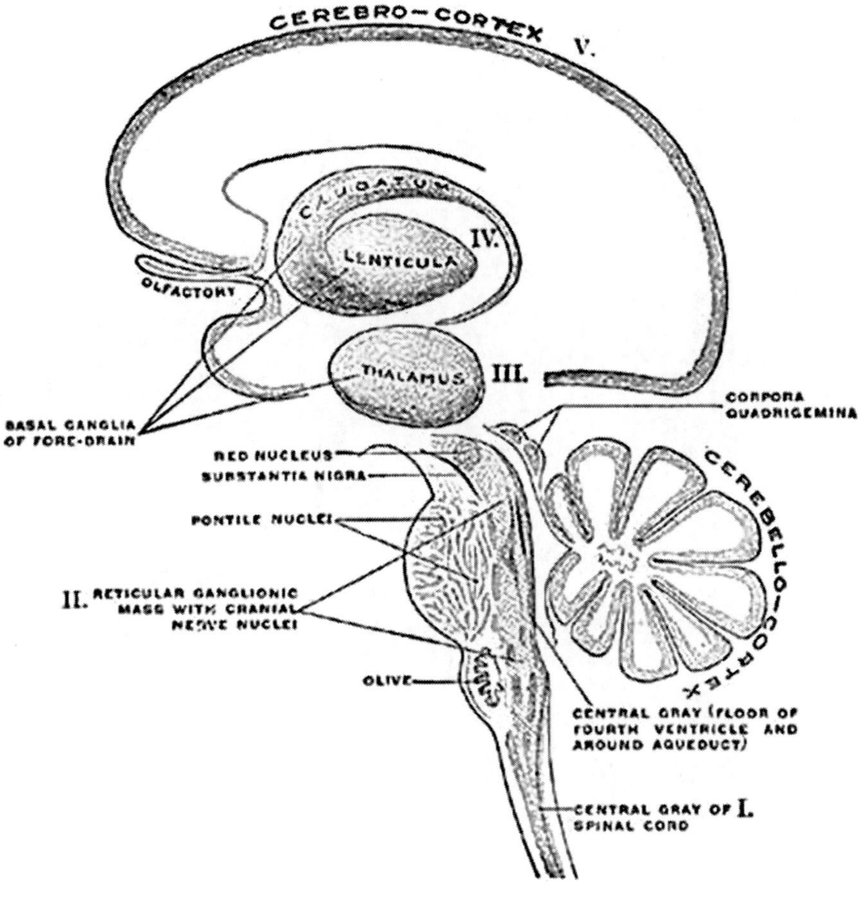

Figure 5.4. Basal ganglia, Brainstem nuclei and their connections. Taken from Gray's anatomy (out of copyright and in the public domain).

The lenticular nucleus is located within the base of the hemisphere, surrounded by white matter tracts. The internal capsule borders it medially whereas the external capsule separates it from the claustrum laterally. The putamen is a large structure that is separated from the caudate nucleus by the anterior limb of the internal capsule. The putamen is connected to the caudate head by bridges of cells that cut across the internal capsule. Because of the striated appearance of these cell bridges, the caudate and putamen are collectively referred to as the striatum or neostriatum, and the nucleus accumbens is often called the ventral striatum.

Functionally, the caudate nucleus and the putamen are considered equivalent to each other; indeed, most mammals have only a single nucleus called the striatum. It is unclear whether there is any functional significance of the separation of the striatum into the caudate and putamen in primates. The putamen and the globus pallidus are collectively called the lenticular nucleus, or lentiform nucleus. The globus pallidus (GP) is divided into two segments by sheets of dorsoventrally oriented white matter: the internal (or medial) segment and the external (or lateral) segment. The GP is also separated from the Putamen by a thin layer of white matter. Refer to figures 4.4-4.5, 4.14 and 5.5-5.7.

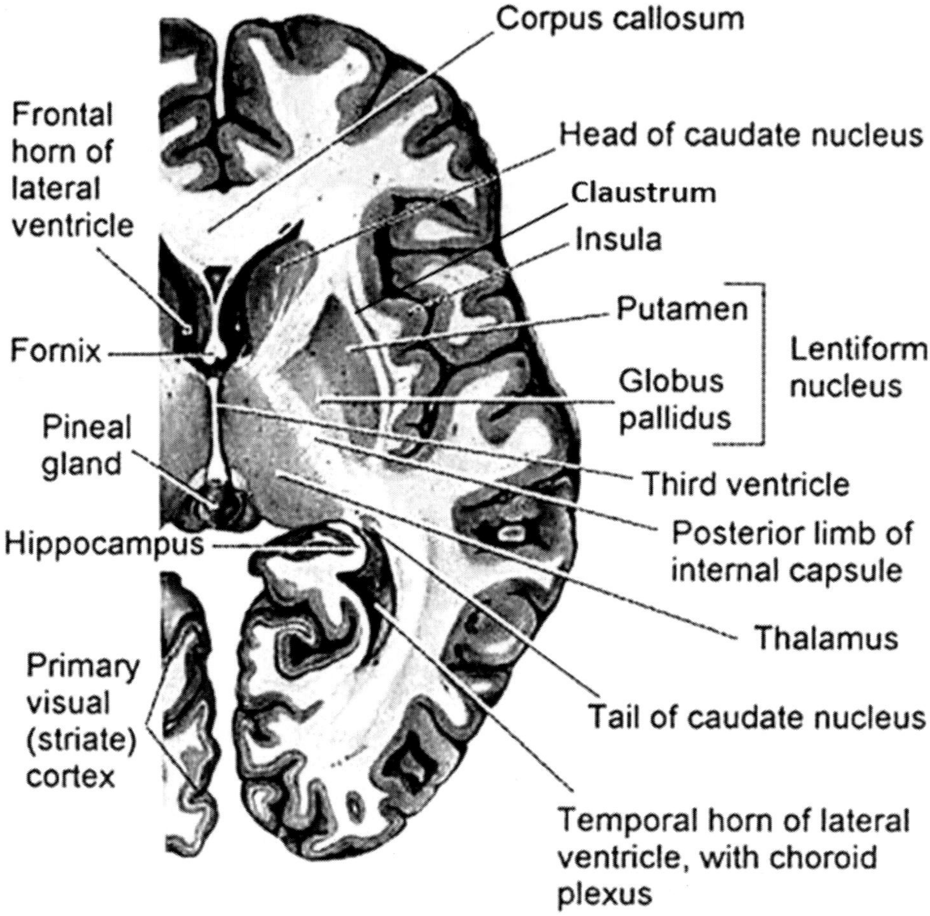

Figure 5.5. An axial section at the level of foramen of Monro and the third ventricle showing the different basal ganglia structures and spatial relations. Taken with permission from www.radiopaedia.org.

5.3.2. Nucleus Accumbens

The nucleus accumbens is found in an area of the brain called the basal forebrain. There is a nucleus accumbens in each hemisphere. It is situated rostrally-ventrally in the hemisphere, where the putamen is continuous with the head of the caudate nucleus. It is also closely opposed to the septal nuclei, and the nucleus of diagonal band. The nucleus accumbens and the olfactory tubercle collectively form the ventral striatum, which is part of the basal ganglia. The nucleus accumbens itself is separated into two anatomical components: the shell and the core. These two contiguous areas have overlapping connections, but may make different contributions to the functions of the nucleus accumbens.

The nucleus accumbens has a significant role in the cognitive processing of motivation, pleasure, and reward and reinforcement learning, and hence has significant role in addiction. When we do anything that is considered rewarding (e.g., eat food, have sex, take drugs), dopamine neurons (mainly) in the ventral tegmental area (VTA) of the midbrain are activated.

These neurons project to the nucleus accumbens, and when they are activated it results in an increase in dopamine levels in the nucleus accumbens. The nucleus accumbens is an important component of a major dopaminergic pathway in the brain called the mesolimbic pathway, which is stimulated during rewarding experiences. It plays a lesser role in fear, impulsivity, and the placebo effect. It is involved in the encoding of new motor programs as well.

Major inputs to the nucleus accumbens include prefrontal association cortices, basolateral amygdala, and dopaminergic neurons located in the midbrain ventral tegmental area (VTA), which connect via the mesolimbic pathway. Thus the nucleus accumbens is often described as one part of a cortico-striato-thalamo-cortical loop. Another major source of input comes from the CA1 and ventral subiculum of the hippocampus (refer to chapter 7) to the dorsomedial area of the nucleus accumbens. The sole source of histamine neurons in the brain, the tuberomammillary nucleus, projects to the nucleus accumbens as well.

The output neurons of the nucleus accumbens send axon projections to the basal ganglia and the ventral analog of the globus pallidus, known as the ventral pallidum (VP). The VP, in turn, projects to the medial dorsal nucleus of the dorsal thalamus, which projects to the prefrontal cortex as well as the striatum. Other efferents from the nucleus accumbens include connections with the tail of the ventral tegmental area, substantia nigra, and the reticular formation of the pons.

5.3.3. Substancia Innominata

The substantia innominata (literally "unnamed substance") also termed as the basal nucleus of Maynert, is a stratum in the human brain consisting partly of gray and partly of white substance. It is located at a slightly more caudal level, below the anterior part of the thalamus and lentiform nucleus, internal to anterior perforated substance and ventral to anterior commissure. In Alzheimer disease, a noticeable loss of larger neurons here is seen.

5.3.4. The Subthalamic Nucleus and Substancia Nigra

The subthalamic nucleus is a part of the diencephalon (refer to chapter 4), capped by a thin layer of fibers, the lenticular fasciculus. Substancia nigra is a part of the midbrain, located dorsomedially to crus cerebri, caudal to subthalamic nucleus, and is divided into a reticulated part (pars reticulate), and a compact part (pars compacta, having many melanin containing nerve cell bodies). In Parkinson's disease, a selective degeneration of this region triggers the extrapyramidal signs and is the etiology and the base for therapeutic intervention.

5.3.5. The Claustrum

The claustrum is a thin strip of gray matter between the lentiform nucleus and the insular cortex. It is separated from adjacent structures by the external capsule medially and the extreme capsule laterally. It receives projections from lateral hypothalamus, centromedian (CM) thalamic nucleus and the locus ceruleus of the brainstem. Refer to figures 5.5 - 5.7.

5.3.6. Stepwise Dissection

As shown in figure 5.6a, the anteroinferior part of the caudate and lentiform nuclei blends without clear demarcation into the large mass of gray matter above the anterior perforated substance and adjacent part of the orbital surface of the frontal lobe that also includes the nucleus basalis and accumbens. The extreme capsule separates the claustrum and insula, and the external capsule separates the claustrum and lentiform nucleus (figure 5.6b). The lateral medullary lamina separates the putamen from the outer segment of the globus pallidus and the medial medullary lamina separates the medial and lateral segments of the globus pallidus. At the level of the foramen of Monro, the caudate nucleus is considerably smaller than anteriorly. The globus pallidus has a clearly defined inner and outer segment. The anterior part of the roof of the temporal horn has been removed to expose the amygdala and anterior part of the hippocampus. The amygdala, at its upper margin, blends into the globus pallidus. The combination of the globus pallidus and amygdala seem to wrap around the lateral aspect of the optic tract. The claustrum is located between the insula and the lentiform nucleus (figure 5.6c).

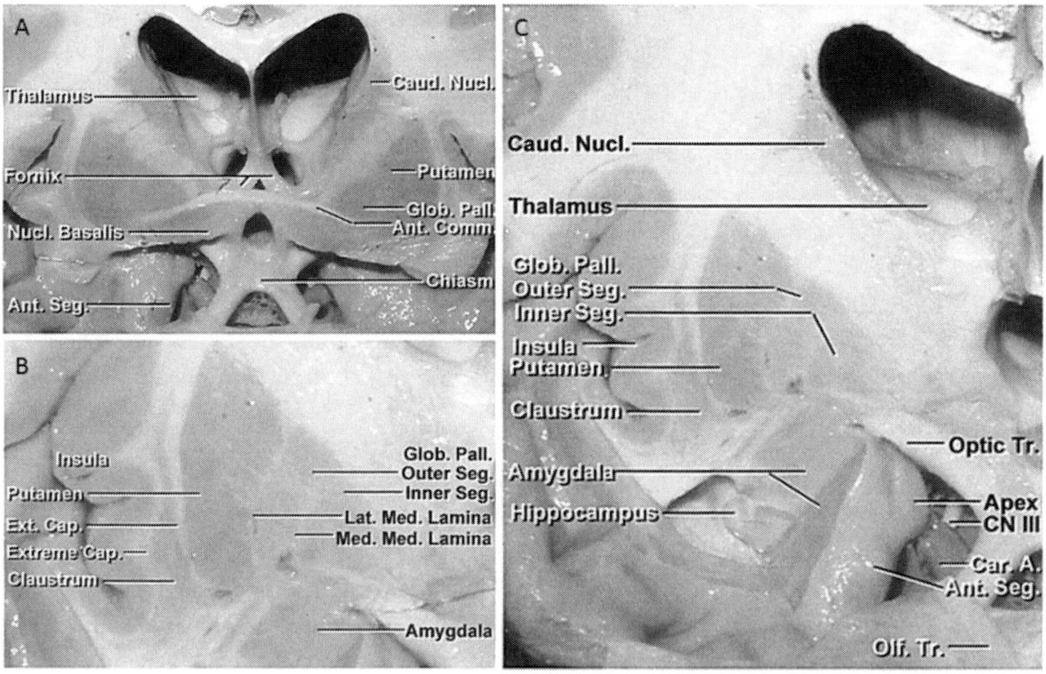

Figure 5.6. A Stepwise dissection of the cerebral hemispheres. A, The anterior limb of the internal capsule separates the caudate and lentiform nuclei. B, Enlarged view of the lentiform nucleus and amygdala. C, Coronal section at the level of the foramen of Monro. Ant., anterior; Cap., capsule; Car., carotid; Caud., caudate; CN, cranial nerve; Ext., external; Glob., globus; Inf., inferior; Int., internal; Lam., lamina; Lat., lateral; Lent., lentiform; Nucl., nucleus; Olf., olfactory; Pall., pallidus; Post., posterior; Seg., segment; Sup., superior; Tr., tract; Vent., ventricle. Taken with permission from the Rhoton Collection.

The external and extreme capsule and the claustrum fill the interval between the insula and the lentiform nucleus (figure 5.7a). The anterior limb of the internal capsule is separated from the frontal horn by the caudate nucleus and the posterior limb is separated from the body of the ventricle by the thalamus, but the genu reaches the ventricular surface lateral to the foramen of Monro. At higher levels, the lentiform and caudate nuclei are separated by the anterior limb of the internal capsule, but at the level below the anterior limb of the internal capsule (figure 5.7b), the two nuclei blend into a mass of gray matter located above the anterior perforated substance and adjacent part of the orbital surface of the frontal lobe. The caudate and lentiform nuclei blend into the nucleus basalis located below the anterior commissure and the nucleus accumbens situated anterior to the nucleus basalis to form a massive collection of gray matter in the basal part of the hemisphere.

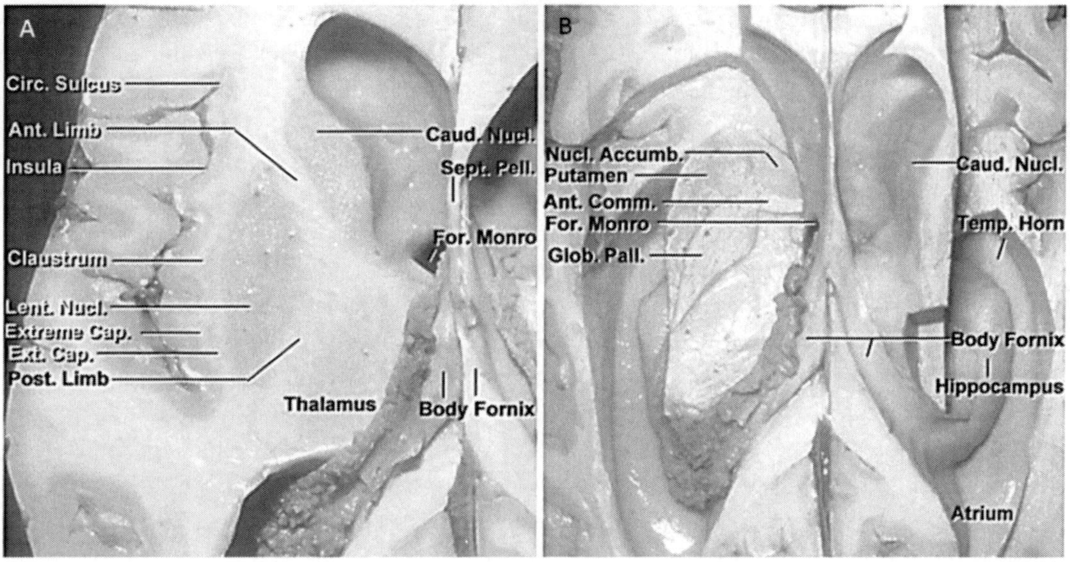

Figure 5.7. Axial cross sections of the cerebral hemisphere and central core. A, The axial section in the left hemisphere extends through the internal capsule just above and lateral to the foramen of Monro where the genu of the capsule reaches the ventricular surface. B, the section through the left hemisphere has been extended downward below the frontal horn to the level of the anterior commissure. The anterior part of the section extends through the deep gray matter below the frontal horn anterior limb of the internal capsule. Accumb., accumbens; Ant., anterior; Cap., capsule; Caud., caudate; Cent., central; Cer., cerebral; Circ., circular; CN, cranial nerve; Ext., external; For., foramen; Glob., globus; Hippo., hippocampal; Inf., inferior; Lent., lentiform; Nucl., nucleus; Post., posterior; Sept., septum; Temp., temporal; Vent., ventricle. Taken with permission from the Rhoton Collection.

5.4. Major Connections of the Basal Ganglia

All inputs to the basal ganglia arrive via the striatum and all (most) output leaves via the internal segment of the globus pallidus and substancia nigra pars reticulate. The basal ganglia function in general include motor control, eye movements control, cognitive functions, emotional functions etc. Inputs are received mainly from the cerebral cortex through putamen (mostly excitatory, glutamate mediated), from the substancia nigra pars compacta (dopamine mediated), from thalamic intralaminar nuclei (mainly glutamate mediated) and from the raphe nuclei of the brainstem (mainly serotonin mediated). The basal ganglia output is directed inly to the substancia nigra pars reticulate for head and neck and globus pallidus internal segment for the rest of the body. Generally speaking, the output is inhibitory mainly (GABA mediated). Output is also directed to thalamic nuclei (VL, VA, thalamic fasciculus), reticular formation, superior colliculus (substancia nigra projects to it) etc.

5.4.1. Basal Ganglia Afferents

The striatum is the main recipient of afferents to the basal ganglia. These excitatory afferents arise from the entire cerebral cortex and from the intralaminar nuclei of the thalamus (primarily the centromedian nucleus and parafascicularis nucleus). The projections from different cortical areas are segregated, such that the frontal lobe projects predominantly to the caudate head and the putamen; the parietal and occipital lobes project to the caudate body; and the temporal lobe projects to the caudate tail. The primary motor cortex and the primary somatosensory cortex project mainly to the putamen, whereas the premotor cortex and supplementary motor areas project to the caudate head. Other cortical areas project primarily to the caudate. Thus, generally speaking, along the C-shaped extent of the caudate nucleus, the caudate cells receive their input from the cortical regions that are close by. The enlarged head of the caudate reflects the large projection from the frontal cortex to the caudate. In addition, the nucleus accumbens (ventral striatum) receives a large input from limbic cortex.

In the motor regions of the basal ganglia, there is a motor homunculus similar to that seen in the primary motor cortex. Thus, the projections from the medial wall of the anterior paracentral lobule (the part of M1 that contains a representation of the legs and torso) innervate regions of the striatum that are next to the recipient zones from the dorsal surface of the precentral gyrus (the part of M1 that contains a representation of the arms and hands, refer to chapter 7). Similarly, the projections from the lateral surface of the precentral gyrus (the part of M1 that contains a representation of the face) innervate regions that are next to the arm and hand representation. This topography of projections is maintained in the intrinsic circuitry of the basal ganglia.

5.4.1.1. Pathways for Movement, Eye Movement, Cognition and Emotions

Four parallel pathways are described, each passing through different pathway projecting to different regions of the frontal lobes (refer to figure 5.8). Three of these circuits (all except the limbic one) are termed dorsal striatal pathways. The limbic circuit is termed as the ventral striatal pathway. Briefly speaking, with this topic being quite diverse and not in the scope if this book, refer to figure 5.8 for the scheme. The motor pathway channel encompasses the cortical input, putamen, globus pallidus internal segment, and substancia nigra pars reticulate, as well as the thalamic VL and VA nuclei, supplementary motor cortex, premotor cortex, and the primary motor cortex. The oculomotor pathway channel encompasses input from the body of the caudate nucleus, frontal and supplementary eye field (frontal lobe). The prefrontal pathway channel encompasses input from the head of the caudate nucleus and output to prefrontal cortex. The limbic pathway channel refers to input from different limbic regions (e.g., the limbic cortex, hippocampus, and amygdala), nucleus accumbens, and the ventral striatum regions. Output emerges from the ventral pallidum, the mediodorsal nucleus of thalamus, anterior cingulated gyrus and medial orbital frontal gyrus.

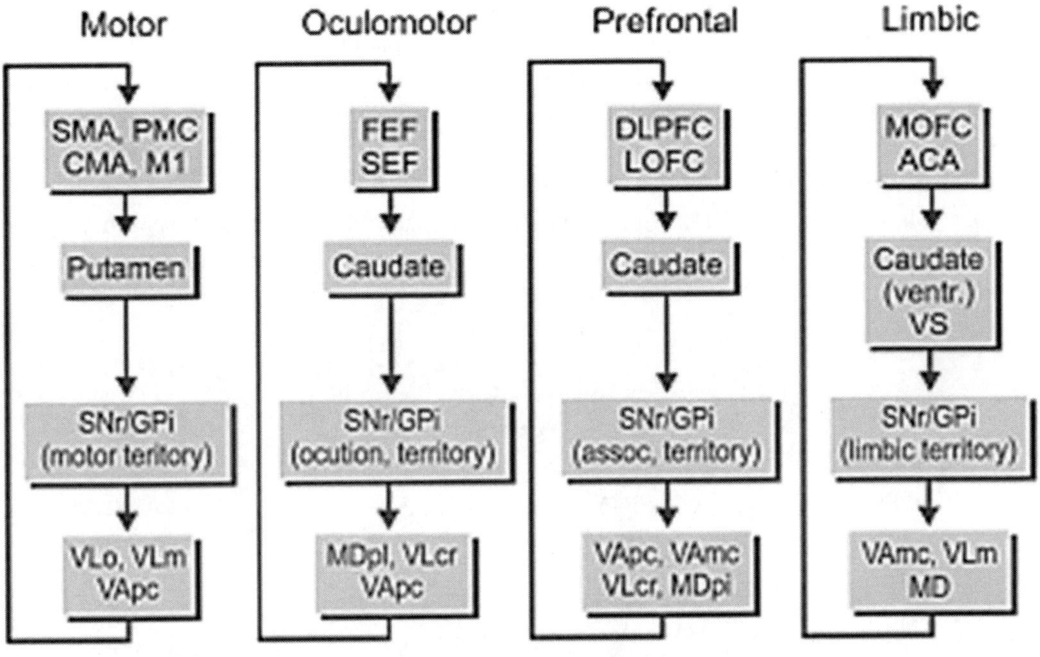

Figure 5.8. Anatomy of the Cortex–Basal ganglia–Thalamocortical circuits. Refer to text. ACA, anterior cingulate area; CMA, cingulate motor area; DLPFC, dorsolateral prefrontal cortex; FEF, frontal eye fields; GPi, globus pallidus interna; HD, Huntington's disease; LOFC, lateral orbitofrontal cortex; M1, primary motor cortex; MDpl, mediodorsal nucleus of the thalamus, pars lateralis; MOFC, medial orbitofrontal cortex; OCD, obsessive-compulsive disorder; PD, Parkinson's disease; PMC, premotor cortex; SMA, supplementary motor area; SEF, supplementary eye field; SNr, substantia nigra pars reticulata; TS, Tourette's syndrome; VApc, ventral anterior nucleus of the thalamus, pars parvocellularis; VAmc, ventral anterior nucleus of the thalamus, pars magnocellularis; VLm, ventrolateral nucleus of the thalamus, pars medialis; VLo, ventrolateral nucleus of the thalamus, pars oralis; VLcr, ventrolateral nucleus of the thalamus, pars caudalis, rostral division; VS, ventral striatum. Modified with permission from Focused Neurosurgery textbook.

5.4.2. Basal Ganglia Efferents

The major output structures of the basal ganglia are the globus pallidus internal segment (GPint) and the substantia nigra pars reticulata (SNr). Both of these structures make GABA as a neurotransmitter and thus have inhibitory effect on their targets. The GPint projects to a number of thalamic structures by way of two fiber tracts; the ansa lenticularis and the lenticular fasciculus. The loop that processes sensorimotor information from the motor cortex and the somatosensory cortex projects to the ventral anterior (VA) and ventral lateral (VL) nuclei of thalamus. The loop that processes other neocortical information projects to the dorsomedial nucleus (DM), intralaminar nuclei, and parts of the VA nucleus of thalamus. The SNr projects to the superior colliculus, which is involved in eye movements, as well as to the VA/VL thalamic nuclei. Refer to figure 4.7, 5.9.

The lenticular fasciculus leaves the globus pallidus, traverses the posterior limb of internal capsule and forms a sheet between the subthalamic nucleus and the zona incerta. These fibers loop around the medial aspect of the zona incerta, and pass laterally as the thalamic fasciculus. The ansa lenticularis fibers originate at more rostral levels. These fibers arch around the anterior-ventral aspect of the internal capsule, and pass caudally to join the fibers of the lenticular fasciculus, as they enter the thalamic fasciculus. Refer to figure 5.9.

Two smaller bundles, also termed as the subthalamic fasciculi are bidirectional connections between globus pallidus and the subthalamic nucleus. The subthalamic fasciculi are also termed as the fields of Forel (Haubenfelder (H) of Forel). H1 (field number one) marks the thalamic fasciculus, H2 (field number two) marks the lenticular fasciculus, and the H field of Forel marks the location where ansa lenticularis and the lenticular fasciculus join (i.e., the thalamic fasciculus). Refer to figure 5.9.

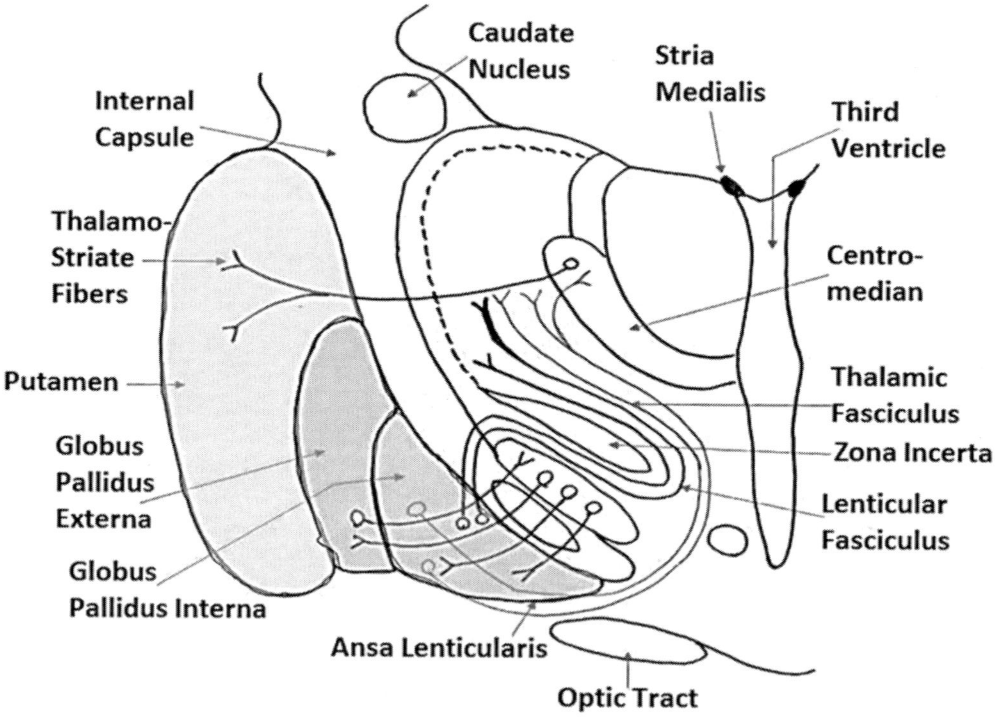

Figure 5.9. A scheme showing the basal ganglia afferent and efferent pathways. Refer to text.

5.4.3. Basal Ganglia Intrinsic Connections

A number of intrinsic pathways interconnect various basal ganglia structures:

1) The striatopallidal pathway is a GABAergic, inhibitory connection between the striatum and both segments of the globus pallidus.
2) The striatonigral pathway is a GABAergic, inhibitory connection between the striatum and the SNr.
3) The globus pallidus external segment makes a GABAergic, inhibitory connection to the subthalamic nucleus.

4) The subthalamic nucleus makes glutamatergic, excitatory connections onto both segments of the globus pallidus and the SNr. This pathway is the only purely excitatory pathway among the intrinsic pathways of the basal ganglia.
5) The nigrostriatal pathway makes a dopaminergic synapse onto striatal neurons. This is a mixed pathway, with excitatory effects on some striatal neurons and inhibitory effects on others.

5.4.4. The Direct and Indirect Pathways

There are two distinct pathways that process signals through the basal ganglia: the direct pathway and the indirect pathway. These two pathways have opposite net effects on thalamic target structures. Excitation of the direct pathway has the net effect of exciting thalamic neurons (which in turn make excitatory connections onto cortical neurons). Excitation of the indirect pathway has the net effect of inhibiting thalamic neurons (rendering them unable to excite motor cortex neurons). The normal functioning of the basal ganglia apparently involves a proper balance between the activities of these two pathways. One hypothesis is that the direct pathway selectively facilitates certain motor (or cognitive) programs in the cerebral cortex that are adaptive for the present task, whereas the indirect pathway simultaneously inhibits the execution of competing motor programs. An upset of the balance between the direct and indirect pathways results in the motor dysfunctions that characterize the extrapyramidal syndrome (Parkinsonism).

5.5. Vasculature of the Basal Ganglia and Related Structures

The caudate nucleus and the putamen are supplied by branches of the anterior and medial lenticulostriate arteries. The anterior lenticulostriate arteries, coming off the anterior cerebral artery first segment (A1) supply in most the head of the caudate nucleus. A large notable such branch is the recurrent artery of Heubner, termed for its course, going "back" laterally along the A1 segment towards the terminal internal carotid artery (ICA), so it often looks like a small artery running alongside and above the much bigger A1. It is simply one of the larger medial perforator arteries arising from A1 segment to head towards the basal ganglia. The lateral lenticulostriate branches coming off the middle cerebral artery first segment (M1) supply the lenticular nucleus and surrounding capsule. The anterior choroidal artery contributes branches as well. Refer to figure 5.10. The lenticulostriate branches are most commonly involved in the very common hypertension Induced hemorrhagic stroke. Refer to figure 5.11.

The subthalamic nucleus and substancia nigra are supplied via posteromedial striate branches of the posterior cerebral artery first segment (P_1) and lenticulostriate branches of the posterior communicating artery, penetrating the brain at the midbrain-diencephalon junction. For a detailed discussion in the arterial blood supply to cerebral and basal ganglia structures refer to chapter 9.

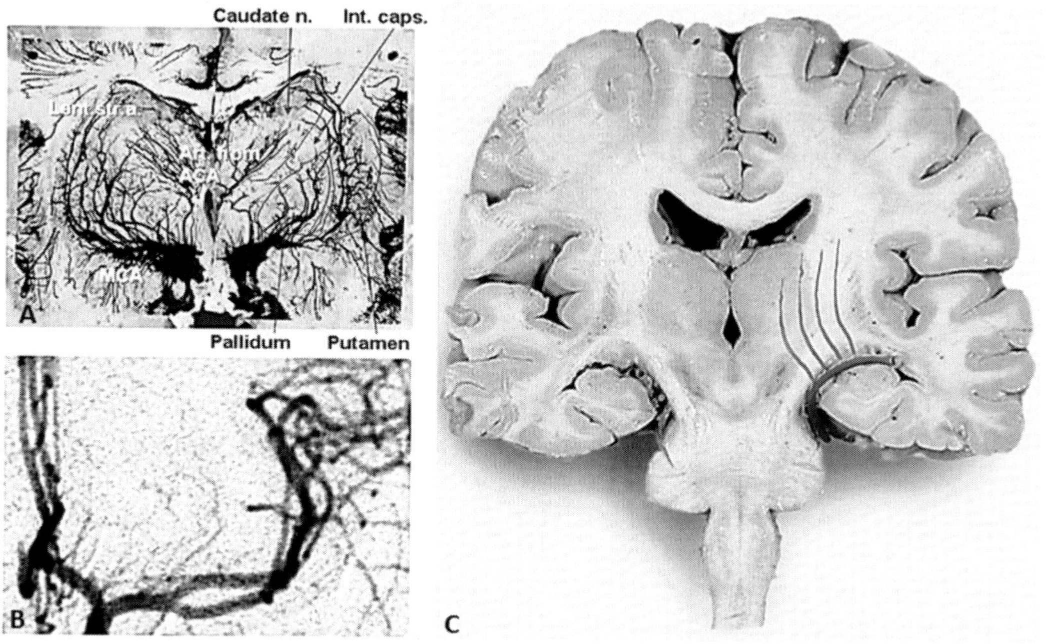

Figure 5.10. The lenticulostriate arteries. A+B Angiographic presentation of the lenticulostriate arterial system. These are straight end arteries (vasa rectae). Taken with permission from www.neuroangio.org. C, coronal section presenting the lenticulostriate arterial path. Taken with permission from www.radiopaedia.org.

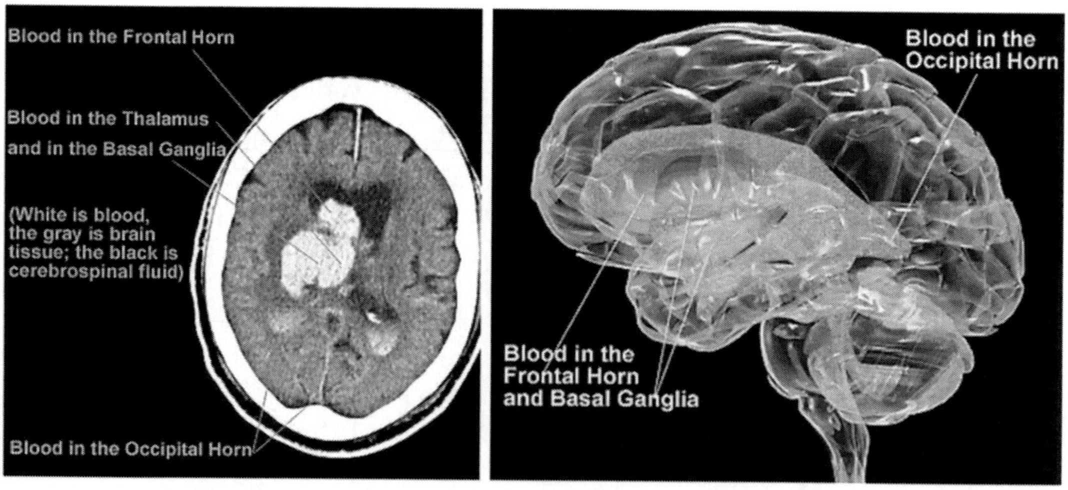

Figure 5.11. Hemorrhagic stroke, most commonly caused by hypertension induced rupture of a lenticulostriate artery. A, axial non-contrast enhanced CT showing the parenchymal hemorrhage with a ventricular breakthrough component. B, 3-dimensional reconstruction of the CT. Taken with permission from www.radiopaedia,org.

Chapter 6

The Cerebellum

6.1. Abstract

The cerebellum is a unique part of the CNS, connected directly to the brainstem at the level of the pons, but not considered a part of the brainstem. It is an important component of the motor circuit but has no direct connections to lower motor neurons. This chapter begins with a short embryological description of cerebellar development, followed by an overview of the gross anatomical features important for the clinician and for the medical student. The cerebellum is commonly described grossly as composed of three surfaces, each is described separately. Next, the taxonomy around cerebellar sections, lobes, lobules and zones is presented and integrated for the ease of understanding. The cerebellar nuclei, histological highlights and cellular components are discussed next. Afferent and efferent systems are presented along with the different modules, i.e., the spinocerebellar and the pontocerebellar modules. The topographic representation and concept is presented as well. The chapter ends with a short concise overview of the vascular territories and supply to the cerebellum.

6.2. Neuro-Embryology

6.2.1. Neuro-Embryology of the Rhombencephalon

The myelencephalon is the most caudal part of the central nervous system. It gives rise to the medulla oblongata, and differs from the spinal cord in that its lateral walls are everted. Alar and basal plates (separated by the sulcus limitans) are clearly seen. The basal plate, like the spinal cord, contains motor nuclei. The alar plate contains 3 groups of sensory relay nuclei. The roof plate is a single layer of ependymal cells, covered by the pia (together called in the developed brain the tela choroidea. The metencephalon has also both basal and alar plates, but two other new components are formed from these. These are the cerebellum (the coordination center for posture and movement) and the pons. Refer to chapter 3 and to the development of the brainstem.

6.2.2. Neuro-Embryology of the Cerebellum

The dorsolateral parts of the alar plate form the rhombic lips that in its caudal portion of the metencephalon are widely separated, but approach each other in the midline below the mesencephalon. With further deepening of the pontine flexure, the lips become compressed, forming the cerebellar plate. This plate has a vermis process (midline), hemispheres (two lateral masses).

A transverse fissure separates the nodule from the vermis, and the lateral flocculus from hemispheres, forming a flocculonodular lobe, which is (phylogenetically) the most primitive part of the cerebellum. Initially the plate consists of neuroepithelial, mantle and marginal layers, but cells from the neuroepithelial layer migrate to the surface of the cerebellum, to form the external granular layer.

This layer forms the proliferative zone on the surface of the cerebellum, retaining dividing ability. The granular layer will give rise to granule cells, basket cells and stellate cells. Deep cerebellar nuclei (Dentate nucleus) reach their final position before birth. Refer to figure 6.1. The Madrid collection studied 20 human embryos and fetuses between 6 weeks to 16 weeks. Refer to table 6.1 and to figure 6.2 for a short description of developmental time points.

Table 6.1. Developmental landmarks in Cerebellum Neuro-Embryology

6 weeks (CRL 14mm)	The cerebellum can first be identified as a pair of thickenings on the lateral site of the alar plate that faced the fourth ventricle.
7-9 weeks (CRL 28mm)	The rhombic lip (a pair of thickenings of the alar plate) protrudes dorsally, bent laterally, extends ventrolaterally and fuses with the medially located midbrain. During that process, the primitive choroid plexus appear to become involved in the cerebellar hemisphere to form a centrally located eosinophilic matrix. At that stage, the inferior olive had already developed in the thick medulla. Thus, the term 'bulbo-pontine extension' may represent an erroneous labeling of a caudal part of the rhombic lip. The cerebellar vermis develop much later than the hemisphere possibly from a midline dark cell cluster near the aqueduct.
11–12 weeks (CRL 80mm)	The cerebellar hemispheres become as thick as the midbrain. In the hemisphere, a laminar configuration becomes evident but the central eosinophilic matrix remained present. Fissures of the future vermis appear in the midline area. The developing fissures provide island-like structures in horizontal sections. The hemisphere and vermis, including the surfaces of the fissures, are covered by the external germinal cell layer.
15–16 weeks (CRL 120mm)	The cerebellar hemispheres contain the primitive dentate nucleus. The nodule and flocculus are identified, and the vermis becomes as thick as the hemisphere and it accompanied several deep fissures.

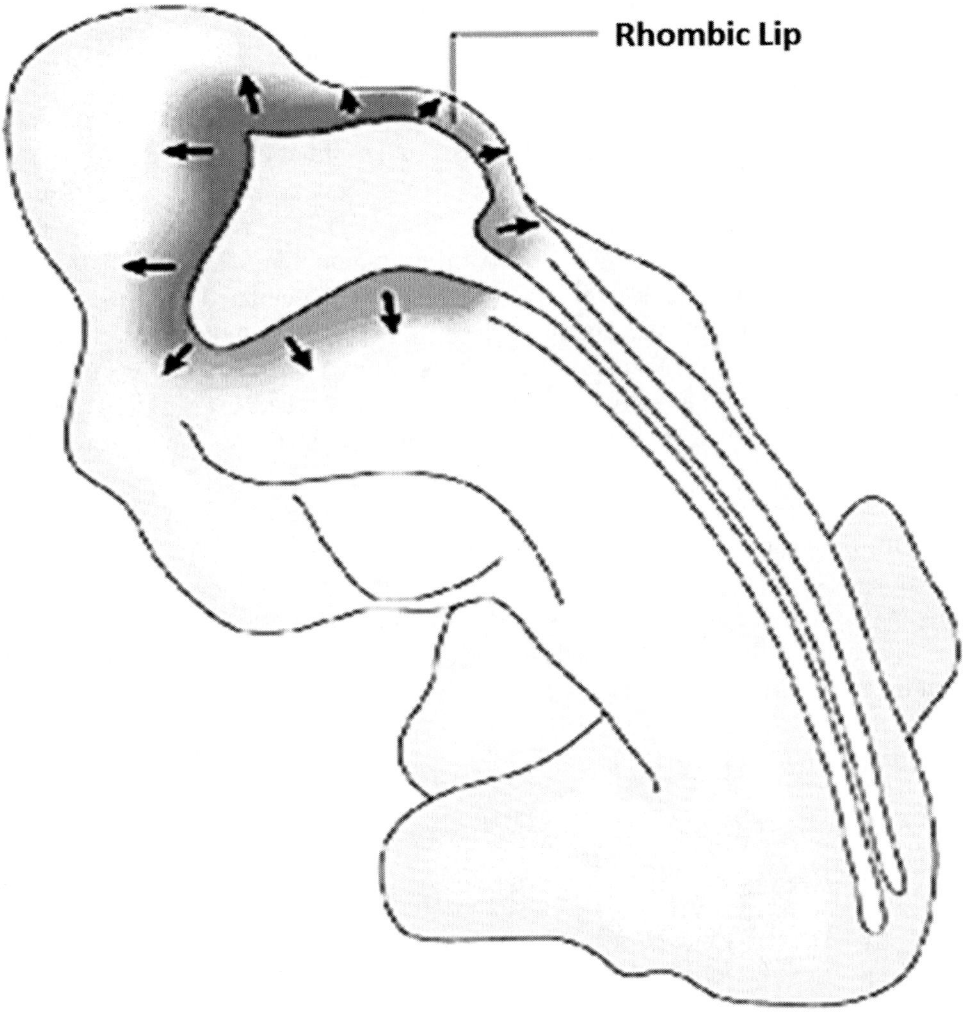

Figure 6.1. Cerebellar development, early stages (week 7-8). Refer to text.

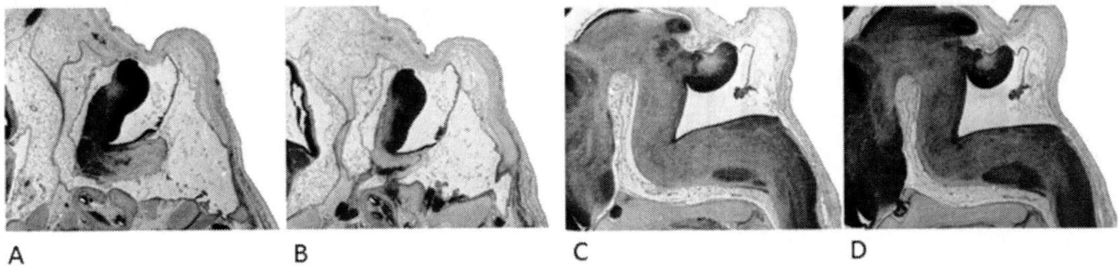

Figure 6.2. Sagittal images of a 10week human embryo. A, median. B, medial. C, Lateral. D, most Lateral. Modified from the Madrid collection. Taken with permission from www.radiopaedia.org.

6.3. Overview of Cerebellar Anatomy

6.3.1. Introduction

The internal organization of the cerebellum is similar to that of the cerebral hemispheres, namely the cerebellar cortex has surface gray matter, sulci & folia and a white matter core, containing internal cerebellar Nuclei (four, discussed later). The cerebellum, like the basal ganglia, has no direct connections to LMN (lower motor neurons). Several regions are defined within the cerebellum. The inferior vermis and flocculonodular lobes coordinate balance and eye movements. The lateral regions control lateral motor systems and distal appendicular muscles. The cerebellar hemispheres are involved in motor planning. A few major fissures are present. The tentorial (primary) fissure is the deepest of fissures, separating the anterior and posterior cerebellar lobes. The posterolateral fissure, found in the ventral surface, separates the posterior lobe from the flocculonodular lobe.

Before diving into the gross anatomical details of the cerebellum, a short clinical correlation to the anatomy is due. Ataxia (defined previously as cerebellar dysfunction by definition manifesting by either abnormal gait, posture or walking and movement) is ipsilateral to the side of lesion (because of a double decussation, not the lack thereof, discussed in chapter 3 and mentioned later). Midline lesions cause unsteady gait (i.e., truncal ataxia) and eye movement abnormalities, accompanied with vertigo and vomiting. Lesions lateral to vermis manifest with appendicular ataxia (lack of coordination and reduced ability to perform repetitive proprioceptive actions).

6.3.2. Gross Anatomical Organization of the Cerebellum

The cerebellar cortical surfaces are divided on the basis of the structures they face, or along which they may be exposed, to make this description more readily applicable to the operative setting (refer to figure 6.3). The first surface, the tentorial surface, faces the tentorium; the second surface, the suboccipital surface, is located below and between the lateral and sigmoid sinuses; and the third surface, the petrosal surface, faces forward toward the posterior surface of the petrous bone. Each of the surfaces has the vermis in the midline and the hemispheres laterally and is divided by a major fissure named on the basis of the surface that it divides. The hemispheric lobules forming each of the three surfaces commonly overlap onto and form a part of the adjacent surfaces. The fissures dividing the three cortical surfaces are to be distinguished from the fissures between the cerebellum and the brainstem.

6.3.2.1. The Tentorial Cerebellar Surface

As shown in figure 6.3a, in the tentorial surface, facing the lower surface of the tentorium, the anterior vermis is the most superior part. This surface slopes downward to its posterior and lateral margins. The vermian subdivisions of this surface are superior to their corresponding hemispheric parts. The culmen and quadrangular lobules correspond to the anterior part of the tentorial surface, and the declive, simple lobules, and part of the superior semilunar lobules correspond to the posterior part of the tentorial surface. The fissure separating the tentorial surface into anterior and posterior parts is referred to as the tentorial fissure (or primary fissure in older nomenclature). This fissure separates the hemispheric surface between the quadrangular and simple lobules and the vermis between the declive and culmen. The anterior part of the superior surface of the cerebellum surrounds the posterior half of the midbrain to form the cerebellomesencephalic fissure.

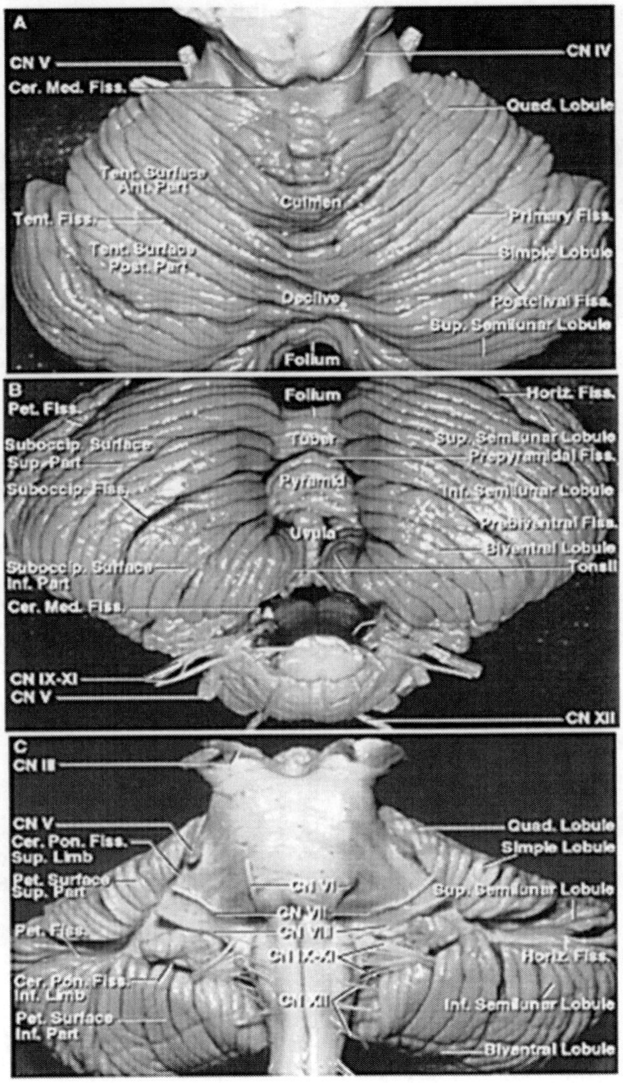

Figure 6.3. Tentorial, suboccipital, and petrosal cerebellar surfaces. A, The tentorial surface. The classical nomenclature applied to the vermian and hemispheric subdivisions of the tentorial surface is listed on the right, and a simplified nomenclature is listed on the left. B, The suboccipital surface. The classical nomenclature applied to this surface is shown on the right, and a simplified nomenclature is on the left. C, The petrosal surface. The classical nomenclature applied to this surface is shown on the right, and a simplified nomenclature is on the Left. Ant., anterior; Cer.Med., cerebellomedullary; Cer.Pon., cerebellopontine; CN, cranial nerve; Fiss., fissure; Horiz., horizontal; Inf., inferior; Pet., petrosal; Post., posterior; Quad., quadrangular; Suboccip., suboccipital; Sup., superior; Tent., tentorial. Taken with permission from the Rhoton Collection.

The cerebellomesencephalic fissure, which extends downward between the midbrain and the cerebellum, is shown in figure 6.4. The superficial part of the posterior lip is formed by the culmen in the midline and the quadrangular lobule laterally. The quadrigeminal cistern extends caudally from the pineal into the cerebellomesencephalic fissure. The central lobule and its wings form part of the posterior lip of the cerebellomesencephalic fissure. The lower half of the roof is formed in the midline by the nodule and laterally by the inferior medullary velum, which passes laterally above, but is separated from the rostral pole of the tonsils by the cerebellomedullary fissure.

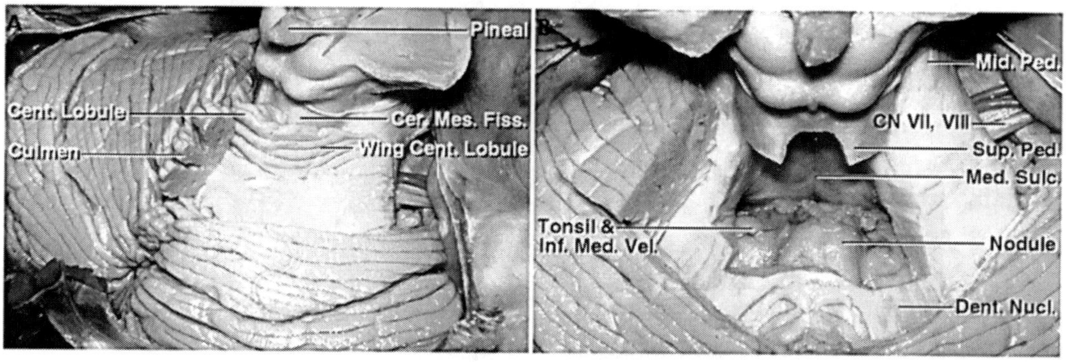

Figure 6.4. The Tentorial surface and cerebellomesencephalic fissure. A, The culmen has been removed, exposing the central lobule and its wings, which form part of the posterior lip of the cerebellomesencephalic fissure. B, The central lobule and its wings, the lingula, the superior medullary velum, and medial part of the superior cerebellar peduncles have been removed to expose the fourth ventricle. Cent., central; Cer., cerebellar; Cer.Mes., cerebellomesencephalic; CN, cranial nerve; Dent., dentate; Fiss., fissure; Inf., inferior; Mid., middle; Med., median, medullary; Nucl., nucleus; Ped., peduncle; Sulc., sulcus; Sup., superior. Taken with permission from the Rhoton Collection.

6.3.2.2. The Suboccipital Cerebellar Surface

The suboccipital surface located below and between the lateral and sigmoid sinuses, is the most complex of the three surfaces. The suboccipital surface, as shown in figure 6.3b, is located below and between the sigmoid and lateral sinuses. The vermis sits in a large median depression, the posterior cerebellar incisura, between the cerebellar hemispheres. According to classical nomenclature, the portions of the vermis within the incisura from above to below are the folium, tuber, pyramid, and uvula. The parts of the hemispheric surface from above to below are the superior and inferior semilunar and biventral lobules and the tonsils. These lobules extend beyond the suboccipital surface to the other surfaces of the cerebellum. The prebiventral fissures between the inferior semilunar and the biventral lobules separate the hemispheres into superior and inferior parts, and the prepyramidal fissure between the pyramid and tuber separates the vermis into superior and inferior parts.

A simplified terminology in referring to the union of the prebiventral and the prepyramidal fissures (dividing the suboccipital surface into superior and inferior parts) is as the suboccipital fissure. From below to above the corresponding vermian and hemispheric parts are the uvula and the tonsils, the pyramid and the biventral lobules, the tuber and inferior semilunar lobules, and the folium and the superior semilunar lobules. The petrosal (horizontal) fissure, the most prominent fissure on the petrosal surface, extends onto the suboccipital surface and divides the superior half of the suboccipital surface between the superior and inferior semilunar lobules. The cerebellomedullary fissure extends superiorly between the cerebellum and medulla.

The anterior surface of each tonsil faces and is separated from the posterior surface of the medulla by the cerebellomedullary fissure (refer to figure 6.5). The medial surfaces of the tonsils face each other across a narrow cleft, the vallecula, which leads into the fourth ventricle. The ventral aspect of the superior pole of each tonsil faces the three structures (tela choroidea, inferior medullary velum, and nodule) forming the lower half of the roof of the fourth ventricle. The superior pole is separated from the surrounding structures by a posterior extension of the cerebellomedullary fissure, called either the telovelotonsillar or the supratonsillar cleft. The nodule on which the velum arises is hidden in front of the uvula. The uvula hangs downward between the tonsils, thus mimicking the situation in the oropharynx. The choroid plexus arises on the inner surface of the tela and extends through the foramen of Luschka behind the glossopharyngeal and vagus nerve. The inferior medullary velum arises on the surface of the nodule, drapes across the superior pole of the tonsil, and blends into the flocculus laterally.

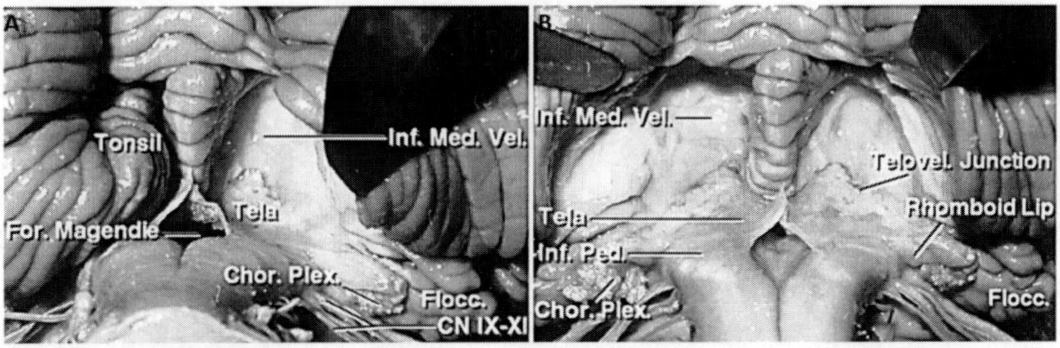

Figure 6.5. The Suboccipital surface of the cerebellum and the cerebellomedullary fissure. A, the right tonsil has been removed to expose the lower part of the roof formed by the inferior medullary velum and tela choroidea. B, both tonsils have been removed to expose the inferior medullary velum and tela choroidea bilaterally. Chor., choroid; CN, cranial nerve; Fiss., fissure; Flocc., flocculus; For., foramen; Inf., inferior; Med., medullary; Ped., peduncle; Plex., plexus; Sup., superior; Telovel., telovelar; Vel., velum. Taken with permission from the Rhoton Collection.

6.3.2.3. The Petrosal Cerebellar Surface

The petrosal surface, as shown in figure 6.3c, faces forward toward the petrous temporal bone. The petrosal fissure divides the petrosal surface into superior and inferior parts. The superior part is formed by the quadrangular, simple, and a small part of the superior semilunar lobules. The inferior part is formed by the inferior semilunar and biventral lobules and the tonsil. The cerebellopontine fissures are V-shaped fissures formed where the cerebellum wraps around the pons and the middle cerebellar peduncles. These fissures have a superior and an inferior limb, which meet at a lateral apex. The petrosal fissure extends laterally from the apex of the cerebellopontine fissures.

6.3.2.4. Cerebellar Cisterns

Several subarachnoid space enlargements, i.e., cisterns, surround the cerebellum. These are discussed in depth in chapter 8. A brief overview of clinically important cisterns include the cisterna magna located between the cerebellar hemispheres on the suboccipital surface, the cerebello-pontine cistern, located on the petrosal surface and the quadrigeminal plate cistern and superior cerebellar cisterns, located on the tentorial surface of the cerebellum.

6.3.3. The Cerebellar Peduncles

The cerebellar peduncles are white matter bundles, connecting both functionally and physically the cerebellum to the brainstem at the level of the pons, forming the lateral walls of the fourth ventricle. As shown in figure 6.6, the inferior Cerebellar peduncle is composed of the Restiform body and the juxtaRestiform body. The restiform body contains fibers arising from the spinal cord and medulla oblongata. Proprioceptive information arriving via the spinocerebellar tracts is one such tract entering the spinal cord through it. The juxta-restiform body (the name meaning the body near to the restiform body) is located in the wall of the fourth ventricle. Its fibers form reciprocal connections between the cerebellum and vestibular structures. Exiting fibers of the trigeminal nerve, at lateral mid-pons, represent the gross anatomical border between the basilar pons and the middle cerebellar peduncle.

The middle cerebellar peduncle is the largest of the cerebellar pedunculi, conveying fibers from the basilar pons into the cerebellum. These are mainly cerebellar afferents. The superior cerebellar peduncle, also termed brachium conjunctivum, courses into the midbrain, just caudally to the exit point of the trochlear nerve (CN-IV). This superior bundle contains efferent fibers that originate from neurons of cerebellar nuclei, destined to the diencephalon and brainstem. The white matter tracts and connections of the cerebellum can be beautifully demonstrated in the timeless Gray's Anatomy illustration shown in figure 6.7.

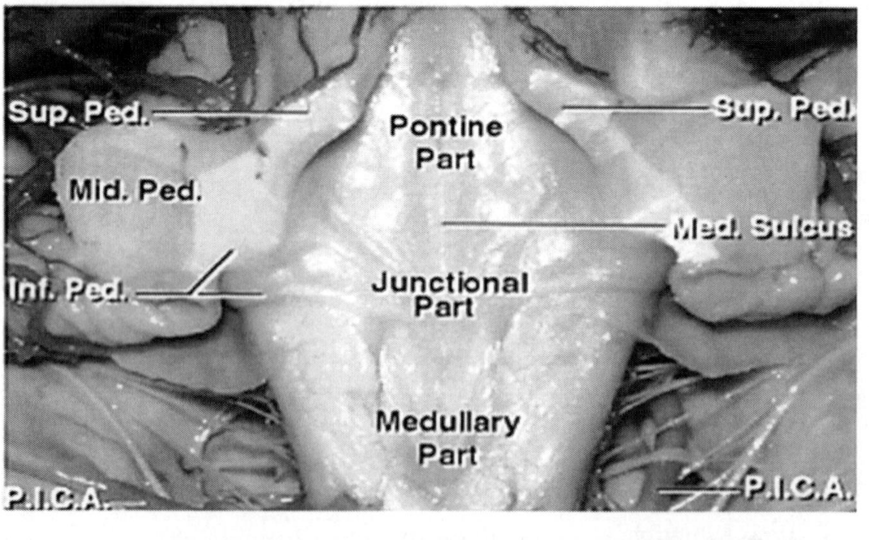

Figure 6.6. Posterior view of the brainstem with the cerebellum removed. The nodule and the inferior medullary velum have been removed to expose the full length of the floor of the fourth ventricle, which is divided in the midline by the median sulcus and craniocaudally into pontine, junctional, and medullary parts. The superior and inferior peduncles face the ventricular surface. The middle cerebellar peduncle is separated from the ventricular surface by the superior and inferior peduncles. Dent., dentate; Inf., inferior; Med., median, medullary; Mid., middle; P.I.C.A., posteroinferior cerebellar artery; Ped., peduncle; Sup., superior. Taken with permission from the Rhoton Collection.

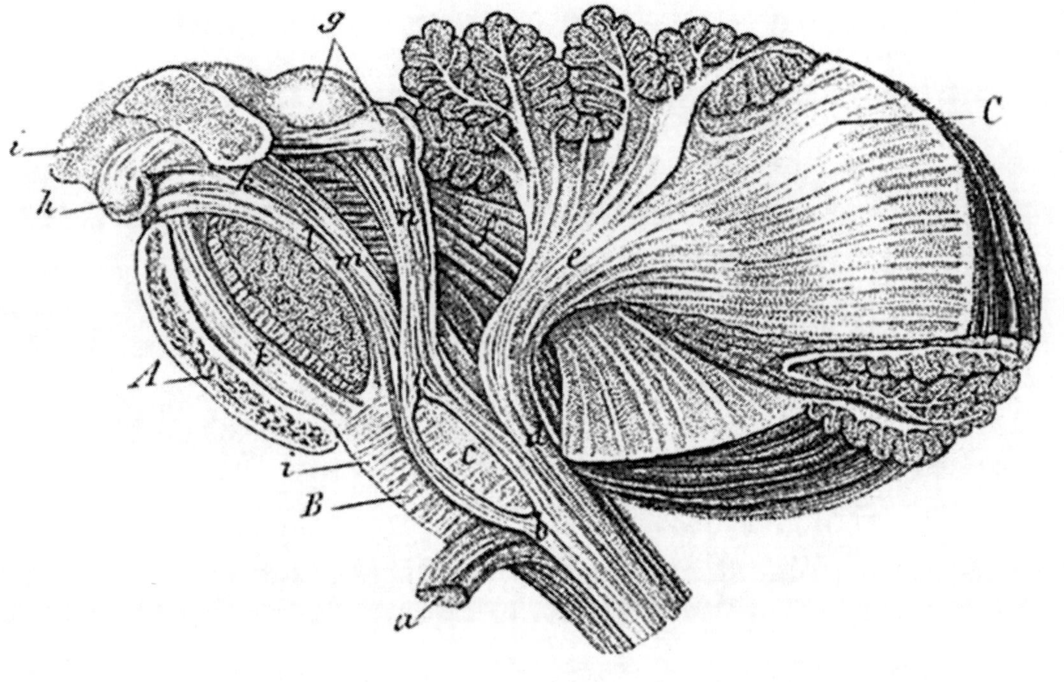

Figure 6.7. Cerebellar dissections, showing the white matter tracts. Refer to the text for details. The original terminology has been kept. A, pons varoli. B, Medulla oblongata. C, cerebellum left hemisphere. a) Left pyramid (cut across). b) Left olivary fascicle. c) Inferior olivary nucleus. d) left restiform body (inferior cerebellar peduncle). e) Inferior cerebellar peduncles. f) Brachium conjunctivum (superior cerebellar peduncle). g) Corpora quadrigemina. h) corpora mammilare (mamillary bodies). i) Horizontal fibers of the right pyramid. k) Lateral lemniscus. l) Medial lemniscus. n) Amiculum olivae. o) Cerebral peduncles. p) Fibers of the cerebral peduncles. Taken from Gray's anatomy (out of copyright and in the public domain).

6.3.4. Cerebellar Lobes, Lobules, Zones

There are many different schemes to the organized view of the cerebellum. Three common, superimposed organizational schemes, each having merits and disadvantages are the cerebellar division into lobes, lobules or zones. The lobar segmentation, the simplest of the three, yet the most commonly used clinically, segregates the cerebellar into a narrow midline vermis (associated functionally with truncal coordination and gait) and two large laterally located hemispheres (engaged mainly with appendicular coordination, motor memory and other functions).

The lobules segregation (presented in figures 6.8-6.9) describes the cerebellum as composed of ten different lobules. These lobules are divided into anterior and posterior groups, separated by the tentorial (primary) and posterolateral fissures. The anterior group comprises lobules I-V; the posterior group comprises lobules VI to IX. The flocculonodular lobule, the tenth lobule, is formed by the flocculus and nodulus. Each lobule is composed of individual ridges (folia), which are continuous from one hemisphere to the other, across the midline. This pattern is disrupted on the inferior surface by the enlargement of the lateral masses and the subsequent infolding of the midline area.

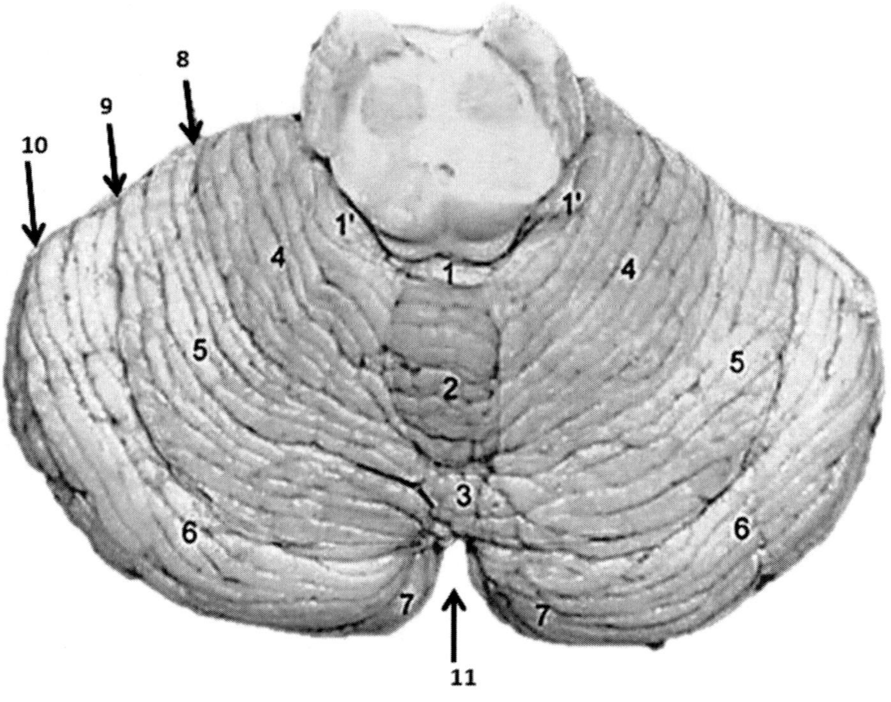

Figure 6.8. Cerebellar lobules, superior view. Refer to text. 1-Central lobule, 1'-Wing of the central lobule, 2-Culmen, 3-Declive, 4-Quadriangular lobule, 5-Simple lobule, 6-Superior semilunar lobule, 7-Inferior semilunar lobule, 8-Primary fissure, 9-Superior posterior fissure, 10-Horizontal fissure, 11-Posterior cerebellar incisura. Taken with permission from www.radioloassistent.org.

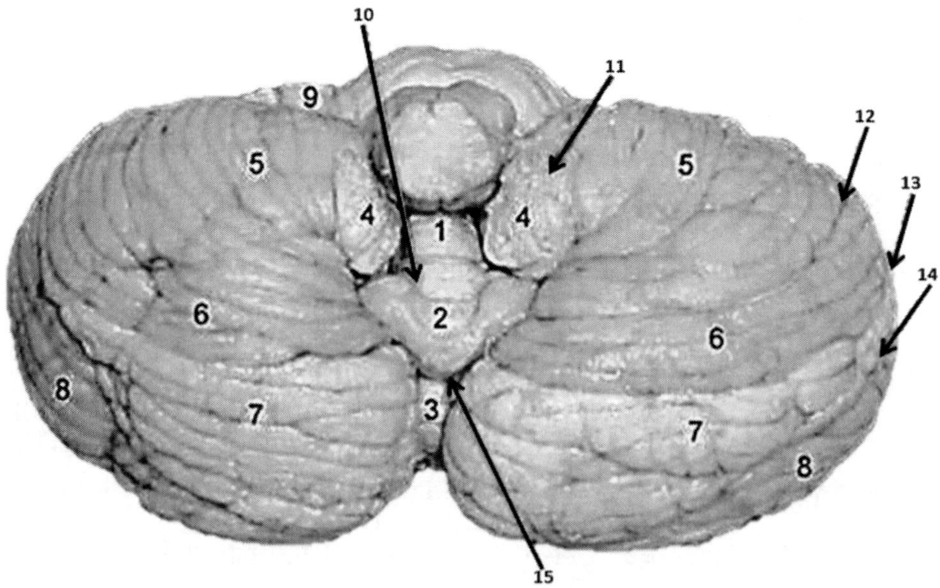

Figure 6.9. Cerebellar lobules, inferior view. Refer to text. 1-Uvula, 2-Pyramis, 3-Tuber vermis, 4-Tonsils, 5-Biventer lobule, 6-Gracile lobule, 7-Inferior semilunar lobule, 8-Superior semilunar lobule, 9-Flocculus, 10-Secondary fissure, 11-Retrotonsillar fissure, 12-Inferior anterior fissure, 13-Inferior posterior fissure, 14-Horizontal fissure, 15-Postpyramidal fissure. Taken with permission from www.radioloassistent.org.

The zonal division of the cerebellum can be superimposed on the lobes and lobules segregation. Zones are oriented rostrocaudally, defined on the basis of their connections (refer to figure 6.10). On each cerebellar side, three major zones are defined. The medial (vermal) zone is divided to smaller zones (zones A, B). It is located adjacent to the midline, extending through the anterior and posterior lobes and includes the nodulus. It is widest in lobule-VI and tapers rostrally and caudally. The intermediate (paravermal) zone is subdivided into three smaller zones (C_1, C_2, and C3). It is located adjacent to the medial zone, extending throughout the anterior and posterior lobes, but has little representation in the flocculonodular lobe. The lateral (hemisphere) zone is subdivided into two smaller zones (D_1, D_2). It occupies the largest parts of the cerebellar cortex, anterior and posterior lobes as well as the flocculus. Refer to figure 6.10.

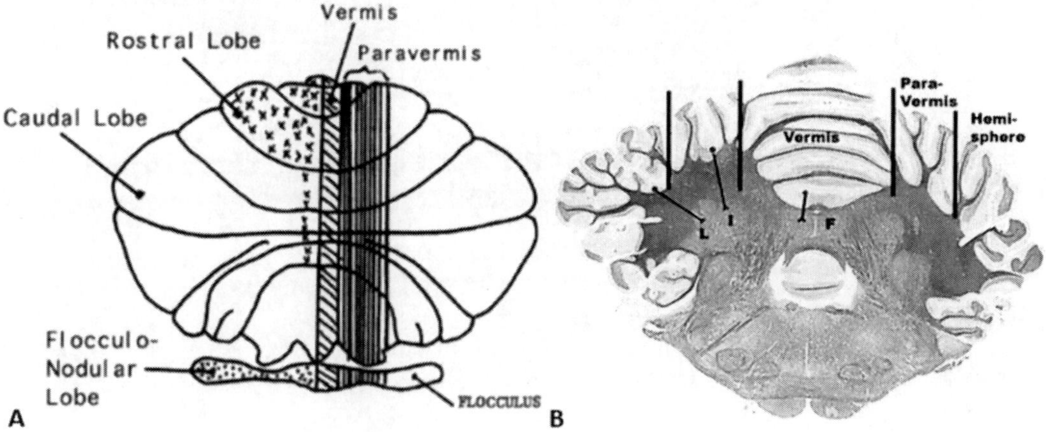

Figure 6.10. A+B The zonal segregation of the cerebellum. A, Illustration. B, Section. Refer to text. Taken with permission from www.radioloassistent.org.

6.3.5. The Cerebellar Nuclei

Similarly to the cerebral hemispheres, these nuclei are gray matter islands embedded within the white mater core of the cerebellar hemispheres. The cerebellar nuclei play a crucial role in modulating the cerebellar cortical processing prior to projecting it outside the cerebellum. As discussed later, most of the cerebellar output passes and is modified to some extend by these nuclei. Four nuclei are commonly defined (refer to figure 6.11):

1) The fastigial nucleus is located more medially within the cerebellar hemispheres, functionally related to the overlying medial zone of the cerebellar cortex. It generally projects bilaterally to the brainstem through the juxta-restiform bodies.
2) The globose nucleus is more posteriorly interspread.
3) The emboliform nucleus is more anteriorly interspread (the globose and emboliform nuclei are interspread laterally by the fastigial nucleus).
4) The dentate nucleus is located lateral to the emboliform nucleus. It is a large undulating sheet "C" shaped like crumpled paper bag. the dentate hilus, the opening of the nucleus is directed rostromedially. It is functionally related to lateral cortical zone.

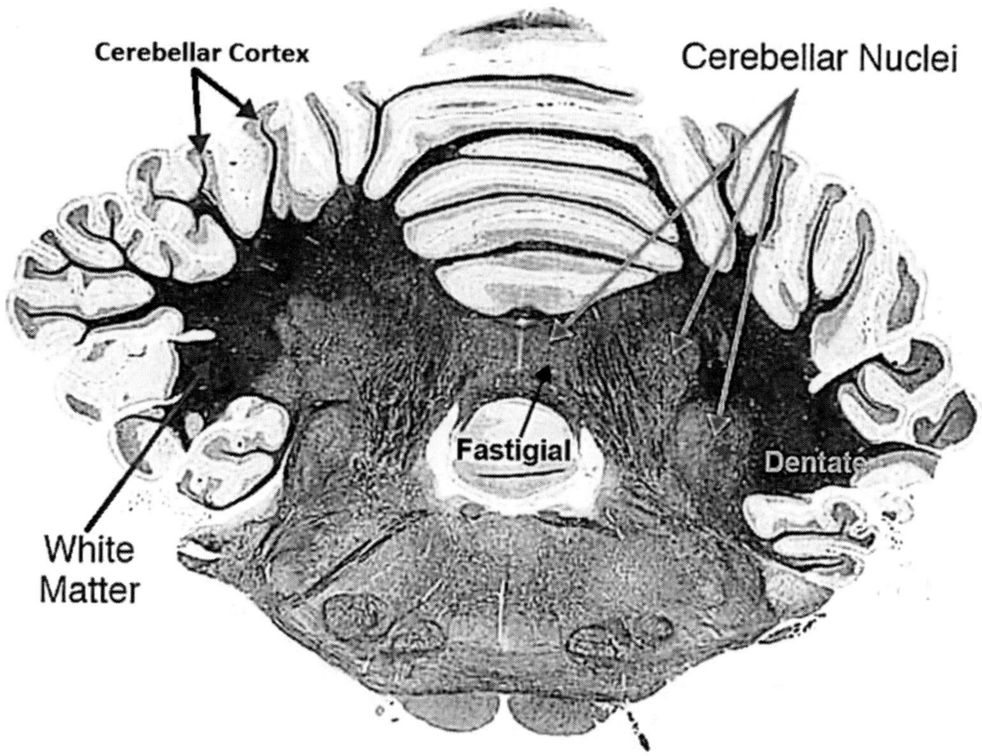

Figure 6.11. The Cerebellar nuclei. Refer to text. Taken with permission from www.radioloassistent.org.

6.4. Cerebellar Histology and Internal Architecture

6.4.1. Cellular Components and Organization

The cerebellar internal architecture can be described as composed of three major layers. These are the superficial cellular layer, the cortex proper layer composed of three sub layers (the molecular, the Purkinje and the granular layers) and a myelinated fibers core, containing the cerebellar afferents or efferents fibers. Refer to figure 6.12. Although not in the scope of this book, a short description of these layers is provided.

The molecular layer is characterized by less cell bodies (somata) than the granular layer, but more cell processes (parallel fibers, Purkinje cell dendrites, golgy cell dendrites, climbing fibers, processes of intrinsic cells etc.). Stellate cells are found in the outer regions of the layer, referred to as superficial or outer stellate cells. Basket cells are also found here with their stomata above that of the Purkinje cells. Basket cells axons travels in the sagittal plane giving rise to descending branches forming baskets around the Purkinje cells. The two cell types are similar in general shape, but the extent of dendritic and axonal fields is much larger for the basket cells (thus they influence much larger numbers of Purkinje cells). These cells receive excitatory input from parallel fibers, but themselves are GABA-ergic (inhibitory).

The Purkinje cell layer is a single cell layer of these large soma cells (large cell body), located at the interface of the granular and molecular layers. Each Purkinje cell gives rise to an elaborate dendritic tree, radiating into the molecular layer (this tree is fan-shaped, with its widest part oriented perpendicular to the long axis of the folium). Synaptic contacts are formed on short terminal branches emerging from the secondary and tertiary dendrites. These are the only efferents fibers of the cerebellar cortex. Their axons arise from the base of their body, and may give recurrent branches. Axon traverses the granular layer and subcortical white matter to terminate in cerebellar and vestibular nuclei.

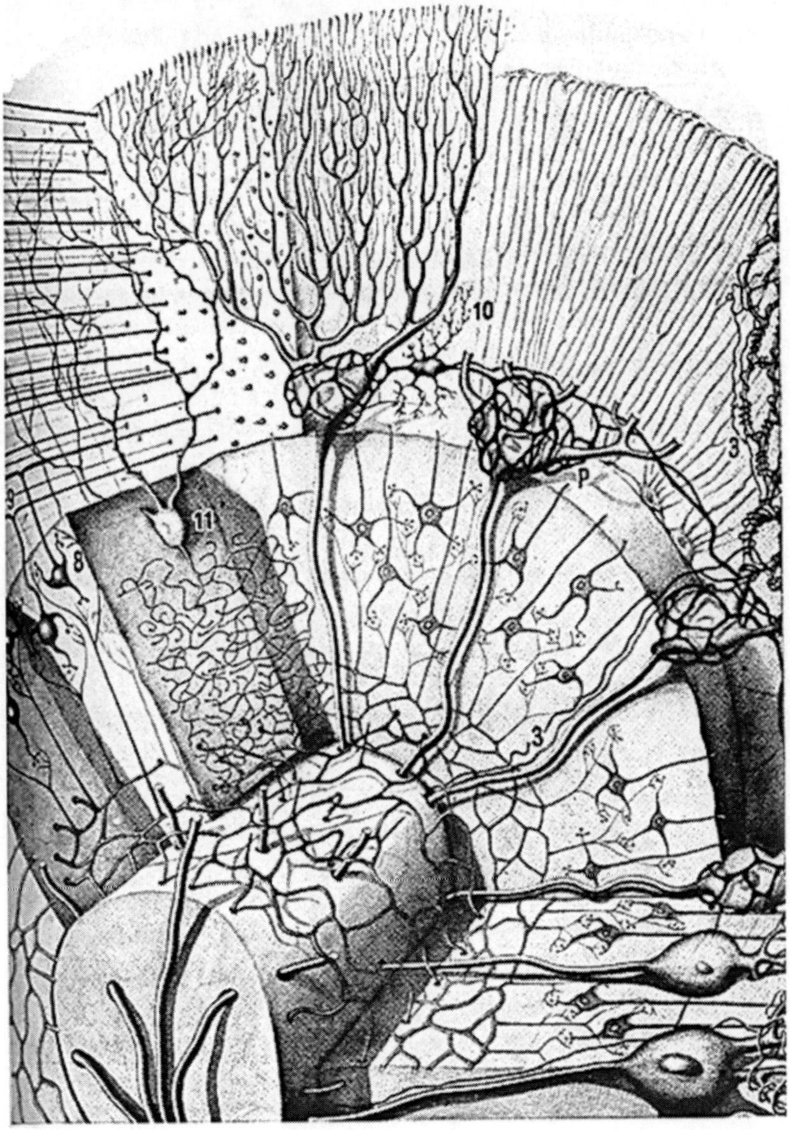

Figure 6.12. The cerebellar architecture and histology. Refer to text. Taken from Gray's anatomy (out of copyright and in the public domain).

The granular layer contain mostly small granule cells (5~8μm), whose dendrites form clawlike endings (dendritic digits). Their axons ascend into the molecular layer, where they bifurcate to form parallel fibers (parallel to the long axis of the folium). Thus, these fibers pass through the dendritic tree of the Purkinje cells, and during this passage make synaptic contact on them. These cells use mainly glutamate, thus have an excitatory effect on their target cells, and are the only excitatory neurons of the cerebellar cortex. Golgy cells have a large soma and are usually found adjacent to the Purkinje cells layer. The golgy cell dendrites branch in the granular layer, but extend mainly to the molecular layer. It uses GABA (hence inhibitory).

The cerebellar glomerulus is a synaptic complex found in the neuropil of the granular layer. It is composed of dendrites and axons of both granule and golgy cells, and a specialized synaptic segment of a mossy fiber (discussed next).

6.4.2. Cerebellar Afferent Fibers

Affarent fibers to the cerebellar cortex are grouped to three types, based on their morphology and connections of their nerve terminals in the cortex. These are mossy fibers, climbing fibers and multilayered fibers. Mossy fibers have their axon originate from cell bodies in the cerebellar nuclei (or extra-cerebellar in the spinal cord, medulla, and pons). On route to the cerebellar cortex, many of these fibers send collaterals to the cerebellar nuclei. In the granular layer, these fibers branch and their large terminals contact other cells at irregular intervals (the so called mossy fibers rosettes). The mossy fiber rosette is a major element of the cerebellar glomerulus, giving it the mossy appearance. A single mossy fiber may form up to 50 rosettes (each existing in a synaptic contact with 10~15 different granule cells). These cells use glutamate as a neurotransmitter and are thus excitatory to granule and golgy cells.

Climbing fibers arise only from the inferior olivary nuclei. These fibers terminate in the molecular layer, by entwining up the dendritic trees of Purkinje dendrites. Each Purkinje cell is innervated by a single climbing fiber, but one climbing fiber may serve several Purkinje cells. These cells use aspartate as a neurotransmitter and are thus excitatory to the Purkinje cells and cerebellar nuclei neurons.

The multilayered fibers are non-aminergic neurons originating from the cells of locus ceruleus, raphe nuclei (serotonin), hypothalamus etc. These fibers enter the cerebellum mostly via the peduncles (or in case of some hypothalamo-cerebellar fibers through the periventricular gray matter). In the cerebellar cortex, these fibers branch diffusely and terminate in the molecular and granular layers, influencing all major cell types. Generally speaking, these fibers modulate the output of the cortex either by decreasing the spontaneous discharge rate of the Purkinje cells or directly and via interneurons alter the responsiveness of the Purkinje cells to excitation by climbing fibers and mossy fibers.

As a rule of thumb, in the cerebellum, axons projecting upward are excitatory (mossy, climbing, granule cell parallel fibers) whereas axons projecting downward are inhibitory (Purkinje, satellite, basket, Golgy cells).

6.4.3. Cerebellar Efferent Pathways

The cerebellar efferent pathways are organized around the three functional regions of the cerebellum: the lateral hemispheres, the intermediate zones and the vermis and flocculonodular lobule. The lateral hemispheres, in which lesions affect mainly distal limb coordination, project to the dentate nucleus mainly. The intermediate hemispheres, coordinating ongoing movements of distal extremities, project to the emboliform and globose nuclei of cerebellum. From these nuclei, projections arise reaching the red nucleus magnocellular division (midbrain) to affect the rubrospinal tract and lateral motor systems. The vermis and flocculonodular lobule, in which lesions affect mainly trunk control, posture, balance and gait, as well as the vestibule-ocular reflex, affecting proximal trunk muscles on the one hand and extra-ocular muscles on the other. These regions project mainly to the vestibular nuclei. Vestibule-cerebellum is a term used for the flocculonodular lobule and the inferior vermis, since these projects mainly to the vestibular nuclei.

As a rule of thumb, deficits in coordination occur ipsilateral to the lesion, since pathways are double crossed (decussate twice). The first decussation occurs at the decussation of superior cerebellar peduncle (exit from cerebellum) at midbrain level. The second decussation occurs as the corticospinal and rubrospinal tracts descend to the spinal cord (at the pyramidal decussation). Each cerebellar hemisphere receives information about the ipsilateral limbs. In contrast, midline lesions in the vermis have effects on the medial motor system, influencing the proximal trunk muscles bilaterally.

6.4.3.1. The Spinocerebellar Module

The vermis and the intermediate zones receive input mainly via the dorsal and ventral spinocerebellar tracts, and are collectively termed as the spinocerebellum. The dorsal spinocerebellar and cuneocerebellar fibers enter the cerebellum via the restiform body, while ventral fibers enter the cerebellum via the superior cerebellar peduncle (the exception to the rule). Thus, fibers entering into the vermis zone send collaterals to the fastigial nucleus, while those entering to intermediate zone, branch into the emboliform and globose nuclei. The spinocerebellum output functions in the control of axial musculature through the vermis cortex and fastigial efferents and controls limb musculature through efferents of the globus and emboliform nuclei. The dorsal spinocerebellar and cuneocerebellar fibers inform the cerebellum on limb position and movement, and after processing, through connections with the motor cortex through the thalamus, influence movements and tone. Spinal cord cells (in ventral horn) receive primary sensory input and are also under the influence of descending reticulospinal and corticospinal fibers.

The fastigial nucleus projections include projections bilaterally to vestibular and reticular nuclei (these in turn, via their spinal projections influence axial muscles), projections to the contralateral medial accessory olivary nucleus, and projections to medial areas of the ventral horn in upper spinal cord (fastigiospinal fibers) and to the ventrolateral nucleus of the thalamus. The emboliform and globus nuclei projections include projections to the magnocellular part of the red nucleus, and to the ventrolateral nucleus of thalamus.

6.4.3.2. The Pontocerebellar Module

Since most fibers enter the cerebellum via the middle cerebellar peduncle, the lateral pontine zone is termed as the pontocerebellum. Pontine nuclei receive many important projections from the ipsilateral cortex, thus this lateral zone may be also be termed as the cerebro-cerebellum or the neocerebellum part. The pontocerebellum functions in the planning and control of precise dexterous movements of limbs, particularly in the arm, forearm and hand, and in the timing of these movements. The dentate nucleus modulates activity in cortical regions via direct connections to motor cortical areas, projecting to the contralateral spinal cord. The inferior olivary nucleus is another affarent fiber source for the cerebellum with fibers entering via through the restiform body, sending collaterals to the dentate nucleus, ending (synapsing) in the molecular layer. The dentate nucleus gives off efferent fibers that exit the cerebellum via the superior cerebellar peduncle (through its decussation). Fibers passing rostrally, project to the parvocellular part of the red nucleus, and to the intralaminar and ventrolateral (VL) nuclei of thalamus.

6.5. Topographic Localization

Input to the cerebellum may be direct (via the spinocerebellar or vestibulocerebellar tracts), or indirect, passing through many integration centers before reaching the cerebellum (after visual, auditory, or sensorimotor stimuli for example). Visual and auditory cortices project to the cells of basilar pons, which provide mossy fibers to areas of the cerebellar cortex where the eye and ear are represented. Sensorimotor cortex, also via projections through the basilar pons, influences cerebellar cortices regions containing body representations. Body parts are not represented continuously over a large area of cerebellar cortex, like seen in the different homunculi of the cerebral cortex. Rather, the different body parts are broken into smaller discontinuous patches. A small area receiving sensory input from the arm (via mossy fibers-granule cell connections), may be located adjacent to an area receiving input from a noncontiguous region of the same upper limb. Furthermore, each body part is represented in several locations, related more to the type of information rather than to the body region. This is termed fractured somatotopy.

6.6. Cerebellum and Motor Learning

The cerebellum is largely involved in the learning of simple reflexive motor behaviors. Modifications in certain reflexes are performed by the cerebellum as well, like the adaptation of the vestibuloocular reflex, classic (Pavlovian) conditioning of reflexes evoked by aversive stimuli (eye blink, withdrawal reflexes) etc. The cerebellar role in voluntary complex motor skills is still not clear to some extent. Under normal conditions, the cerebellum plays a role in the acquisition component of the motor learning process. The cerebellum however is not essential for the memory storage for volitional movements (retention of previously learned complex motor behaviors). The complex interaction the cerebellum has with different other components of the motor circuitry (i.e., basal ganglia, cerebellum, red nucleus, substancia nigra, reticular formation, different cortical regions) adds to the complexity in isolating its specific roles. Current day view looks at the motor system regions of the brain as a network and not as isolated functionally unique structures. Other functions are attributed to the cerebellum, manifested by different clinical phenomena unexplained by current knowledge. One such phenomenon is cerebellar mutism seen mostly in children after cerebellar surgery (or approach to the 4th ventricle).

6.7. Vascular Supply to the Cerebellum

The vascular supply to the cerebellum was largely discussed with the brainstem vascular supply in chapter 3, and reviewed in chapter 9. Briefly summarizing, the cerebellum is supplied by branches of the vertebral and basilar arteries. Refer to figure 6.13 for a simplified view and to figure 6.14 for dissection details. The posterior inferior cerebellar artery (PICA) supplies the lateral medulla and inferior half of cerebellum and inferior vermis. Its occlusion results in the Wallenberg syndrome (also termed as lateral medullary syndrome, refer to chapter 3).

The anterior inferior cerebellar artery (AICA) supplies the inferior-lateral pons, middle cerebellar peduncle, a strip of the anterior cerebellum and the flocculus. The superior cerebellar artery (SCA), supplies the upper lateral pons, the superior cerebellar peduncle, the superior half of the cerebellar hemisphere including the deep nuclei and the superior vermis. Refer to figure 6.15 for the different cerebellar vascular territories.

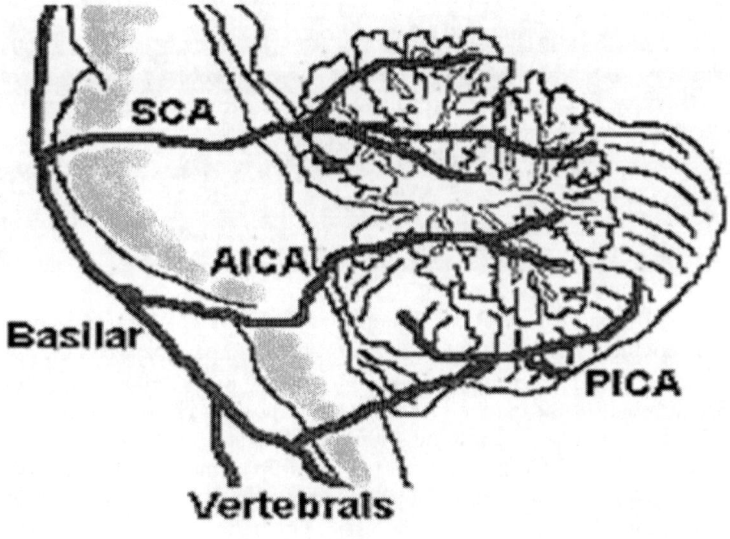

Figure 6.13. The cerebellar blood supply, simplified view. Taken with permission from www.radiopaedia.org.

The SCAs are intimately related to the superior half of the fourth ventricular roof and the cerebellomesencephalic fissure. The AICAs are intimately related to the cerebellopontine fissures and the lateral recesses. The PICAs are intimately related to the caudal half of the roof and the cerebellomedullary fissure. The SCAs pass around the midbrain above the trigeminal nerve and divide into rostral and caudal trunks. The branches of these trunks loop deeply into the cerebellomesencephalic fissure and give off the precerebellar arteries, which pass along the superior cerebellar peduncles to the dentate nuclei. The PICAs arise from the vertebral arteries and pass between the glossopharyngeal, vagus, and accessory nerves to reach the cerebellomedullary fissure.

After passing near the caudal pole of the tonsils, where they form a caudal loop, they ascend through the cerebellomedullary fissure, where they are intimately related to the caudal part of the ventricular roof. They pass around the rostral pole of the tonsil and through the telovelotonsillar cleft, where they form a cranial loop. In their course around the tonsils, they divide into medial and lateral trunks. They give off branches to the dentate nuclei near the superior pole of the tonsils. Refer to figure 6.14.

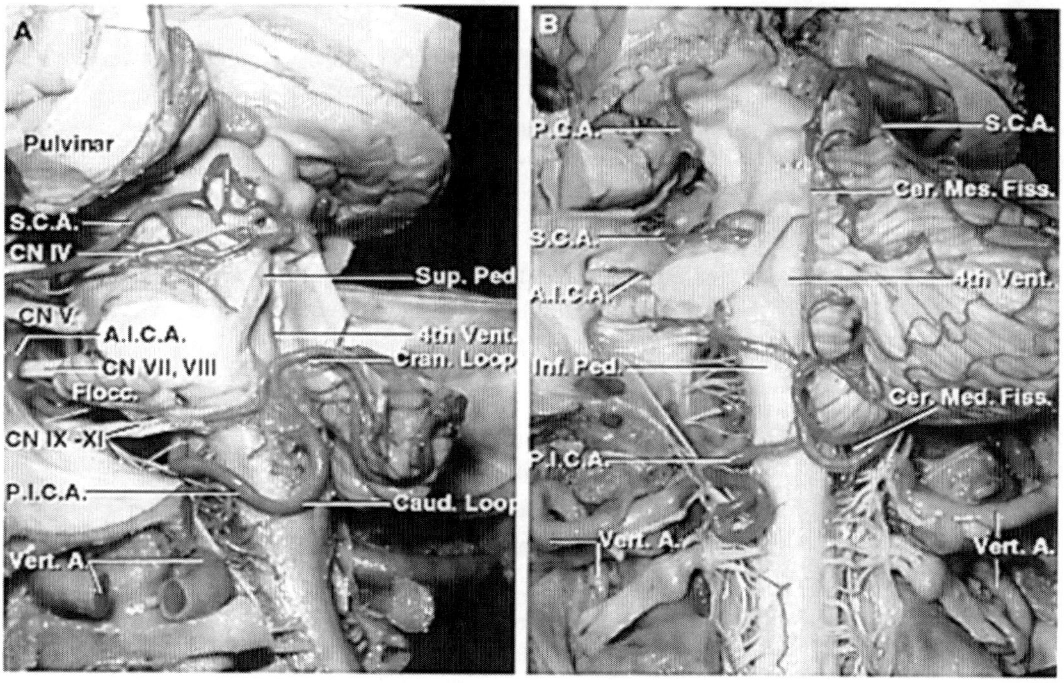

Figure 6.14. Cerebellar blood supply. A, Posterolateral view. The AICA loops around the flocculus and the facial and vestibulocochlear nerves. The left PICA is shown to pass between the rootlets of the nerves entering the jugular foramen, turning caudally around the lower pole of the left tonsil, which has been removed. B, The left half of the cerebellum has been removed. The SCA passes around the midbrain below the PCA in the lower part of the ambient and quadrigeminal cisterns, enters the cerebellomesencephalic fissure, and loops over the posterior lip of the fissure to supply the tentorial surface. The AICA passes laterally around the pons and above the flocculus. A., artery; A.I.C.A., anteroinferior cerebellar artery; Caud., caudal; Cer. Med., cerebellomedullary; Cer. Mes., cerebellomesencephalic; Chor., choroid; CN, cranial nerve; Cran., cranial; Dent., dentate; Fiss., fissure; Flocc., flocculus; Inf., inferior; Mid., middle; Nucl., nucleus; P.C.A., posterior cerebral artery; Ped., peduncle; P.I.C.A., posteroinferior cerebellar artery; Plex., plexus; S.C.A., superior cerebellar artery; Sup., superior; Vent., ventricle; Vert., vertebral. Taken with permission from the Rhoton Collection.

The AICAs arise from the basilar artery and pass near or between the facial and vestibulocochlear nerves and are intimately related to the cerebellopontine fissures, the flocculi, and the lateral recesses (refer to figure 6.16). The AICAs divide into rostral and caudal trunks before reaching the facial and vestibulocochlear nerves. The rostral trunk passes between the nerves and along the middle cerebellar peduncle near the cerebellopontine fissure.

The caudal trunk passes below the nerves and near the lateral recess to supply the lower part of the petrosal surface. The AICA and the PICA give rise to the choroidal arteries, which supply the tela choroidea and attached choroid plexus.

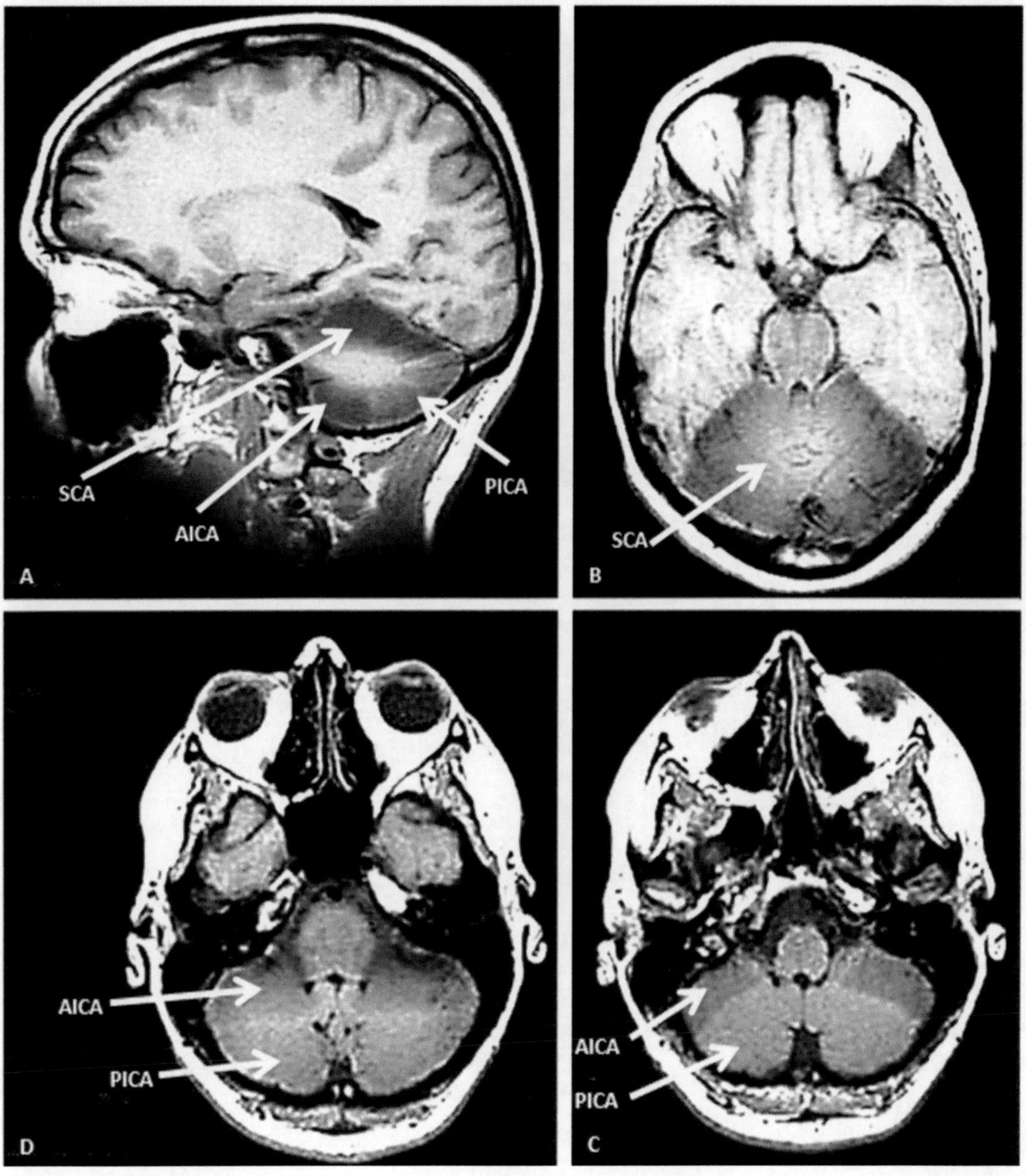

Figure 6.15. Cerebellar vascular territories. A, Parasagittal view. B, Superior cerebellum. C, Mid-cerebellum. D, Inferior cerebellum. Image created by Frank Gaillard and made available under Creative Commons license of Raidopaedia.org.

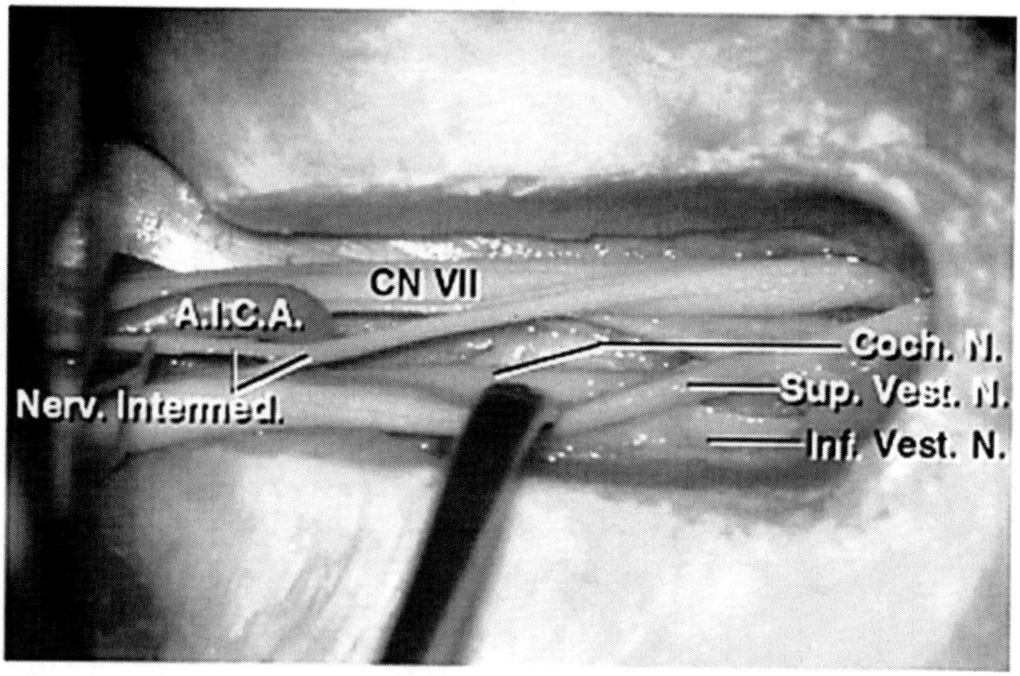

Figure 6.16. The AICA relationships in the right cerebellopontine angle (CPA). The cleavage plane between the superior and inferior vestibular nerves has been developed. The cochlear nerve is located anterior to the inferior vestibular nerve. A.I.C.A., anterior inferior cerebellar artery; CN, cranial nerve; Coch., cochlear; Inf., inferior; Intermed., intermedius; N., nerve; Nerv., nervus; Sup., superior; Vest., vestibular. Taken with permission from the Rhoton Collection.

Chapter 7

The Cerebrum and the Cerebral Cortex

7.1. Abstract

This topic, maybe more than others in CNS anatomy, captures the imagination. The discussion on the matter that forms one's soul and personality is fascinating, since the essence of human behavior is processed and formed in the cerebral hemispheres. The chapter begins with a neuro-embryology overview. Telencephalon development, the histogenesis of the cerebral cortex and the commissures development are presented in brief. Next, a short discussion on cerebral cortex histology and cytoarchitectural features, followed by the introduction of the laminar and columnar cortical organization schemes is given. The gross neuroanatomy is presented next, focusing on brief concise descriptions of the different structures and connections. Gray and white matter anatomy is described separately. The limbic system is discussed separately next, presenting its different components and intricate relationships its different structures share. Higher order cerebral functions, the classification of memory and memory disorders and dominant hemispheral syndromes are presented next in a focused clinically oriented manner.

7.2. Neuro-Embryology of the Cerebrum and Cerebral Cortex

A discussed in chapter 1 in the frame of the general embryology, as cerebral vesicles enlarge in all directions, they pull along portions of the neural canal, until it forms the lateral ventricles, the cavity of the telencephalon. Portions of the lateral ventricle are found in the frontal, parietal, temporal, and occipital lobes. Refer to table 7.1 for developmental milestones.

Table 7.1. Major CNS Developmental Milestones

Gestation (Weeks)	Major Developmental Events
3	Neural tube invaginates.
4	The anterior and then posterior ends of the neural tube close.
	The brain and head represent 50% of the total body length
	Rapid neuronal division into bipolar neuroblasts at rates up to 250,000 / min.
	Radial glia appear and migration begins
5	Lens placodes of eye develop
	Forebrain, midbrain and hindbrain become evident
	Neuronal migration largely complete
	Dorsal and ventral horns of the spinal cord appear, peripheral nerves appear.
6-8	Migration of neurons, ears develop, limbs develop
	All major organs are under development
9-12	Gross brain structure is established
	Glial development and migration appears
	Very rapid growth of axons and synapses
	Muscle contractions begin
13-20	Rapid brain growth, cranial nerves appear and myelination begins
	Alpha-feto-protein elevates in the amniotic fluid and maternal serum if there is failure for proper neural tube closure.
21-40	Primary cerebral fissures appear, followed by secondary sulci
	Myelination and synaptic development continues
Birth	The head is 25% of the total body length
	Peripheral nerves myelination is almost complete but the CNS myelination continues through age two years.

7.2.1. Development of the Telencephalon

The telencephalon, a subset of the prosencephalon is the most rostral vesicle. It forms the hemispheres (laterally), and the lamina terminalis (medially). The lateral ventricles (hemispherical cavities) communicate with the diencephalic lumen through the interventricular foramina of Monro. The cerebral hemispheres start developing on the fifth week of gestation. These arise as bilateral outgrowths of the lateral telencephalic vesicle wall. By the Middle of the second month of development, their basal part (the part that forms first) enlarges, causing it to bulge into the lumen of the lateral ventricle. The cerebral cortex develops from the pallium and is divided to two regions: the paleopallium (or archipallium, located lateral to corpus striatum) and the neopallium (lying between the hippocampus and paleopallium) which is formed by migratory waves of neuroblasts, the most superficial layer is the youngest.

7.2.1.1. Histogenesis of the Cerebral Cortex

By the end of the first month of gestation, the telencephalic pallium (cortex), in the human fetus consists of a germinal layer and an ependymal layer, which together form the stratified cellular wall of the neural tube. By the end of the second month, medullary differentiation is well advanced, and the cells migrate toward the surface to form the mantle layer. Thus, the wall of the hemisphere has the general primitive structure of the neural axis with the germinal or mantle layer on the interior and the marginal or future molecular layer on its exterior. During the third month of gestation, the cortical layer is formed by cells from the mantle layer migrating toward the surface. This cortical layer is thin in the archi- and paleopallial regions and thick in the neopallial region. Various cortical regions differentiate from the cortical layers. The primordial olfactory cortex begins first between the second and third months, manifesting with the hippocampus (archeocortex) and paleocortex. A three layer cortex forms in these areas.

Differentiation of the neocortex extends from the beginning of the third month to the end of the sixth month of gestation. It is characterized by extensive cellular migrations, resulting in the formation of 6 cellular layers. In the adult, the cerebral cortex forms a layer of gray matter approximately 3 to 5 mm thick. The cellular migration and layering of cells are first seen at the level of the insula and parietal cortex. Thus, the somesthetic system, which ends in the ascending parietal convolutions of the brain, is functional in the fetus very early, before the special senses like sight and hearing. Cellular migrations then appear at the level of the frontal and occipital cortices. In the sixth month, the neurons form their processes and in the seventh month, the various types of cortical structures are established, motor, sensory, associative, and intermediary, according to the proportion of specialized cells they contain. In contrast to other regions of the nervous system, the germinal layer is active for only several months after birth (Refer to figure 7.1).

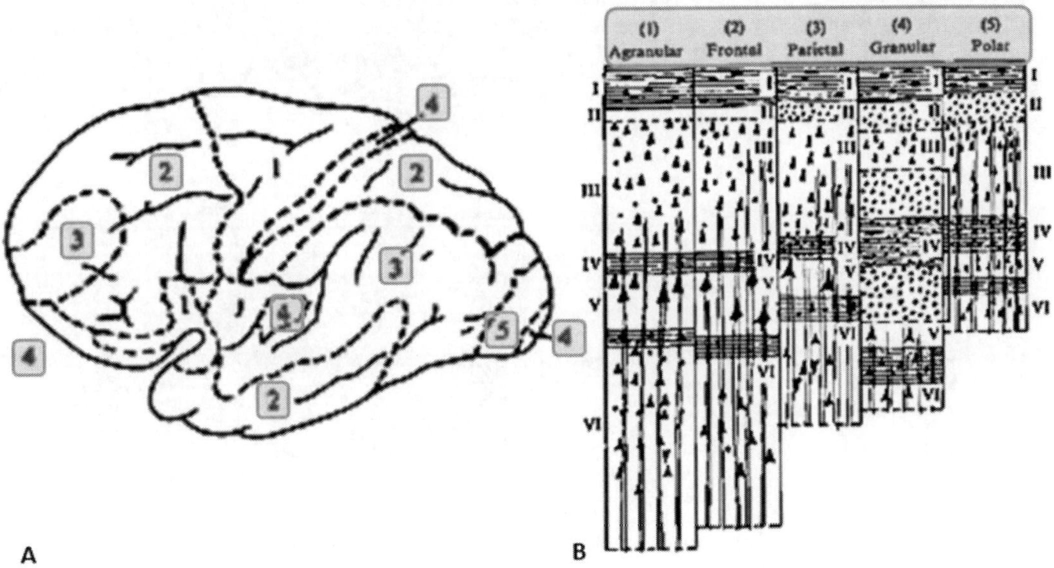

Figure 7.1. Histogenesis of the cerebral cortex. Distribution of the five major types of cerebral cortex. A, cortical surface showing the different histological types according to position. B, Illustrative representation of the different histological cortical types. Refer to text.

7.2.2. Development of the Commissures

A number of fiber bundles connecting in a mirror fashion the right and left hemispheres, crossing the midline, some using the lamina terminalis. Those developed in the lamina terminalis include the anterior commissure, the hippocampal and the corpus callosum commissures (all discussed later in details). The anterior commissure is the first to appear, having fibers connecting the olfactory bulbs and related brain areas of the two sides. The hippocampal or fornix commissure is the second to appear. It develops within the hippocampus, passing close to the diencephalic roof. The fibers form arches outside the choroid fissure to the mamillary body and hypothalamus. The corpus callosum, the most important commissure, originates from the area of the lamina terminalis, connecting non-olfactory areas, arching over the thin diencephalic roof. Failure of the corpus callosum to develop is sometimes accompanied by an absence of the anterior or hippocampal commissures.

Other commissures, non-lamina terminalis originated, include the posterior commissure, the habenular commissure and the optic chiasm. The posterior commissure is considered a part of the limbic system (discussed later); the habenular commissure is located below and rostral to pineal gland stalk. The optic chiasm is located in the rostral wall of diencephalon, conveying fibers from the medial half of retina (Refer to figure 7.2).

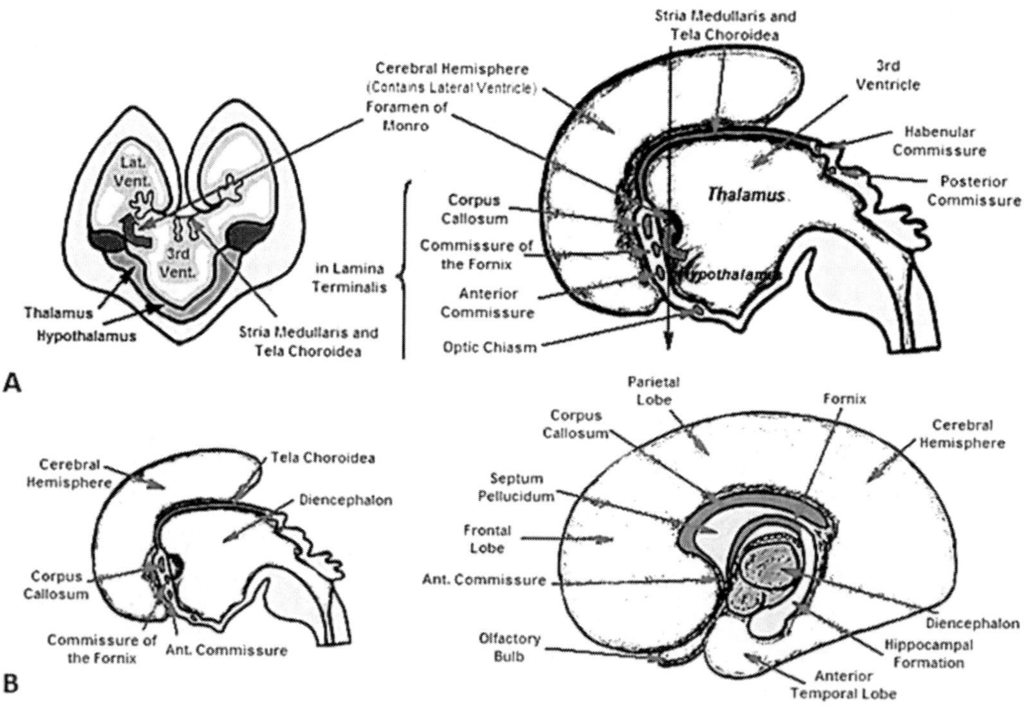

Figure 7.2. Development of the commissures. A, left is a coronal section of the right image at the assigned line. Right is a midsagittal view. B, left is an earlier time point. Refer to text. Taken with permission from www.radiopaedia.org.

7.3. Cerebral Cortex Histology

7.3.1. Introduction

The cerebral cortex is a dense aggregation of nerve cell bodies (measuring 2~4mm in thickness), forming the surface of each cerebral hemisphere. The total cortical area is estimated to be about 2500cm^2. Input from the different subcortical areas reaches the cortex via thalamic relays. Information also reaches the cortex from other regions of the cortex via association fibers. These in turn project to many neural structures (other cortical areas, thalamus, basal ganglia, cerebellum via pontine nuclei, brainstem nuclei, spinal cord etc). the cerebral cortex can be segregated into three functional areas: Those devoted to processing incoming sensory information, those involved in the organization of motor activity and those regions devoted to "higher intellectual functions" (i.e., memory, planning, language, mathematics etc).

7.3.2. Basic Connections of a Given Cortical Region

The basic connections of a given cortical region include projections fibers, commissural fibers and association fibers. The projections fibers reach, by definition, subcortical structures (diencephalon, basal nuclei, brain stem, and spinal cord). Commissural fibers, by definition, connect symmetric regions in the two hemispheres (aka corpus callosum fibers). Association fibers terminate at cortical regions within the same hemisphere. These association fibers connect cortical areas in same (short) or different (long) lobes of the same hemisphere. Since almost all neural input to the cortex that originates in non-cortical regions arises from the thalamus, the thalamocortical fibers term was coined as a subtype of projection fibers.

7.3.3. Cortical Cytoarchitecture

A described in the embryology section, most cerebral cortex regions have six distinct layers of neurons, and are classified as neocortex. Some regions, i.e., the hippocampal formation, have only three layers and are defined as archicortex. The paleocortex has three to five cortical and includes the olfactory sensory area and the nearby entorhinal and periamygdaloid cortices. The layers are numbered from the pia inward into the molecular layer, the external granular layer, the external pyramidal layer, the internal granular layer, the internal pyramidal layer and the multiform layers (refer to figure 7.1). The molecular layer has very few nerve cell bodies and consists primarily of axons running parallel (horizontal) to the surface of the cortex. The external granular layer is a mixture of small neurons called granule cells and slightly larger neurons named pyramidal cells (based on the shape of their soma). The external pyramidal layer contains small to medium sized pyramidal cells and other type neurons. The internal granule layer is composed exclusively of smooth (a-spiny) stellate neurons, and spiny stellate neurons, both are sometimes classified as "granule cells". The internal pyramidal layer is composed of medium to large pyramidal cells. The sixth, innermost multiform layer contains an assortment of neuron types, including some with pyramidal and fusiform shaped cell bodies.

The neocortex myelinated fibers has some unique features: the so called outer and Inner bands of Baillerger are horizontally running myelinated fibers located in layers IV, V. The outer layer-V is greatly expanded in the primary visual cortex (bordering the calcarine sulcus) and is seen in the naked eye (where it is termed as the Stria/band of Gennari). Another feature, seen in most regions of neocortex, is the many radially oriented bundles of axons, passing between the subcortical white matter and different parts of the cortex.

7.3.4. Neuron Types in the Cerebral Cortex

Pyramidal cells are the most common cell type in cerebral cortex, found in all its layers (except the molecular layer), and are the major cellular elements in layers II, III, V, ranging 10~50μm in height. These cells are roughly triangular cell body, having a single large apical dendrite, arising from the apex of the cell body. This dendrite usually extends towards the molecular layer, giving branches along the way. Pyramidal cells have an array of basal dendrites running horizontally and an axon that originates from its base, leaving the cortex to run through the white matter. Betz cells are giant pyramidal cells, found mainly in the primary motor cortex of the precentral gyrus, whose somata can reach up to 100μm in height. These are most common in the region of the motor cortex that project to the anterior horn of the lumbar spinal cord. Dendritic spines appear in both apical and basal dendrites. These are small outgrowths from the dendrites, onto which the vast majority of synaptic contacts are received (rather than on the dendritic shaft or soma).

The laminar organization will be discussed later, but a pertinent point at time is the concept that the cell bodies in a given cortical layer project to specific nerve targets. Neurons in layers II, III generally give rise to association and callosal fibers. Neurons in layer V mainly project to subcortical structures (including to the spinal cord). Neurons in layer VI have axons reaching many different targets. Axon collaterals are located within the cortex, terminating in all cortical layers, extending through horizontal area of a few millimeters, around the cell body.

Local circuit neurons are another cellular subgroup. These are intrinsic cortical neurons (interneurons), whose axons do not leave the immediate region of the cell body. Although until recently all of these cells were termed as stellate, there are in fact three cell types receiving thalamocortical axons in layer-IV. These are the small spiny stellate cells (which are probably excitatory), the aspiny stellate cells (which are inhibitory, using GABA as a neurotransmitter) and the dendrites of the large basket cells (also inhibitory, using GABA as a neurotransmitter).

7.3.5. The Laminar Cortical organization

The laminar cortical organization refers to the intrinsic circuitry of the cerebral cortex. The thalamocortical axons terminate primarily in layer-IV, and to a lesser extent in layers III and VI on inhibitory/excitatory interneurons. This dedicated arrangement is maintained throughout the different cortical regions. Local processing culminates in connections to pyramidal cells (which carry the information to other cortical or subcortical regions). Corticocortical axons have their laminar pattern of termination quite different from that of thalamocortical axons, in that they branch repeatedly and make synaptic contact on neurons in all layers of cortex. A third set of input to the cortex is the diffuse input, in which fibers branch extensively and end diffusely over a wide area of cortex, with no respect to cytoarchitectural boundaries. These neurons subtype regulate the overall levels of cortical excitability, associated with the arousal, sleep, wakefulness phenomena (parallel in function to the reticular formation of the brainstem).

The laminar cortical organization also manifest in the cytoarchitectural features of the different regions. This cytoarchitectural differences from one area to the other, are correlated to the function of that specific cortical region. Thus, the primary sensory cortex has its layer IV which is the major input layer, very thick and developed; Its layer V, which is the major projection layer, is thin and indistinct. In sharp contrast, within the primary motor cortex, this pattern is reversed, with layer IV being almost invisible, while layer V is thick and seems to merge directly with layer III.

7.3.6. The Columnar Cortical Organization

The columnar cortical organization is a second vertical pattern of organization, superimposed on the layered organization. Neurons are often grouped together, so that their cell bodies, axons and apical dendrites form clusters that are oriented at right angles to the surface of the cortex. The basis of columnar organization in primary sensory cortices is selective input from relay nuclei of the thalamus. Naturally, the signals from the respective sensory receptors (different modalities of the same area, or same modality of different regions division), must have been continuously segregated all the way from the periphery through dorsal column nuclei and the vertebrobasal complex of the thalamus, to terminate in the cortex (This is best understood in the visual cortex). Connections of different regions of the cortex, may also be arranged in columns (like fibers from inferior parietal lobule terminating in many columns in the ipsilateral and contralateral cingulate cortex). Another example of such a columnar organization are the homunculi (discussed later).

7.4. The Cerebral Cortex Neuroanatomy

7.4.1. Overview

The Cerebrum is the largest part of the brain, in which highest level of processing occurs. It is the final destination of sensory information, the Source of voluntary motor commands and the seat of high brain functions (language, memory, personality). The paired cerebral hemispheres constitute the largest part of the brain. They are separated by the longitudinal fissure, interconnected by the corpus callosum, and merged with the diencephalon to establish continuity with the brainstem and the spinal cord. They encase the lateral and third ventricles. The cerebral hemispheres have three surfaces: lateral, medial, and basal; three margins: superior, inferior, and medial; three poles: frontal, temporal, and occipital; three types of white matter fibers: projection, commissural, and association; and five lobes: frontal, parietal, temporal, occipital, and the hidden insula.

The convoluted surface is composed of gyri and sulci. Gray matter outer cortex and a white matter core (opposite to the spinal cord). Most cell bodies reside in a thin layer of gray matter, the cerebral cortex. The core is mainly composed of white matter (axons and myelin). Within the white matter reside deep brain nuclei – the basal Nuclei (ganglia), amygdala, Claustrum etc. The most important landmarks for orienting are the three borders, the three poles, the sylvian and interhemispheric fissures, and the central sulcus. The cerebral hemispheres have their greatest transverse diameter across the parietal lobes. The longitudinal fissure, the deep cleft separating the upper part of the paired hemispheres, contains a sickle-shaped process of dura called the falx cerebri that separates the anterior and posterior parts of the hemispheres (figure 7.3-7.4).

The anterior portion of the falx cerebri is not as wide as its posterior part, leaving a wide space anteriorly between the free falx margin and the corpus callosum, where the medial surface of the hemispheres faces each other and not the falx (refer to chapter 8). Further posteriorly, the free margin slopes toward and becomes closely applied to the corpus callosum. The anterior part of the cingulate gyrus is below the free margin of the falx cerebri and is free to shift across the midline, whereas the middle and posterior parts have progressively less of the gyrus below and more above the free margin, where its displacement across the midline is limited by the rigidity of the falx (refer to herniation syndromes in chapter 8).

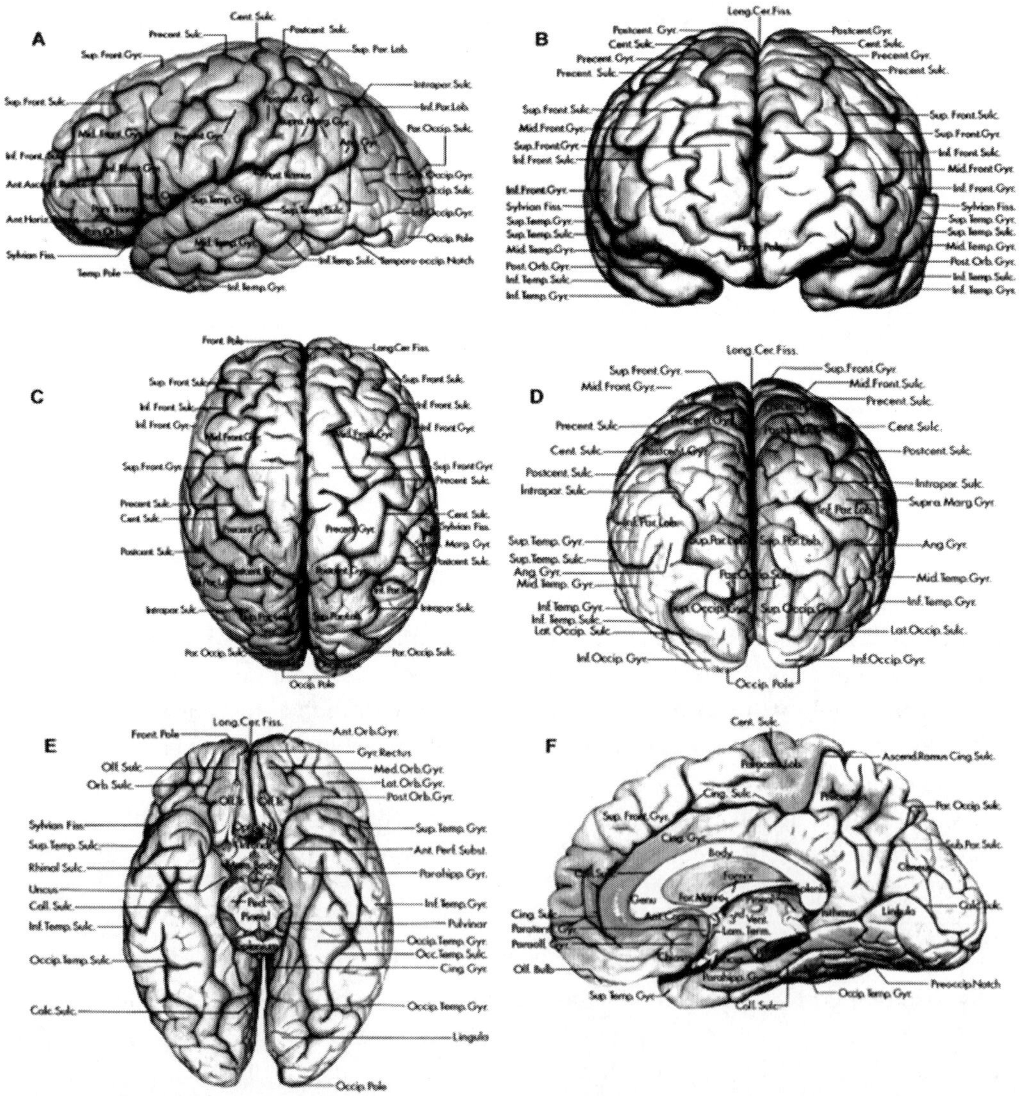

Figure 7.3. Lateral, medial, and inferior surfaces of the cerebral hemispheres. A–D, lateral surface (A, lateral view; B, anterior view; C, superior view; D, posterior view). E, inferior surface. F, medial surface. Taken with permission from the Rhoton Collection.

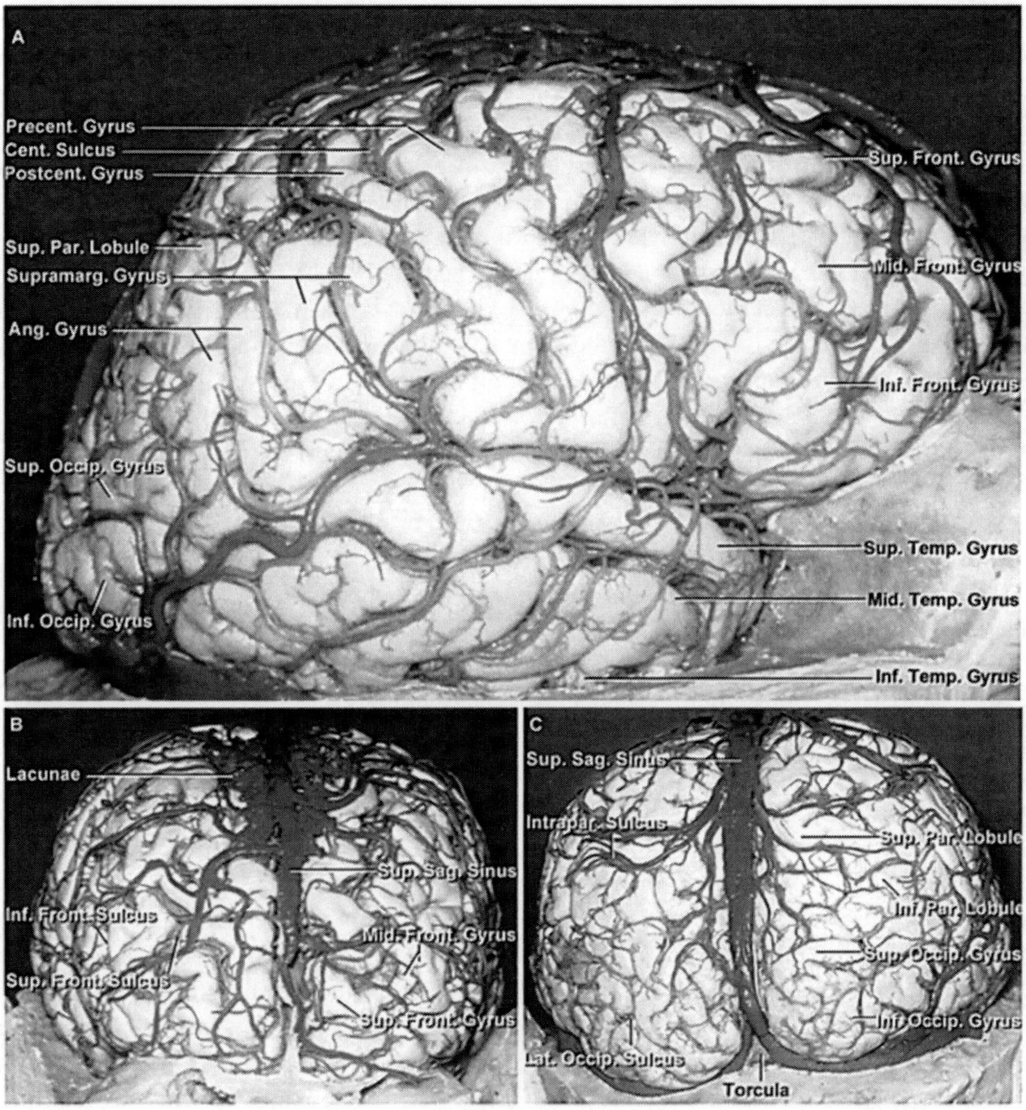

Figure 7.4. Lateral view of the right cerebral hemisphere. A, the brain exposed carefully. B, anterior view. C, posterior view of the hemisphere. Ang., angular; Cent., central; Front., frontal; Inf., inferior; Intrapar., intraparietal; Lat., lateral; Mid., middle; Occip., occipital; Par., parietal; Postcent., postcentral; Precent., precentral; Sag., sagittal; Sup., superior; Supramarg., supramarginal; Temp., temporal. Taken with permission from the Rhoton Collection.

7.4.2. Gross Neuro-Anatomy

The cerebral hemispheres have three surfaces: lateral, medial, and basal (Figure 7.3-7.5). The lateral surface, referred to as the convexity, faces the cranial cap. The medial surface of the frontal, parietal, and occipital lobes faces the falx cerebri medially, and the medial surface of the temporal lobe faces the lateral aspect of the midbrain. The basal surface faces the floor of the anterior and middle cranial fossae and the tentorium. The three borders separate the three cerebral surfaces. The superior border follows along the course of the superior sagittal sinus and upper edge of the interhemispheric fissure from the frontal to the occipital pole and separates the lateral convexity from the medial surface. The lateral border has anterior and posterior parts. The anterior part extends from the frontal pole along the lateral border of the basal surface of the frontal lobe to the sylvian fissure and separates the lateral and orbital surfaces of the frontal lobe. The posterior part of the lateral border has a gentle upward convexity that extends along and conforms to the lateral edge of the middle fossa floor and tentorium, and anteriorly turns upward around the temporal pole to reach the sylvian fissure. It separates the lateral surface of the temporal and occipital lobes from the basal surface that rests on the cranial base and tentorium.

The medial border extends from the frontal to the occipital pole and has frontal and occipital parts. The frontal part extends in a straight line from the frontal pole to the lamina terminalis and separates the medial from the orbital surface of the frontal lobe. The occipital part of the medial border lies in the angle between the falx cerebri and tentorium cerebelli and extends parallel to the straight sinus from the occipital pole to just below the splenium of the corpus callosum, separating the medial and basal surfaces of the occipital lobe. Refer to tables 7.2-7.4 for gross anatomical features of each surface.

Although differences in the gyri and sulci can be identified between any two hemispheres, close inspection reveals a basic arrangement within which variations exist. The sylvian fissure and central sulcus are the most important landmarks on the lateral surface. The sylvian fissure is the most distinct and consistent landmark on the lateral surface. It is a complex fissure that carries the middle cerebral artery and its branches and provides a surgical gateway connecting the cerebral surface to the anterior part of the basal surface and cranial base. The sylvian fissure is not a simple longitudinal cleft as its name implies (Figure 7.3-7.5). It crosses both the basal and lateral cerebral surface and has a superficial and a deep part. The superficial part is visible on the surface of the brain and the deep part, often referred to as the sylvian cistern, is hidden below the basal surface. The central sulcus, which separates the motor and sensory areas and the frontal and parietal lobes, follows in constancy after the sylvian fissure. It begins at the superior border of the lateral surface extending onto the medial surface of the hemisphere in nearly 90% of cases. It intersects the upper hemispheric border approximately 2 cm behind the midpoint between the frontal and occipital poles. Below, it usually ends approximately 2.0 to 2.5 cm behind the anterior ascending ramus of the sylvian fissure without intersecting the sylvian fissure.

The frontal convexity is made up of the superior, middle, and inferior frontal and precentral gyri. The parietal convexity is composed of the postcentral gyrus and the superior and inferior parietal lobules. The inferior parietal lobule is made up of the supramarginal and angular gyrus. The temporal convexity is composed of the superior, middle, and inferior temporal gyri. The occipital convexity is formed by the superior and inferior occipital gyri. The superior and middle frontal gyri are separated by the superior frontal sulcus. The inferior frontal sulcus courses between the middle and inferior frontal gyri. The veins from the anterior part of the hemisphere are directed backward to reach the superior sagittal sinus. The lateral occipital sulcus divides the lateral aspect of the occipital lobe into the superior and inferior occipital gyri. The posterior part of the parietal lobe is divided by the intraparietal sulcus into the superior and inferior parietal lobules.

Table 7.2. Gross Neuroanatomy - Lateral Cerebral Hemispheral Surface

<table>
<tr><td rowspan="2">Lateral sulcus</td><td colspan="5">Begins inferiorly in the sylvian fossa, extending obliquely posteriorly, separating the frontal and temporal lobes. Caudally it separates portions of the parietal and temporal lobes. It has anterior, ascending and posterior rami.
Its terminal posterior ramus, extends into the parietal lobe</td></tr>
<tr><td>Opercular portion</td><td colspan="4">The portions of the frontal, parietal and temporal lobes adjacent to it, overlying the insular region.</td></tr>
<tr><td>Central sulcus</td><td colspan="5">Running from the superior margins down and forward towards the lateral sulcus, usually bowed in two locations. Superiorly, it does not extend onto the medial surface of the hemisphere. It constitutes the border between frontal and parietal lobes</td></tr>
<tr><td rowspan="7">Frontal lobe</td><td colspan="5">Largest lobe, extending rostrally from the central sulcus. Its inferior border is the lateral sulcus</td></tr>
<tr><td>Precentral gyrus</td><td colspan="4">Parallel to the central sulcus, bordered anteriorly by the precentral sulcus. Regions rostral to it are the premotor and prefrontal areas.</td></tr>
<tr><td rowspan="5">Horizontal Gyri</td><td colspan="4">Superior gyrus</td></tr>
<tr><td>Middle gyrus</td><td colspan="3">Broad, divided by a shallow sulcus into upper and lower tiers.</td></tr>
<tr><td rowspan="3">Inferior gyrus</td><td rowspan="3">Divided by the anterior and ascending rami of the lateral sulcus into three:</td><td colspan="2">Pars orbitale</td></tr>
<tr><td>Pars triangularis</td><td rowspan="2">In the dominant hemisphere it is referred to as Broca's speech area</td></tr>
<tr><td>Pars opercularis</td></tr>
<tr><td rowspan="8">Parietal lobe</td><td colspan="5">Less defined borders except the anterior central sulcus.</td></tr>
<tr><td rowspan="2">Posterior border</td><td colspan="4">It is the parieto-occipital sulcus on medial aspect of the hemisphere</td></tr>
<tr><td colspan="4">On lateral surface surface it is a line projecting from the superior limit of the parieto-occipital sulcus to the small indentation on the inferior surface, the preoccipital notch.</td></tr>
<tr><td rowspan="2">Postcentral gyrus</td><td colspan="4">Parallel and caudal to central sulcus, usually not continuous and broken into Superior and inferior segments. The sulcus demarcates the caudal limit of the paracentral lobule. It is the primary sensory cortex.</td></tr>
<tr><td colspan="4">Most neurons here deal with fixed receptive fields, which are place specific, modality specific, relating to discriminative aspects of sensation.</td></tr>
<tr><td rowspan="3">Inferior lobule</td><td colspan="2">Supramarginal gyrus</td><td colspan="2">At banks of posterior ramus of lateral sulcus.</td></tr>
<tr><td colspan="2">Angular gyrus</td><td colspan="2">Surrounds ascending terminal of superior temporal sulcus.</td></tr>
<tr><td colspan="4">It represents a cortical association area, where multisensory signals from parietal, temporal, occipital regions converge.</td></tr>
<tr><td rowspan="6">Temporal lobe</td><td colspan="5">Lies inferior to lateral sulcus and has three oblique convolutions (superior, middle and inferior gyri)</td></tr>
<tr><td colspan="3">Superior sulcus</td><td colspan="2">Its posterior ascending ramus terminates in the angular gyrus.</td></tr>
<tr><td colspan="3">Transverse gyrus of Heschl</td><td colspan="2">The primary auditory cortex</td></tr>
<tr><td rowspan="3">Inferior surface</td><td colspan="2">Inferior temporal gyrus</td><td colspan="2">Lateral</td></tr>
<tr><td colspan="2">Occipitotemporal gyrus</td><td colspan="2">Has lateral and medial gyri</td></tr>
<tr><td colspan="2">Parahippocampal gyrus</td><td colspan="2">Its medial protrusion (uncus) is separated by the collateral sulcus from the occipitotemporal gyrus.</td></tr>
</table>

Table 7.2. (Continued)

			Uncus	With the lateral olfactory stria forms the pyriform lobe (primary olfactory cortex).
Occipital lobe	Rests on the tentorium cerebelli, constitutes the caudal pole, bounded rostrally by the parieto-occipital sulcus. Its lateral surface is not clearly separated from the parietal lobe, has irregular occipital gyri, separated to groups by more constant lateral occipital sulcus.			
	Calcarine sulcus	On medial aspect, divides the lobe into the cuneus and lingual gyri. It joins the parieto-occipital sulcus in a "Y"-shaped form.		
		Cortex on both its banks is the primary visual cortex.		
	The visual cortex receives inputs from the temporal half of the ipsilateral retina and nasal half of contralateral retina, concerned with perception from contralateral half of the visual field.			
	Upper ½ of retina	fibers terminate on superior bank of the calcarine sulcus		
	Lower ½ of retina	fibers terminate on inferior bank of the calcarine sulcus		
Insula	Invaginated cortical area, buried in the depths of the lateral sulcus, covered by the temporal, parietal and frontal opercular regions. A triangular cortical area, whose apex is directed antero-inferiorly to open into the lateral fossa, the limen Insula.			
	Gyrus breves & gyrus longus	Cover the surface, course parallel to the lateral sulcus		

Table 7.3. Gross Neuroanatomy – Medial Cerebral Hemispheral Surface

Corpus Callosum	The most prominent structure, composed of myelinated fibers, reciprocally interconnects nearly all cortical regions of the two hemispheres. Callosal fibers projecting to parts of frontal and occipital lobes form the Anterior and posterior forceps. Forms the floor of the longitudinal fissure and the roof of the lateral ventricle.	
	Parts	Rostrum, genu, body, splenium (see later in the text).
	Its complete sectioning shows a striking independence of the two hemispheres in perceptual, cognitive, mnemonic, learned, volitional activities (information perceived in the non-dominant hemisphere being unable to be communicated in speech/writing, but no problem in speech and analytic capability, if they arise in the dominant hemisphere).	
Callosal sulcus	Separates the corpus callosum from the cingulate gyrus. Posteriorly, it curves around the splenium, to continue as the hippocampal sulcus.	
Cingulate gyrus	Dorsal to callosal sulcus, it encircles the corpus callosum. It consists of two tiers.	
Paracentral lobule	Formed by the precentral and postcentral gyri extending onto medial hemispheral surface.	
Precuneus	The portion of the parietal lobe caudal to the paracentral lobule, and rostral to the Parieto-occipital sulcus.	

Table 7.4. Gross Neuroanatomy – Inferior Cerebral Hemispheral Surface

1.	Larger portion, the inferior surfaces of temporal and occipital lobes (lying on the tentorium cerebelli, while rostral temporal lobe, lies in Mid. Cranial fossa).	
	Gyri	Lingual
		Occipitotemporal
		Parahippocampal and Uncus
		Inferior temporal gyrus lies lateral to occipitotemporal gyrus, while the narrow isthmus of the Cingulate gyrus lies medial-posteriorly to the splenium of corpus callosum.
2.	It has a deep, straight sulcus medially (the olfactory sulcus), containing both the olfactory bulb and tract.	
	Gyrus rectus	Along the ventromedial margin of the frontal lobe, medially to the olfactory sulcus.
	The region laterally to the olfactory sulcus contains the orbital gyri.	
	Caudally is the olfactory trigone, Anterior perforated substance (a region with small openings, through which many small arteries pass to subcortical structures).	

7.4.3.1. Stepwise Dissection of the Cerebral Hemisphere

The inferior frontal gyrus is composed of the pars orbitalis, pars opercularis, and pars triangularis. The precentral gyrus borders the sylvian fissure behind the pars opercularis. As seen in figure 7.5s, the sylvian fissure extends backward and turns up into the supramarginal gyrus at its posterior end. The lower part of the postcentral gyrus is positioned in front of the anterior bank of the supramarginal gyrus. The posterior bank of the supramarginal gyrus is continuous with the superior temporal gyrus. There is commonly a gyral bridge (arrow) connecting the pre- and postcentral gyri below the lower end of the central sulcus, so that the central sulcus does not open directly into the sylvian fissure. The angular gyrus wraps around the upturned posterior end of the superior temporal sulcus. As shown in figure 7.5b, The inferior frontal sulcus is located on the convexity at the deep level of the lower margin of the corpus callosum and roof of the frontal horn. The gray matter of the cingulate sulcus is exposed above the corpus callosum.

The insula (shown in figure 7.5c) is defined at its outer margin by the circular or limiting sulcus. The insular gyri radiate upward and backward from the anteroinferior angle situated just lateral to the limen insulae (figure 7.5d+e). The short gyri are located deep to the pars triangularis and opercularis. Heschl's gyrus, the most anterior of the transverse temporal gyri, faces the lower end of the postcentral gyrus across the sylvian fissure. The pre- and postcentral gyri are located lateral to the body of the ventricle and the splenium of the corpus callosum (figure 7.5f). The foramen of Monro is located deep to a point on the pars opercularis approximately 1 cm above the sylvian fissure and deep to the midlevel of the short gyri of the insula.

In a posterior view of the hemisphere (figure 7.5i), the splenium is seen located deep in the interhemispheric fissure. The parieto-occipital and calcarine sulcus converge behind the splenium to give the medial surface a Y-shaped configuration. The parieto-occipital sulcus separates the pre-cuneus and cuneus, and the calcarine sulcus separates the cuneus and lingula. The lingula, shown in figure 7.5j, forms the lower bank of the calcarine sulcus. The calcar avis is a prominence in the lower part of the medial atrial wall overlying the calcarine sulcus. The ascending ramus of the cingulate sulcus (figure 7.5k) marks the posterior edge of the paracentral lobule, the extension of the pre- and postcentral gyri onto the medial surface of the hemisphere. As shown in figure 7.5l, the outer edge of the choroidal fissure is formed by the body of the fornix in the body of the ventricle, the crus of the fornix in the atrium, and the fimbria of the fornix in the temporal horn.

As shown in figure 7.5m, the body, crus, and fimbria of the fornix, forming the outer margin of the choroidal fissure, have been preserved. The stria medullaris thalami marks the lower edge of the velum interpositum, in which the internal cerebral veins course. In figure 7.5n, the pineal gland and posterior commissure are exposed at the posterior margin and the anterior commissure and columns of the fornix are exposed at the anterior margin of the third ventricle.

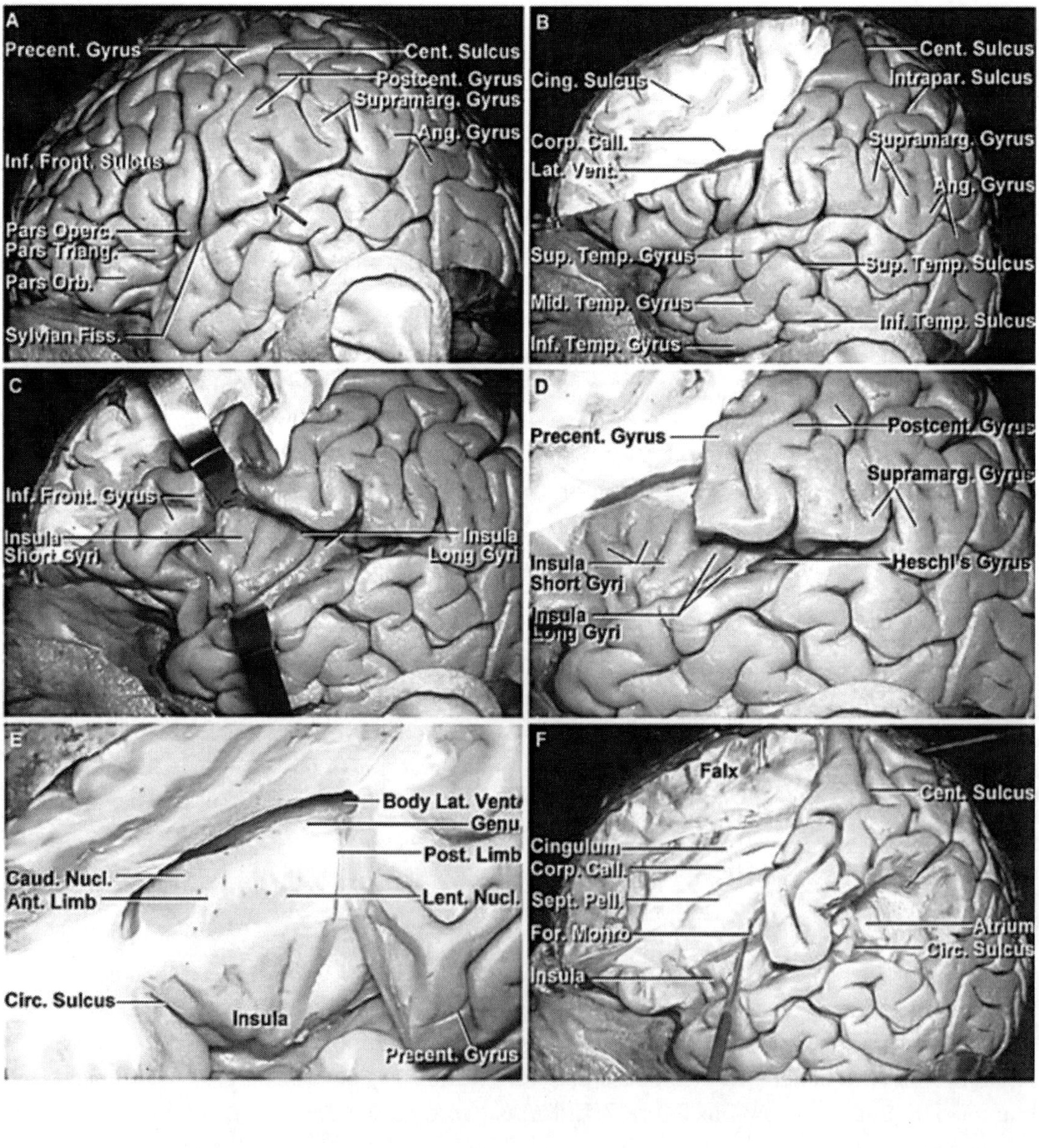

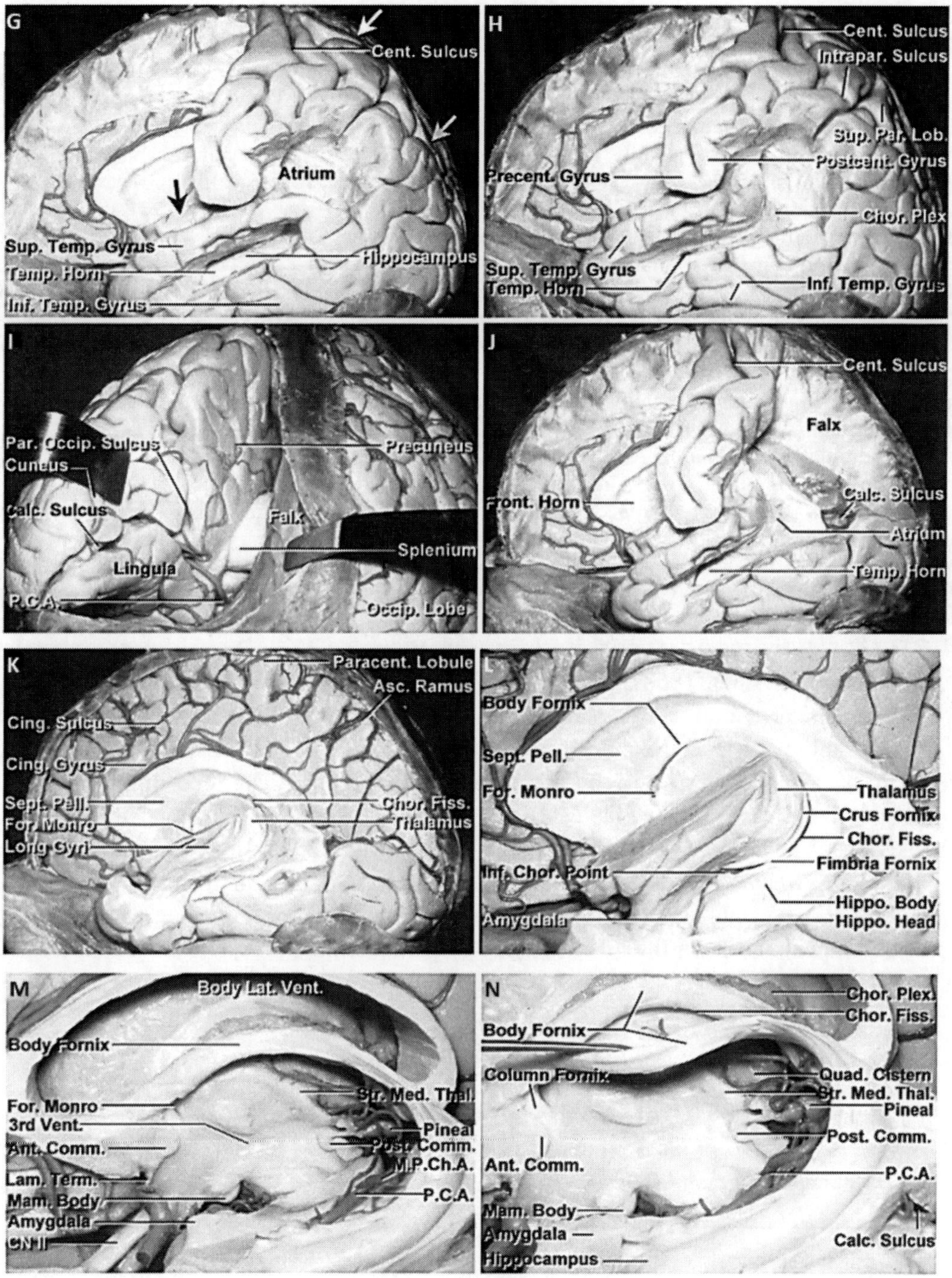

Figure 7.5 A-F. Stepwise dissection of the left cerebral hemisphere. A, Lateral Convexity view. B, the part of the frontal lobe above the inferior frontal gyrus and in front of the precentral sulcus has been removed. C, The opercular lips have been retracted to expose the insula. D, enlarged view with the brain in front of the precentral gyrus removed. E, anterosuperior view of the central core of the hemisphere located deep to the insulae. The circular sulcus surrounds the insula. F, the supramarginal gyrus has been removed to show its location superficial to the atrium. G, The temporal horn and hippocampus are located medial to the middle temporal gyrus, a segment of which has been removed. The black arrow is on the foramen of Monro. The white arrow is located where the upper end of the

ascending ramus of the cingulate sulcus reaches the superior hemispheric border. The light gray arrow is where the upper end of the parieto-occipital sulcus reaches the superior border. H, the remaining bridge of the superior temporal gyrus located superficial to the junction of the atrium and temporal horn has been removed. I, posterior view of the left hemisphere. J, the parietal lobe, above the level of the calcarine sulcus, has been removed. The upper lip of the calcarine sulcus, formed by the cuneus, has been removed to expose the lingula. K, the superior temporal gyrus has been removed. L, enlarged view of the choroidal fissure. The choroid plexus, which attaches along the choroidal fissure, has been removed. M, the thalamus has been removed to expose the third ventricle. The body, crus, and fimbria of the fornix, forming the outer margin of the choroidal fissure, have been preserved. N, the left half of the body of the fornix has been folded downward to expose the right half of the body and medial aspect of the contralateral choroidal fissure located between the body of the fornix and the upper surface of the thalamus. A., artery; A.C.A., anterior cerebral artery; Ang., angular; Ant., anterior; Asc., ascending; Calc., calcar, calcarine; Call., callosum; Caud., caudate; Cent., central; Chor., choroid, choroidal; Cing., cingulate; Circ., circular; CN, cranial nerve; Comm., commissure; Corp., corpus; Fiss., fissure; For., foramen; Front., frontal; Gen., geniculate; Glob., globus; Hippo., hippocampal; Inf., inferior; Intrapar., intraparietal; Lam., lamina; Lat., lateral; Lent., lenticular, lentiform; Lob., lobule; M.P.Ch.A., medial posterior choroidal artery; Mam., mamillary; Med., medullaris; Mid., middle; Nucl., nucleus; Occip., occipital; Operc., opercularis; Orb., orbitalis; P.C.A., posterior cerebral artery; Pall., pallidus; Par., parietal; Paracent., paracentral; Par. Occip., parieto-occipital; Pell., pellucidum; Plex., plexus; Post., posterior; Post-cent., postcentral; Precent., precentral; Quad., quadrigeminal; Sept., septum; Str., stria; Sup., superior; Supramarg., supramarginal; Temp., temporal; Term., terminalis; Thal., thalamic, thalamus; Triang., triangularis; Vent., ventricle. Taken with permission from the Rhoton Collection.

7.4.3.2. The Brodmann Areas

Korbinian Brodmann (1868-1918) was a German neuroanatomist. During the years 1901-1910 Brodmann carried out a systematic study of cerebral cortex histology using brain slices and Nissl staining. Based on subtle differences in cortex histology Brodmann divided the cortex into 47 areas, each given a number accordingly. To this date these numbers are still used, furthermore, many of these areas have since been found to have specific functional characteristics. The 21th century medical student is still in need of a working knowledge of the Brodmann Areas and numbering system due to its rooting in medical language and terminology. Refer to table 7.5 and figure 7.6 for a complete list of the Brodmann areas and at to table 7.6 for a summary of the functional areas of the brain.

Table 7.5. The Brodmann Areas

Area number	Assigned function
1,2, 3	Primary Somatosensory Cortex (frequently referred to as Areas 3, 1, 2).
4	Primary Motor Cortex.
5	Somatosensory Association Cortex.
6	Pre-Motor and Supplementary Motor Cortex.
7	Somatosensory Association Cortex.
8	Includes Frontal eye fields.
9	Dorsolateral prefrontal cortex.
10	Frontopolar area.
11	Orbitofrontal area.
12	Orbitofrontal area.
13	Insular cortex
17	Primary Visual Cortex (V1)
18	Visual Association Cortex (V2)

Area number	Assigned function
19	Visual Association Cortex (V3)
20	Inferior Temporal Gyrus
21	Middle Temporal Gyrus
22	Superior Temporal Gyrus. Its rostral part participates in Wernicke's area
23	Ventral Anterior Cingulate Cortex
24	Ventral Posterior Cingulate Cortex
25	Subgenual Cortex
26	Ectosplenial area
28	Posterior Entorhinal Cortex
29	Retrosplenial Cingular Cortex
30	Part of Cingular Cortex
31	Dorsal Posterior Cingular Cortex
32	Dorsal Anterior Cingulate Cortex
34	Anterior Entorhinal Cortex (on the Parahippocampal gyrus)
35	Perirhinal Cortex (on the Parahippocampal gyrus)
36	Parahippocampal Cortex (on the Parahippocampal gyrus)
37	Fusiform Gyrus
38	Temporopolar area (most rostral part of superior and middle temporal gyri)
39	Angular Gyrus, part of Wernicke's area
40	Supramarginal Gyrus part of Wernicke's area
41, 42	Primary and Auditory Association Cortex
43	Subcentral area (between insula and post/precentral gyrus)
44	Pars Opercularis, part of Broca's area
45	Pars Triangularis Broca's area
46	Dorsolateral Prefrontal cortex
47	Inferior Prefrontal gyrus
48	Retrosubicular area (a small part of the medial surface of the temporal lobe)
52	Parainsular area (Junction of temporal lobe and the insula)

Table 7.6. Functional Areas of the Brain

Functions	Center	Brodmann area
Vision	Primary cortex	17
	Secondary cortex	18, 19, 20, 21, 37
Audition	Primary cortex	41
	Secondary cortex	22, 42
Body sensation	Primary cortex	1, 2, 3
	Secondary cortex	5, 7
	Tertiary cortex	7, 22, 37, 39, 40
Motor	Primary cortex	4
	Secondary cortex	6
	Eye movement	8
	Speech	44
	Tertiary	9, 10, 11, 45, 46, 47

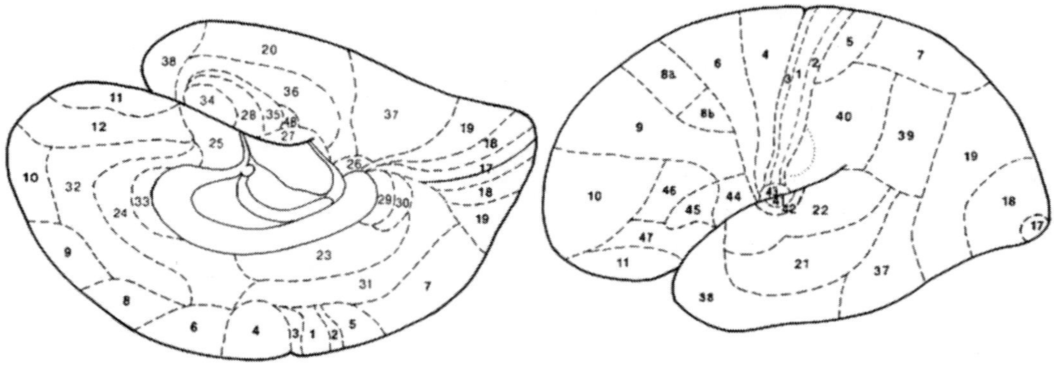

Figure 7.6. The Brodmann areas. Refer to text. Taken from Gray's Anatomy (out of copyright and in the public domain).

7.4.3.3. The Sensory and Motor Homunculi

Wilder Graves Penfield (1891 –1976) treated patients with severe epilepsy by destroying nerve cells in the brain where the seizures originated. Before operating, he stimulated the brain with electrical probes while the patients were conscious and under local anesthesia to more accurately target affected brain regions while minimizing surgery-inflicted damage. This technique allowed him to create maps of the sensory and motor cortices of the brain showing their connections to the various limbs and organs of the body. These maps are still used today, practically unaltered since their original publication in 1951. The relative size of the different body parts in the homunculi is proportional to nerve units to or from that region, and not to actual size. Thus, the palm, in which each motor unit consists of only a few muscle spindles (for better coordination) generates as much motor units almost as the entire trunk. Similarly, sensory receptors for modalities of light touch are tightly arranged in the palm, creating only a very narrow small territory for each receptor and generate many sensory units to the primary sensory cortex, similar in magnitude to the trunk as well. Refer to figure 7.7.

7.4.4. White Matter Hemispheral Anatomy

7.4.4.1. Association Fibers

There are two types of association fibers: short arcuate fibers that interconnect adjacent gyri and long arcuate fibers that interconnect widely separated gyri, at times located in different lobes of the same hemisphere. The long arcuate fibers are situated deep to the short fibers and form several bundles. We will describe a few major association fiber bundles.

Current day functional imaging (diffusion tensor imaging MRI) is able to present these white matter anatomical features, depending on the knowledge of the examiner in defining the anatomy of the tract. Thus, the neuroanatomy of current ages puts much more emphasis on white matter anatomy than before.

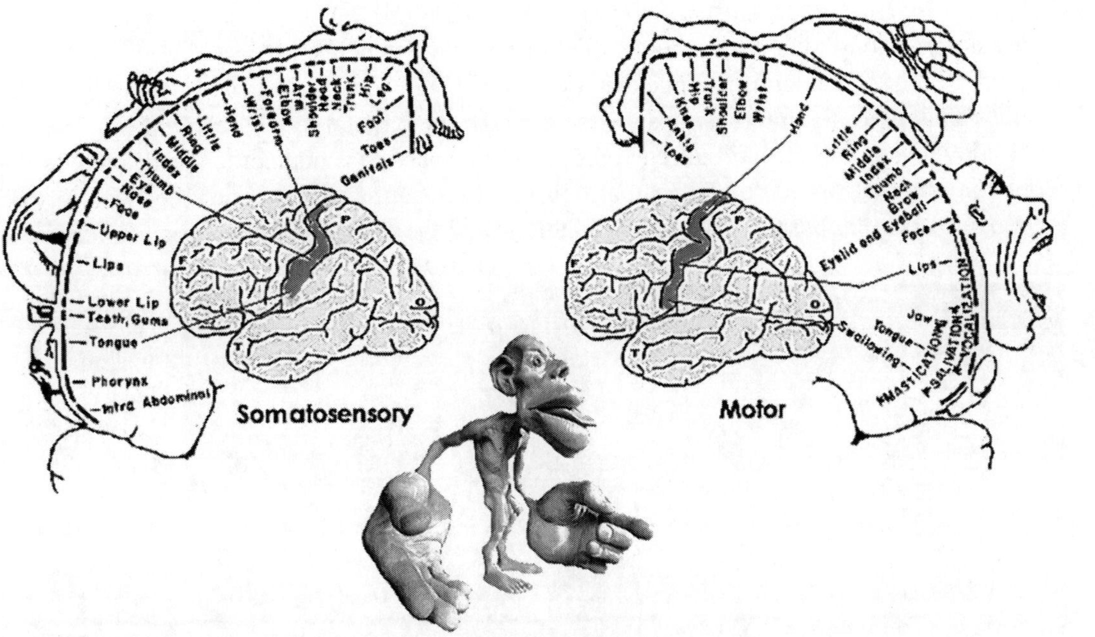

Figure 7.7. The Homunculi. Left – The sensory homunculus in coronal section through the primary sensory cortex with body representation. Right – the motor homunculus in coronal section through the primary motor cortex with body representation. Middle – the disproportionate way the brain perceives the body, based on neural representation. Taken from Gray's Anatomy (out of copyright and in the public domain).

7.4.4.1.1. The Uncinate Fasciculus

The uncinate fasciculus is a hook-shaped bundle of fibers that curves around the stem of the sylvian fissure and connects the frontal and temporal lobes (Figure 7.8). It is located at the lateral edge of the anterior perforated substance bordering the anteroinferior part of the insula. Its fibers course through the limen insulae and produce the prominence at the junction of the sphenoidal and operculoinsular compartments of the sylvian fissure. The uncinate fasciculus has an upper and a lower component. The lower part connects the gyri on the orbital surface of the frontal lobe with the parahippocampal and other gyri on the medial surface of the temporal lobe. The upper component unites gyri on the superolateral part of the frontal lobe with the cortex of the more lateral temporal gyri near the temporal pole.

7.4.4.1.2. The Cingulum

The cingulum courses along the medial aspect of the cerebral hemisphere, following the curve of and forming much of the white matter within the cingulate gyrus (Figures 7.8-7.11). It contains both long- and short-association fibers that follow the curve of the cingulate gyrus and corpus callosum. It interconnects the subcallosal and paraolfactory areas located below the anterior part of the corpus callosum, the cingulate gyrus above the corpus callosum, and the isthmus of the cingulate sulcus and parahippocampal gyri located behind and below the corpus callosum.

7.4.4.1.3. The Superior Longitudinal Fasciculus (SLF)

The superior longitudinal fasciculus, the largest of the bundles, is located along the upper and lateral border of the lentiform nucleus and insula (Figs. 7.8). It arches backward from the frontal lobe lateral to the internal capsule and through the parietal to the occipital lobe, where it arches downward and forward to reach the temporal lobe. Less distinct fasciculi include the inferior longitudinal fasciculus (ILF) that courses near but separated from the walls of the temporal and occipital horns by the optic radiations and the tapetum of the corpus callosum.

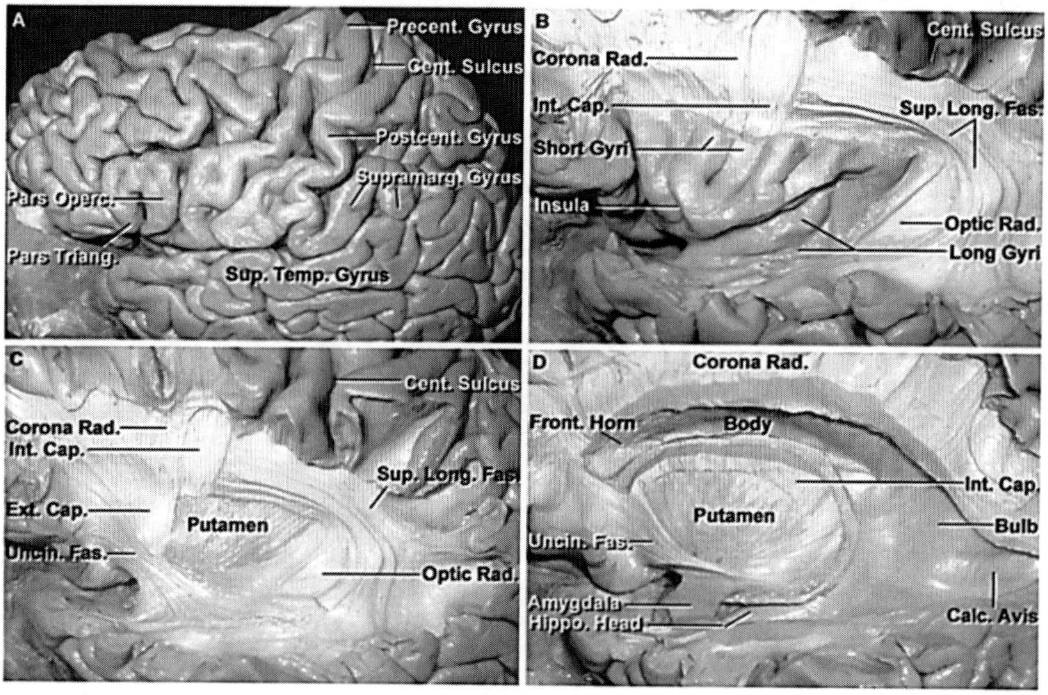

Figure 7.8. Stepwise fiber dissection. A, left cerebral hemisphere. B, the frontal, parietal, and temporal operculi have been removed to expose the insula. C, the claustrum and the posterior part of the external capsule have been removed to expose the putamen. The anterior part of the external capsule has been preserved. D, the frontal horn, body, atrium, and temporal horn of the lateral ventricle have been exposed. The fibers of the external capsule superficial to the putamen have been removed.

7.4.4.2. Projection Fibers

The projection fibers pass up and down the neural axis. Above the level of the thalamus, these projection fibers are arranged in a radiating pattern called the corona radiata (Figures 4.9-4.10). The corona radiate is continuous caudally with the more compact internal capsule whose fibers collect to form the cerebral peduncle. The internal capsule is a thick mass of white matter that is bounded laterally by the lentiform nucleus and medially by the caudate nucleus and the thalamus. The internal capsule has anterior and posterior limbs, a genu, and retro- and sublenticular parts (refer to chapter 4). The internal capsule bends at a right angle around the medial margin of the pallidal part of the lentiform nucleus to form an anterior limb, located between the caudate nucleus medially and the lentiform nucleus laterally, and a posterior limb, interposed between the thalamus medially and the lentiform nucleus laterally. The two limbs join at the genu, where the fibers wrap around the medial apex of the globus pallidus. The medially directed apex is located lateral to the foramen of Monro, where the fibers in the genu reach the wall of the ventricle in the interval between the caudate nucleus and thalamus.

The anterior limb is composed predominantly of fibers that connect the anterior and medial thalamus and the pontine nuclei to the frontal lobe. The genu of the internal capsule, in addition to the corticothalamic and thalamocortical fibers, contains corticobulbar fibers to the motor nuclei of the cranial nerves. The posterior limb, in addition to fibers interconnecting the thalamus and cortex, contains the corticospinal fibers to the motor nuclei of the upper and lower extremity and trunk. The fibers to the arm are nearer the genu than those coursing to the leg. The precentral gyrus is positioned superficial to the posterior limb.

Some fibers of the internal capsule curve around the posterior edge of the lentiform nucleus and are referred to as the retrolenticular fibers and others pass below the lentiform nucleus and are referred to as sublenticular fibers. The sublenticular part of the posterior limb contains the auditory radiation fibers directed from the medial geniculate body to the auditory area in the transverse temporal and adjacent parts of the superior temporal gyri and part of the optic radiations that course from the lateral geniculate to the walls of the calcarine sulcus. Some optic radiation fibers also pass through the retrolenticular part of the internal capsule, but most pass through the sublenticular part.

The optic radiations are separated from the roof and lateral wall of the temporal horn and the lateral atrial wall by only a thin layer of tapetal fibers. The fibers passing to the superior bank of the calcarine fissure leave the upper part of the lateral geniculate body and course almost directly posterior around the lateral aspect of the atrium to reach the striate visual cortex. Fibers from the lower part of the geniculate body destined for the inferior bank of the calcarine fissure initially loop forward and downward in the temporal lobe, forming Meyer's loop, before turning back to join the other fibers in the optic radiations. The fibers of the optic radiation are divided into anterior, middle, and posterior groups (Figure 7.8). The anterior fibers, called Meyer's loop, subserve the upper half of the visual field. The middle fibers, subserving the macula, course laterally above the roof of the temporal horn and turn posteriorly along the lateral wall of the atrium and the occipital horn. The posterior fibers responsible for the lower visual field course directly backward along the lateral wall of the atrium and the occipital horn to end in the upper lip of the calcarine fissure.

7.4.4.3. Stepwise Fiber Dissection

As shown in figure 7.8a+b, The corona radiata and some of the fibers joining the internal capsule are exposed above the insula. The superior longitudinal fasciculus courses around the outer margin of the insula and lentiform nucleus. The retrolenticular part of the optic radiation is exposed behind the insula and deep to the superior longitudinal fasciculus. In figure 7.8c, the claustrum and the posterior part of the external capsule have been removed to expose the putamen. The anterior part of the external capsule has been preserved. The uncinate fasciculus interconnects the frontal and temporal lobes. The retrolenticular part of the optic radiations is exposed behind the lentiform nucleus. The superior longitudinal fasciculus courses superficial to the optic radiations and deep to the extreme and external capsules. In figure 7.8d, the frontal horn, body, atrium, and temporal horn of the lateral ventricle have been exposed. The fibers of the external capsule superficial to the putamen have been removed. The internal capsule courses medial to the lentiform nucleus, the outer segment of which is formed by the putamen. The lower part of the uncinate fasciculus has been removed to expose amygdala and the head of the hippocampus.

7.4.4.4. Commissural Fibers

7.4.4.4.1. The Corpus Callosum

The corpus callosum is located between the hemispheres in the floor of the longitudinal fissure and the roof of the lateral ventricles (Figures 7.8-7.11). The corpus callosum, which forms the largest part of the ventricular walls, contributes to the wall of each of the five parts of the lateral ventricle. Its anterior half is situated in the midline deep to the upper part of the inferior frontal gyrus. Its posterior part, the splenium, is situated deep to the supramarginal gyrus and the lower third of the pre- and postcentral gyri.

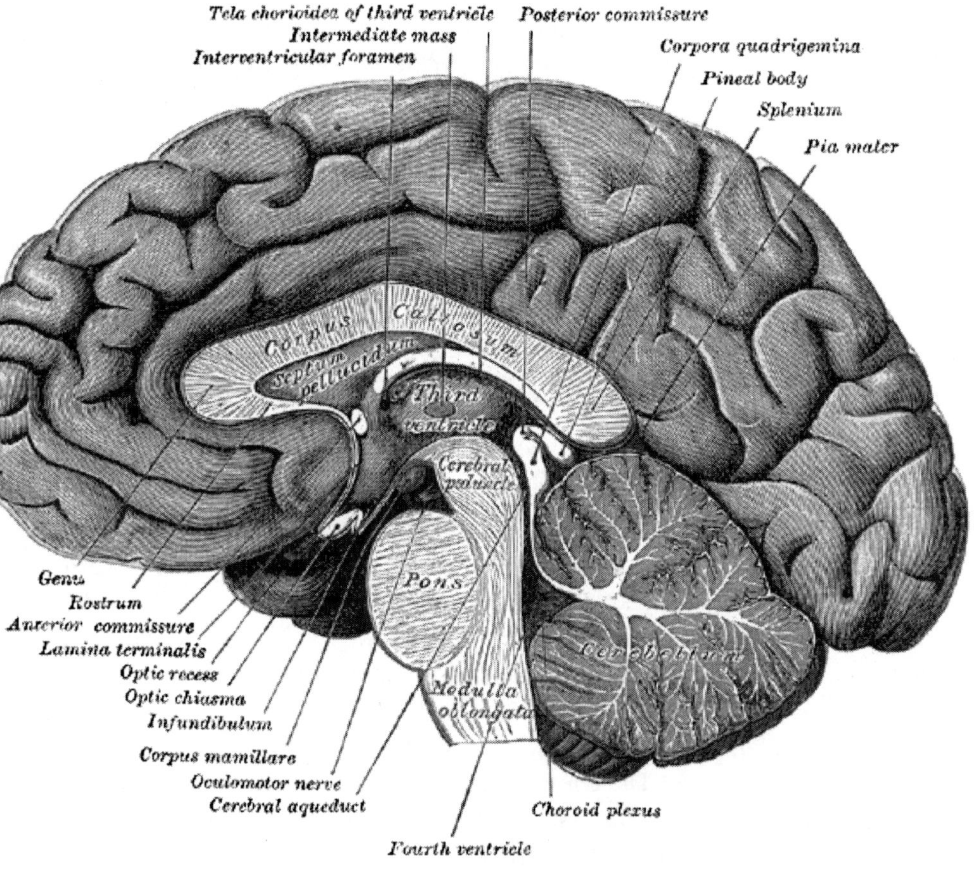

Figure 7.9. Brain (sagittal section). Taken from Gray's Anatomy (out of copyright and in the public domain).

The corpus callosum has five parts: two anterior parts, the genu and rostrum; a central part, the body; and two posterior parts, the splenium and tapetum. The curved anterior part, the genu, wraps around and forms the anterior wall and adjacent part of the roof of the frontal horn. The genu blends below into the rostrum, a thin tapered portion that forms the floor of the frontal horn and is continuous downward, in front of the anterior commissure, with the lamina terminalis. The genu gives rise to a large fiber tract, the forceps minor, which forms the anterior wall of the frontal horn and interconnects the frontal lobes. The forceps minor sweeps obliquely forward and laterally, as does the anterior wall of the frontal horn. The genu blends into the body, located above the body of the lateral ventricle. The splenium, the thick posterior end, is situated dorsal to the pineal body. The splenium gives rise to a large tract, the forceps major, which forms a prominence called the bulb in the upper part of the medial wall of the atrium and occipital horn of the ventricle. Another fiber tract, the tapetum, which arises in the posterior part of the body and splenium, sweeps laterally and inferiorly to form the roof and lateral wall of the atrium and the temporal and occipital horns. The tapetum separates the fibers of the optic radiations from the temporal horn and the atrium.

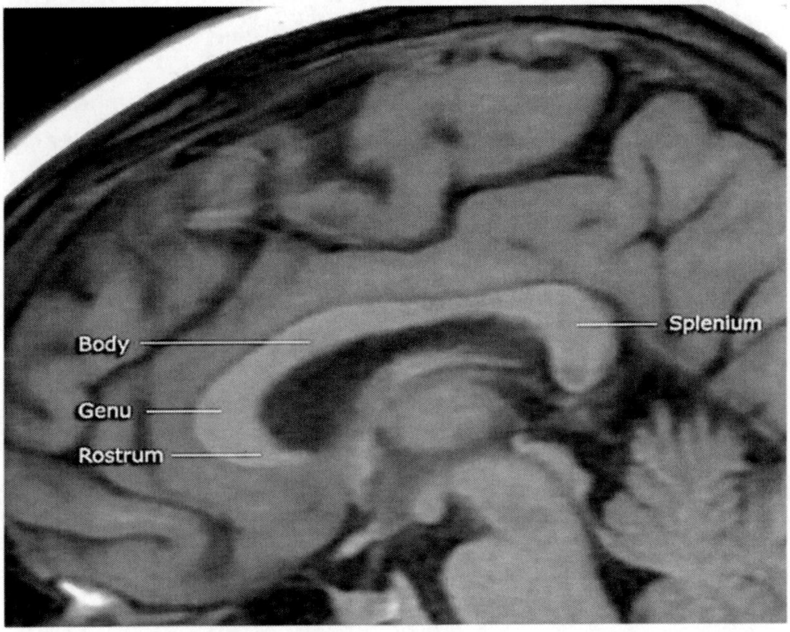

Figure 7.10. The corpus callosum, as seen in a non-gadolinium enhanced T1 weighted image. Taken with permission from www.radiopaedia.org.

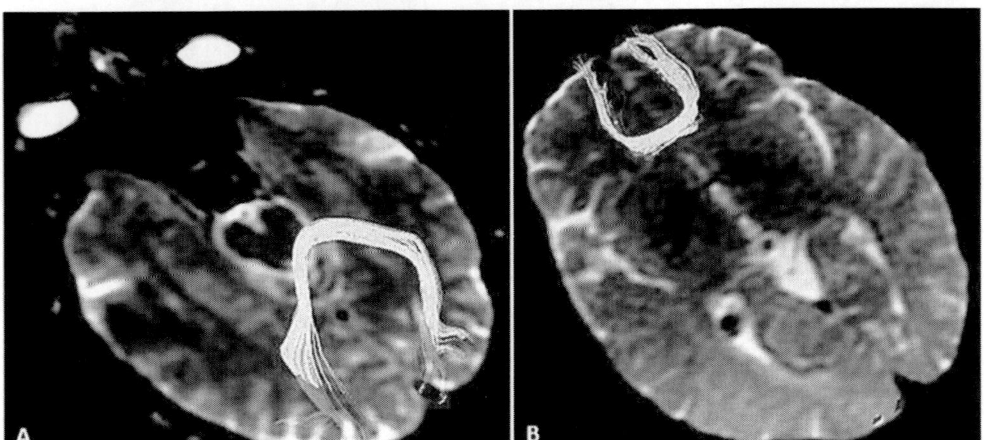

Figure 7.11. The corpus callosum, diffusion tensor imaging MRI superimposed on T2 weighted images. A, Forceps major. B, Forceps minor. Taken with permission from www.radiopaedia.org.

7.4.4.4.2. The Anterior Commissure

The anterior commissure is a small bundle that crosses the midline in front of the columns of the fornix (Figure 4.1, 4.13). It forms part of the anterior wall of the third ventricle. It is shaped somewhat like the handlebars of a bicycle. It interconnects the olfactory structures and temporal gyri on both sides.

7.4.4.4.3. The Fornix

The fornix is the main efferent pathway from the hippocampal formation. It contains both commissural and projection fibers. The fornix is a C-shaped structure that wraps around the thalamus in the wall of the lateral ventricle and has relationships with the cortical surface that are similar to those at the outer edge of the thalamus (Figures 7.12-7.14). The fornix extends from the hippocampus to the mamillary bodies and has four parts: fimbria, crus, body, and columns. It arises in the floor of the temporal horn on the ventricular surface of the hippocampus from fibers that collect along the medial edge of the hippocampus and are directed backward.

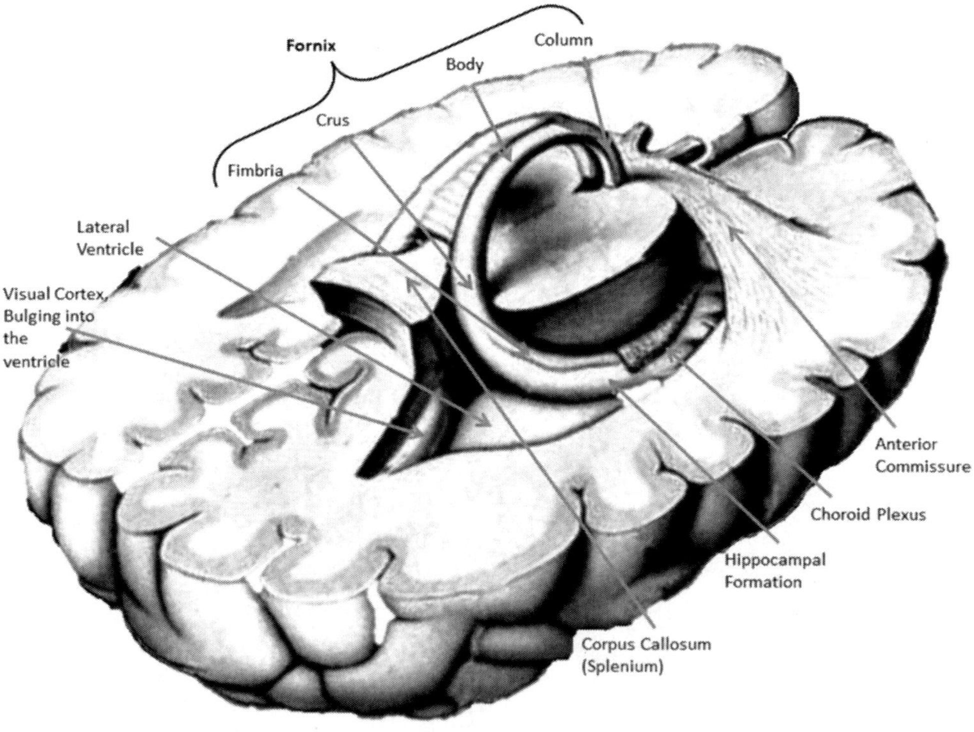

Figure 7.12. The fornix. Axial section with the fornix drawn in 3D to show its C-shaped structure. Refer to text. Taken from Gray's Anatomy (out of copyright and in the public domain).

The fimbria courses along the lateral edge of the lateral geniculate body and is separated from the geniculate body and optic and auditory radiations by the choroidal fissure. Posteriorly, the fimbria blends into the crus of the fornix that wraps around the posterior surface of the pulvinar in the medial part of the antrum and arches superomedial toward the lower surface of the splenium of the corpus callosum. At the junction between the atrium and the body of the lateral ventricle, the paired crura meet to form the body of the fornix, which passes above the thalamus and below the septum pellucidum in the lower part of the medial wall of the body of the lateral ventricle. At the anterior margin of the thalamus, the body of the fornix separates into two columns that arch along the superior and anterior margin of the foramen of Monro and blend into the walls of the third ventricle as they pass behind the anterior commissure and descend to reach the mamillary bodies. In the area below the splenium, a thin sheet of fiber, the hippocampal commissure, interconnects the medial edges of the crura of the fornix. In the body of the lateral ventricle, the body of the fornix is in the lower part of the medial wall; in the atrium, the crus of the fornix is in the medial part of the anterior wall; and in the temporal horn, the fimbria of the fornix is in the medial part of the floor.

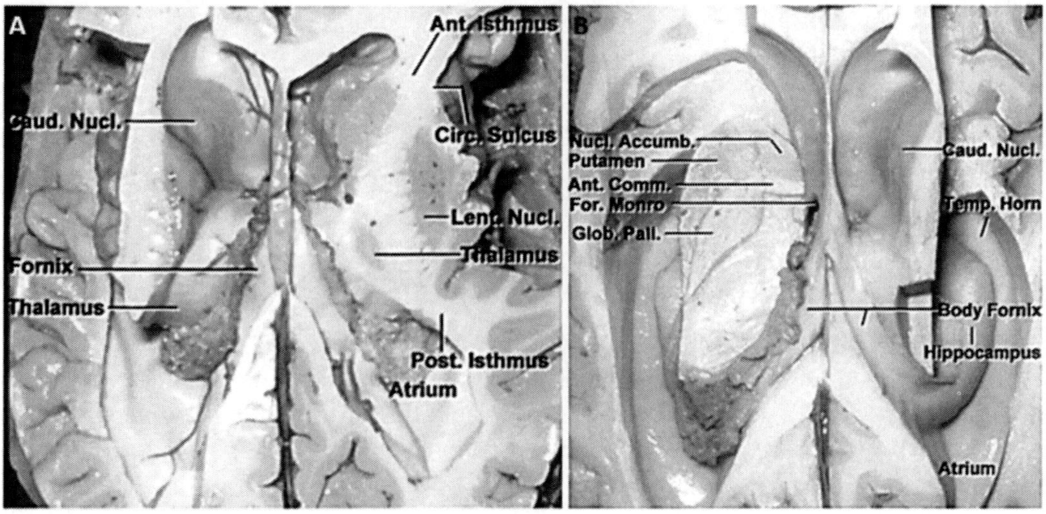

Figure 7.13. Axial cross sections of the cerebral hemisphere and central core. A, the section of the right hemisphere has been extended through the upper part of the lentiform nucleus, thalamus, and caudate head. On the left side, the axial section remains at the level of the upper edge of the circular sulcus. The anterior part of the cerebral isthmus is located between the frontal horn and anterior part of the circular sulcus and the posterior part is located between the posterior part of the circular sulcus and the anterior part of the atrium. B, the section through the left hemisphere has been extended downward below the frontal horn to the level of the anterior commissure. The anterior part of the section extends through the deep gray matter below the frontal horn anterior limb of the internal capsule. Taken with permission from the Rhoton Collection.

7.4.4.4.4. The Septum Pellucidum

The septum pellucidum stretches across the interval between the anterior parts of the corpus callosum and the body of the fornix (refer to figure 4.11). It is composed of paired laminae and separates the frontal horns and bodies of the lateral ventricles in the midline. In the frontal horn, the septum pellucidum is attached to the rostrum of the corpus callosum below, the genu anteriorly, and the body above. In the body of the lateral ventricle, the septum is attached to the body of the corpus callosum above and the body of the fornix below. The septum pellucidum disappears posteriorly where the body of the fornix meets the splenium. There may be a cavity, the cavum septum pellucidum, in the midline between the laminae of the septum pellucidum, often referred to as the fifth ventricle.

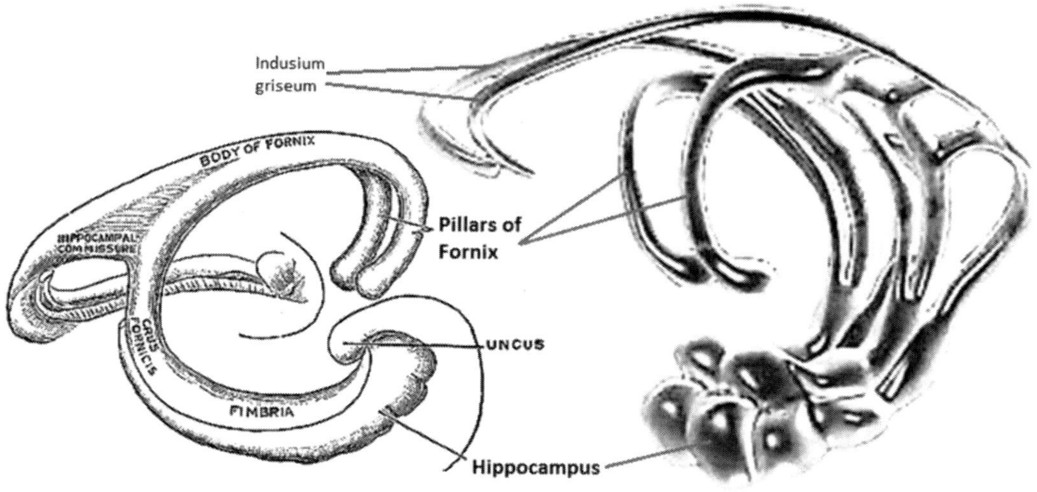

Figure 7.14. The fornix and Indusium griseum. Refer to text. Taken from Gray's Anatomy (out of copyright and in the public domain).

7.5. The Limbic System

The limbic system is a term referring to a functionally unified by anatomically disperse groups of structures. Similarly to the current view of the motor system acting as a circuit, so does the limbic system is viewed as a circuitry system this term refers to a diverse array of cortical and subcortical structures, in medial and ventral regions of the cerebral hemispheres. Evolutionary, these are the more ancient regions of the hemispheres, constituting major portions of the forebrain in many species. The limbic system functions in a diverse but conceptually unified field of neural processing, handling olfaction via the olfactory cortex (the only sense having direct cortical wiring) as well as the HOME mnemonic of functions. This mnemonic stands for memory (via the hippocampal formation), emotions and drives (via the amygdala) and homeostatic, endocrine and autonomic control (via the hypothalamus).

7.5.1. Overview of Limbic Structures

The limbic structures are segregated into a hierarchical system with first and second order limbic structures, as well as dedicated limbic organs versus multifunctional organs having also limbic functions. First order / level limbic organs include the limbic cortex, which forms a ring-like limbic lobe around the edge of the cortical mantle, surrounding the corpus callosum and upper brainstem-diencephalic junction. The structures forming the limbic lobe, on the medial surface of the hemisphere include the structures in the subcallosal area as well as within the cingulate gyrus. Subcallosal area structures include the paraolfactory gyrus and the paraterminal gyrus. The cingulate gyrus, including its isthmus, continues anteriorly and inferiorly as the subcallosal and paraterminal gyri. It than joins the parahippocampal gyrus posteriorly at the isthmus. Additional limbic lobe structures include the parahippocampal gyrus (and uncus) and the hippocampal formation. Limbic cortices share immunologic markers, seen in HSV infection which manifests tropism for the limbic cortex.

Second tier limbic structures include the septum pellucidum with its septal nuclei and nucleus accumbens, hypothalamic nuclei (especially those associated with the mamillary bodies). The amygdaloid complex nuclei and adjacent substancia innominata and parts of dorsal thalamus (mainly the anterior and dorsomedial nuclei). Additional structures include the habenular nuclei, the ventral tegmental area, the periaqueductal gray matter and the prefrontal cortex.

The hippocampal formation is the medial and dorsal continuation of the parahippocampal gyrus, buried within the medial temporal lobe, forming the floor of the temporal horn of lateral ventricle. It is one of several “C”-shaped structures in the limbic system. Unlike the six layered neocortex, the hippocampal formation has only three layers (termed archi-cortex). The Amygdala is a nuclear complex that lies in antero-medial temporal lobe. The posterior amygdaloid complex and the anterior hippocampus lie underneath the uncus (the most medial edge of the temporal lobe). Amygdaloid nuclei include the corticomedial, basolateral and central nuclei. The C-shaped "Bed nucleus of the stria terminalis – BNST" is part of the amygdala. Refer to table 7.7 for other CNS structures sharing limbic functions.

Table 7.7. Limbic System Associated CNS Structures (Second tier limbic organs)

Diencephalon	Hypothalamus, thalamus, habenula	
Basal ganglia	Ventral portions, input reaches the nucleus accumbens, than through the ventral Pallidum to the thalamus.	
Basal forebrain	Structures antero-lateral to the hypothalamus, at the base of the frontal lobe. Although Close to the surface, histologically similar to gray-matter nuclei rather than cortex, hence also termed corticoid structures.	
Substancia innominata	A term used either for the entire basal forebrain or to a nucleus within it called the nucleus basalis of Maynert.	
Other nuclei	Olfactory tubercle, ventral pallidum, nucleus of the diagonal band of Broca.	
Septal nuclei	Near the septum pellucidum, mainly the medial and lateral Septal nuclei.	
Brainstem	Many nuclei have reciprocal connections to limbic structures and at times considered part of the limbic system	
	Examples	Interpeduncular nucleus, superior central nucleus, dorsal tegmental nucleus, parabrachial nucleus, periaqueductal gray, Reticular formation, nucleus solitarius, dorsal vagal nucleus.

7.5.2. Olfactory System

The term rhinencephalon refers to the pathway beginning with the olfactory nerve (cranial nerve-I) linking to the olfactory bulb (within so named sulcus) and to the olfactory cortex. Collateral neurons in the olfactory tract synapse onto scattered neurons forming the anterior olfactory nucleus. The primary olfactory cortex is unique in that it receives direct input from secondary sensory neurons without an intervening thalamic relay. It consists of the piriform cortex and the peri-amygdaloid cortex. Additional connections include the olfactory neurons projections to the corticomedial nucleus of amygdala and the olfactory tubercle located in the anterior perforated substance. Secondary olfactory areas include the anterior entorhinal cortex and the dorsomedial nucleus of the thalamus. These connections provide the anatomical explanation for the ability of odors to evoke intense primary memories.

7.5.3. Hippocampal Formation and Other Memory Related Structures

Two main regions appear to be critical to memory formation, consolidation and retrieval: the medial temporal lobe (i.e., the hippocampal formation and parahippocampal gyrus) and the medial diencephalic memory areas (i.e., the anterior and dorsomedial thalamic nuclei, the internal medullary lamina, the mammillary bodies and other diencephalic structures lining the third ventricle). A complex white matter network constitutes the third component necessary for normal function. Refer to figures 7.13-7.17.

The hippocampal formation has an inverted "S" shape on coronal view (Name means "sea-horse" in Greek). It has three components: the dentate gyrus, the hippocampal gyrus and subiculum. The dentate gyrus has tooth like bumps on its medial surface. Principal neurons in this gyrus are the granule cells. The principle cells within the hippocampus are the pyramidal cells. The Subiculum ("support" in Latin) is continuous with the parahippocampal gyrus. Each of the components has three layers (archicortex): A molecular layer (external, containing affarent axons), a granular (dentate) or pyramidal (hippocampus) layer (its dendrites radiating into the molecular layer) and a polymorphic layer, containing the axons of the pyramidal / granular cells, Glial elements etc.

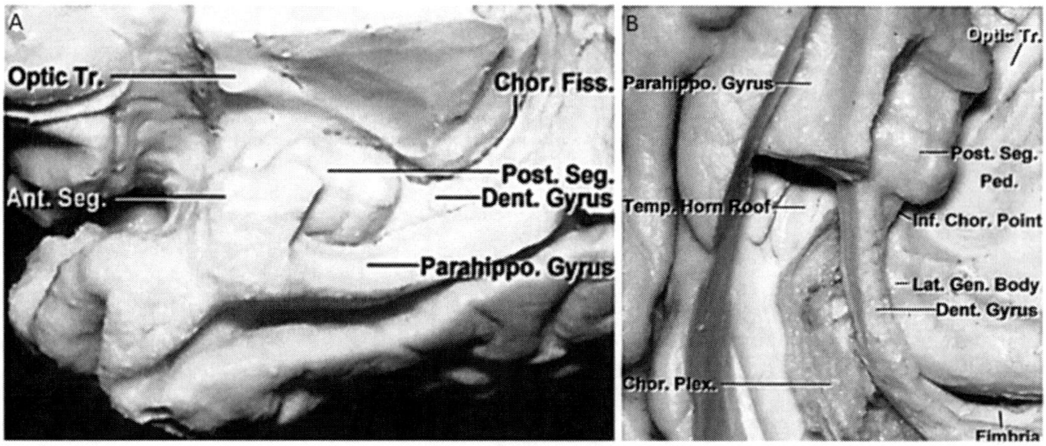

Figure 7.15. The medial surface of the temporal lobe and uncus. A, the medial part of the parahippocampal gyrus and the lower part of the posterior uncal segment have been removed to expose the dentate gyrus and the choroidal fissure. The beaded dentate gyrus blends into the posterior edge of the upper part of the posterior uncal segment and the medial side of the hippocampal head. B The part of the parahippocampal gyrus, lateral to the dentate gyrus, has been removed to expose the roof of the temporal horn, which is formed by the tapetum, the thin layer of fibers from the corpus callosum that separate the optic radiation from the wall of the temporal horn. A.Ch.A., anterior choroidal artery; Ant., anterior; Chor., choroid, choroidal; CN, cranial nerve; Coll., collateral; Dent., dentate; Fiss., fissure; Gen., geniculate; Inf., inferior; Lat., lateral; M.C.A., medial cerebral artery; P.C.A., posterior cerebral artery; Parahippo., parahippocampal; Ped., peduncle; Perf., perforated; Plex., plexus; Post., posterior; Seg., segment; Subst., substance; Temp., temporal; Tent., tentorial; Tr., tract; V., vein; Vent., ventricular. Taken with permission from the Rhoton Collection.

The alveus is the innermost part of the hippocampus, bordering the wall of the lateral ventricle. It is continuous with the fimbriae of the hippocampus (which becomes the fornix). The indusium griseum is a minor remnant of the hippocampal formation, which continues along the dorsal surface of the corpus callosum (refer to figure 7.14). The parahippocampal gyrus has several cortical regions, the most important of which is the entorhinal cortex

(Brodmann 28). The entorhinal cortex lies in the anterior portions of the gyrus, adjacent to subiculum. Its posterior region is called the parahippocampal cortex. Its lateral border is the collateral sulcus, which continues anteriorly as the rhinal sulcus. The perirhinal cortex is present along both sides of the rhinal sulcus (Brodmann 35, 36).

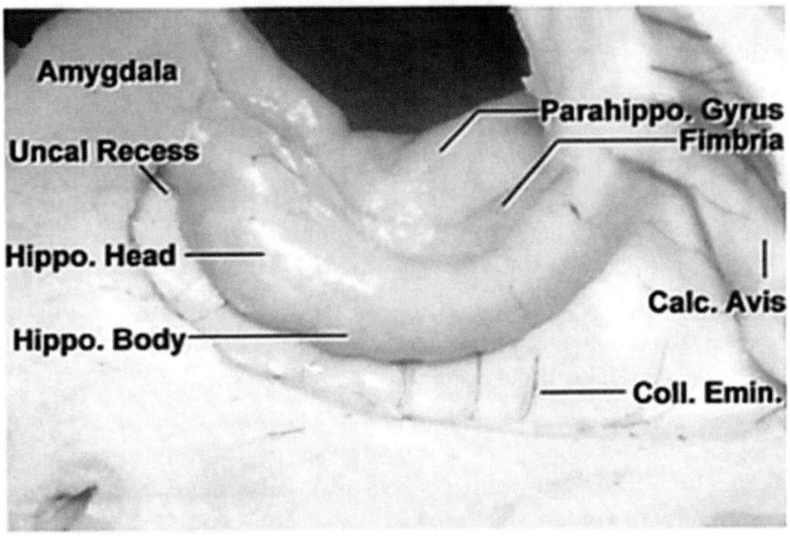

Figure 7.16. Axial section through the temporal lobe and the anterior and posterior segments of the uncus. The amygdala fills the anterior segment and the head of the hippocampus fills the upper part of the posterior segment. The fimbria arises on the surface of the hippocampus. Calc., calcar; Cer., cerebral; Chor., choroid, choroidal; Circ., circular; Coll., collateral; Emin., eminence; Hippo., hippocampal; Inf., inferior. Taken with permission from the Rhoton Collection.

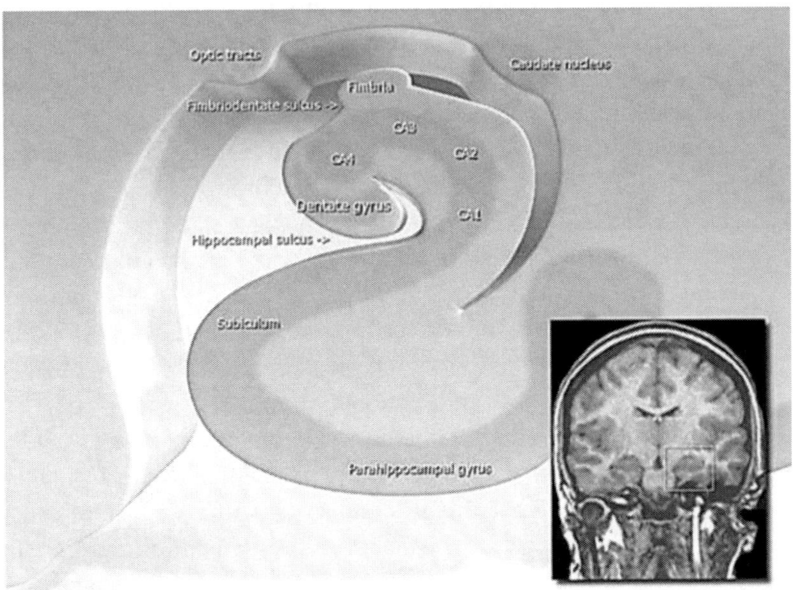

Figure 7.17. Hippocampal anatomy. Refer to text. Taken with permission from www.radiopaedia.org.

7.5.4. Output Connections of the Medial Temporal Lobe Memory System

There are many output connections of the temporal lobe memory system, but three merit special mentioning. The first group of connections is projections from the subiculum to the entorhinal cortex. The second group of connections is the fornix (whose gross anatomy features were previously discussed). The fornix is the output tract to the diencephalon and septal nuclei. As discussed, fibers from hippocampal formation form a white matter layer on the ventricular surface called the alveus. As these sweep medially they form a discrete bundle termed the fimbria of the fornix. The crura (legs) of the fornix leave the hippocampal formation and curve under the corpus callosum, running adjacent in the midline, where they change name to body of fornix. The hippocampal commissure forms between the crura of the fornix. The body of the fornix curves anteriorly to form the columns. Forniceal fibers are destined to different locations: Fibers from subiculum descend behind anterior commissure, in the post-commissural fornix, to reach the mammillary nuclei. A smaller group of fibers from the subiculum and hippocampus, pass anteriorly to reach the anterior commissure and lateral septal nucleus. Some fibers leave the fornix to terminate in anterior thalamic nucleus.

The Papez Circuit, the third output connections merits a separate discussion. Described in **1937**, it is a circuit involving several limbic structures. It was one of the earliest descriptions of this diffuse system later termed as the limbic system. To some extent, based on Papez description was the limbic system defined. The different structures involved in the Papez circuit include the subiculum, the fornix, the mammillary nuclei with related mammillothalamic tract, the anterior thalamic nucleus, the internal capsule, the cingulate gyrus and cingulum, the parahippocampal gyrus and the hippocampal formation.

7.5.5. The Amygdala – Emotions, Drives and Other Functions

The amygdala, as described previously, has three main nuclear groups: the corticomedial nuclei located near the basal forebrain and olfactory areas are involved in olfaction. The basolateral nuclei are the largest amygdaloid nuclear group in humans, involved in both direct and indirect connections. The central nuclear group is the smallest, having connections to the hypothalamus and brainstem important in autonomic control. The bed nucleus of the stria terminalis is also considered a part of the amygdala and has important limbic functions. The functional roles assigned to the amygdala involves emotions and drives functions, with the amygdala considered important for attaching emotional significance to various stimuli perceived by the association cortex. Kluver-Bucy syndrome is a rare syndrome appearing with bilateral lesions of the amygdala. It manifests with a very indolent non-aggressive behavior. When seizures involve the amygdala, these cause powerful emotions of fear and panic. The activity in the amygdala is important for states of fear, anxiety and aggression. In contrast, activity in the septal areas is important in pleasurable states.

Most amygdaloid connections are bidirectional. Important inputs and outputs include cortical fibers passing posteriorly and laterally to reach cortical areas and the uncinate fasciculus which passes anteriorly to connect with the medial orbito-frontal and cingulate cortices (discussed previously). Subcortical connections are important in motivational, autonomic and neuroendocrine aspects, of which two merit mentioning: the stria terminalis (coursing the long way around the fornix of the amygdala) and the ventral amygdalofugal pathway (the "shortcut"). Olfactory inputs from the olfactory bulb through lateral olfactory stria reach the corticomedial nucleus.

7.6. Higher Order Cerebral Functions

7.6.1. Unimodal and Heteromodal Association Cortices

A unimodal association cortex is a modality specific cortex, like the somatosensory cortex, visual or auditory cortex or the motor association cortex etc. A unimodal sensory association cortex receives input from the primary sensory cortex of the specific modality, and performs higher order sensory processing for that sensory modality only. A unimodal motor association cortex projects mainly to the primary motor cortex and is important in formulating the motor program. A heteromodal association cortex in contrast, has bidirectional connections with both motor and sensory association cortices of all modalities, as well as with limbic structures. These bidirectional diverse connections allow for higher order mental functions, which require integration of abstract sensory and motor information from unimodal association cortices with emotional and motivational influences.

7.6.2. Principles of Cerebral Localization and Lateralization

The brain functions both as a collection of specialized areas as well as like a network. Thus, although focal lesions can cause specific deficits localized by a physical examination, false localization may also occur due to the network nature of the brain. Some cerebral neurological functions have a tendency to be lateralized, resulting in hemispheric sub specialization. Handedness is one such example, since although each hemisphere controls simple movements of contralateral limbs, skilled complex motor tasks for both sides are programmed mainly by the dominant hemisphere (Usually left). Thus, dominant hemispheral lesions are usually associated with apraxia (the loss of complex motor memory / functions). Language abilities are another such example of sub specialization. Language functions are lateralized to the dominant hemisphere in most. As stated this is the left hemisphere in >95% of right handed people and over 60~70% of left-handed people. Non-dominant hemisphere is specialized for certain nonverbal functions. It is implicated as important for complex visual-spatial skills, music perception etc. The right hemisphere is significantly involved in attending to both sides. Right hemispheral lesions usually cause marked inattention to the contralateral side (agnosia).

7.6.3. The Dominant Hemisphere

One main dominant hemispheral function is language processing and related functions. Auditory information reaches the primary auditory cortex located on the banks of the sylvian fissure in the temporal lobe. Initial processing occurs in the Wernicke's area (Brodmann 22) in the posterior 2/3 of the dominant superior temporal gyrus. Articulation of sounds depends on the face area of the primary motor cortex, in the inferior precentral gyrus. The planning of the motor program of speech occurs in the nearby motor association cortices termed as Broca's area (Brodmann 44-45), lying in pars-operculum and pars-triangularis of the inferior frontal gyrus. The ability to hear and repeat a word requires proper transfer of information across the sylvian fissure (between Broca's and Wernicke's). The arcuate fasciculus is a part of the superior longitudinal fasciculus subcortical white matter pathway connecting these two speech centers.

There are many other cortical centers and connections relating to language functions beside the Broca's and Wernicke's areas. The premotor, prefrontal and supplementary motor cortices act in concert with Broca's area. The supramarginal and angular gyri act in concert with the Wernicke's area and are important in reading functions. The non-dominant hemisphere, connected via corpus callosum, participates in language processing as well. It is important in the recognition and production of the affective elements of speech. Thus, in right hemispheral lesions, no obvious language disturbance can be shown but difficulty judging the intended expression by a particular tone, or difficulty producing and attaching an emotional expression to a sentence is seen. Subcortical structures involved in language processing and functions to different degrees are the thalamus and basal ganglia. Certain lesions in these subcortical structures can result in subcortical aphasia (lack of normal speech, discussed later).

7.6.4. The Non-Dominant Hemisphere

The Non-dominant hemisphere is important for attention and for an integrated visual-spatial gestalt. Attention has several components: Global attention is manifested in functions such as vigilance and concentration. Selective directed attention is manifested in focusing attention on a particular domain. Attention, like alertness, depends on activating systems such as the ponto-mesencephalic reticular formation, different diencephalic structures, limbic structures etc. Since the right hemisphere is dominant in these functions, hemispheral lesions may lead to prominent and long lasting deficits in attention to the contralateral side. Left hemispheral lesions produce on the other hand a relatively milder contralateral neglect. Under normal conditions, the right hemisphere attends strongly to the left side and less to the right side, while the left hemisphere attends mainly to the right side.

Visuospatial analysis, like other mental functions, is performed by a distributed network and depends on bilateral regions of the frontal and parietal association cortices. Visual information is analyzed by two streams of higher order information Processing. One stream, dealing with the "What?" question is located in the ventral occipital temporal and prefrontal cortex. A second stream, dealing with the "Where?" question is located in the dorsal occipital, parietal and prefrontal cortices. The parietal association cortex, e.g., the cortex located at the junction of the parietal-temporal-occipital lobes, is especially important in visuospatial analysis. The parietal association cortex is part of the dorsal stream, analyzing location and movement of visual objects in space. Spatial analysis encompasses both the surrounding environment and the relative position of the body in space using visual, proprioceptive, vestibular and auditory information.

Hemineglect syndrome appears in patients presenting with profound neglect for the contralateral half of the external world and of their body. Patients are often unaware of the problem, at times not recognizing the left side of the body as theirs. Lesions causing hemineglect symptoms are located in the right parietal or frontal cortex, at times involving the cingulate gyrus, thalamus, basal ganglia or midbrain reticular formation.

7.6.5. The Frontal Lobes – Anatomy and Functions of an Enigmatic Brain Region

More than any other part of the brain, the frontal lobes enable us to function as effective and socially appropriate human beings. There is no single frontal lobe syndrome, and frontal lobe function comprises several different realms, clustering around 3 domains: Restraint, initiative and order. Refer to table 7.9 for some regional brain syndrome. Frontal lobe functions are diverse and at times contradictory, crucial in cognitive functions and social interactions. Restraint is the inhibition of inappropriate behavior. Initiative functions relative to motivation to pursue positive or productive activities. Order refers to the capacity to correctly perform sequencing tasks and other cognitive operations.

Generally speaking, dorsolateral convexity lesions tend to produce an apathetic lifeless abulic state. Orbitofrontal lesions tend to manifest with impulsive, disinhibited behavior and poor judgment. Many exceptions exist, and many lesions occupy both regions. Left frontal lesions are more commonly associated with depression like symptoms. Right frontal lesions are more commonly associated with behavioral disturbances resembling mania.

7.6.6. Attention, Awareness and Other General Network Brain Functions

A discussed previously and in chapter 3 as well, the content of consciousness refers to the human entity, the substrate. This refers to the function of the sensory, motor, emotional and association systems. The level of consciousness is a completely different neurological process and function. It is commonly described in three related processes: Alertness, attention and awareness. The anatomy of attention refers to the widespread projection systems involving both upper brainstem projection systems, thalamic and hypothalamic tracts as well as basal forebrain systems. Other areas involved include the frontal and parietal association cortices, the anterior cingulate cortex and limbic pathways, the midbrain tectum, pretectal area and pulvinar.

7.7. Classification of Memory and Memory Disorders

In classifying memory, one should note the difference between declarative (explicit) memory and non-declarative (implicit) memory. Explicit memory involves the conscious recollection of facts, while implicit memory involves non-conscious learning of skills. The selective loss of explicit memory is typical of bilateral medial thalami or temporal lobe lesions. Part of a more comprehensive understanding of memory is the understanding of related temporal aspects, namely the mechanisms converting memories from short-term to long-term. These mechanisms include cellular mechanisms storing information in the nervous system on different time scales. Another important fact is that different anatomical locations are important for storing memories at different times.

We should also clarify the difference between anterograde and retrograde amnesia. Anterograde amnesia refers to the inability to form new memories from the time of injury.

Retrograde amnesia refers to the loss of memories from the time before the injury. Medial temporal lobe lesions manifest as a combination of anterograde and retrograde amnesia.

7.7.1. Differential Diagnosis of Memory Loss

1) **Infarcts**. Medial temporal lobes are supplied by distal branches Of the PCA (posterior cerebral artery). Medial thalami are supplied by paramedian thalamoperforator branches (from initial PCA).Thus, lesions located at top of the basilar artery may cause bilateral medial temporal or thalamic infarcts (Refer to table 7.9). In addition, bilateral medial thalami are often supplied by a single paramedian thalamoperforator artery (the artery of Percheron), bifurcating shortly after its origin. Its single occlusion results in bilateral lesions.
2) **Basal forebrain lesions**. Anterior-communicating artery aneurysm rupture, tumors.
3) **Wernicke-Korsakoff syndrome**. Thiamine deficiency, with bilateral necrosis of the mammillary bodies. The acute phase of the syndrome manifests with a triad composed of ataxia, eye movement abnormalities and a confusional state. The chronic phase of the disease manifests with Anterograde and retrograde amnesia (bilateral medial temporal lobe), frontal lobe signs. Confabulations are characteristic, related to frontal lobe dysfunction.
4) **Electroconvulsive therapy (ECT)**. Patients develop retrograde and anterograde amnesia.
5) **Transient global amnesia (TGA)**. Lasts 4~12 hours, cause unknown.

7.8. Dominant Hemisphere Syndromes

7.8.1. Aphasia

Aphasia classification is based on three parts of the physical examination: fluency, comprehension and repetition. Refer to table 7.8-7.9 for the different aphasia subtypes. The two major aphasia subtypes are discussed next.

The most common etiology for Broca's (motor) aphasia is an infarct in left middle cerebral artery (MCA) superior division. The most silent feature of motor aphasia is the decreased fluency of spontaneous speech (defined as phrase length less than five words, and the nouns number is more than function words). Prosody (the normal melodious intonation of speech) is characteristically absent in motor aphasia. Decreased fluency is associated with a marked naming difficulty. Repetition is impaired due to the disconnection from Wernicke's. Comprehension is relatively intact (which aggravates the patient's anxiety). Associated features include dysarthria, right hemiparesis, and apraxia (in the non-plegic side). Big Broca's aphasia is the clinical manifestation caused by large lesions (MCA superior division infarct), presenting initially as global aphasia and later settle into Broca's aphasia. Little Broca's aphasia refers to the clinical presentation of smaller lesions confined to frontal operculum, presenting as Broca's aphasia with a partial recovery thereafter.

Most common etiology for Wernicke's (sensory aphasia) is an infarct to left MCA inferior division. It manifests with a marked impaired comprehension. The patient does not follow any commands. Spontaneous speech has normal fluency, normal prosody and normal grammatical structure, but impaired lexical function results in speech that is empty and meaningless. Paraphasic errors (Inappropriate substitutions of a word) and neologism (invented words) may occur. Naming is similarly impaired, as does repetition (due to disconnection from Broca's). Associated features include contralateral visual field cut (right upper ¼), and apraxia. In contrast to Broca's, patients are unaware of their deficit *(anosognosia)*

Table 7.8. Aphasia Classification

Aphasia type	Comments
Broca's	Motor, commonly caused by an infarct in left MCA superior division.
Wernicke's	Sensory, commonly caused by an infarct to left MCA inferior division.
Global	Seen in large CVA. Fluency, comprehension and repetition are all disturbed.
Conduction	Only repetition is disturbed. Caused by an infarct to the arcuate fasciculus.
Transcortical	Only repetition is spared. Commonly caused by a watershed infarct.
Transcortical motor	Impaired fluency, normal comprehension, spared repetition. Commonly caused by an infarct to the ACA-MCA watershed zone.
Transcortical sensory	Normal fluency, no comprehension, spared repetition. Commonly caused by an infarct to the MCA-PCA watershed zone.

7.8.2. Alexia, Agraphia

The impaired reading or writing ability may be caused by deficits in central language processing, not by simple motor or sensory deficits. These deficits may occur in isolation or together._When these occur with aphasia, the clinical manifesting abnormalities tend to parallel those of the aphasic syndrome for spoken language (thus, fluency and comprehension mirrors the spoken language).

The syndrome of alexia without agraphia is caused by a lesion in the dominant occipital cortex extending to the posterior corpus callosum. This is often a PCA infarct. Right hemianopia is usually present as well. The clinical manifestation, putting it simply is a patient that can write but not read. Gerstmann's syndrome refers to the presence of four seemingly unrelated symptoms, each having very little localizing power by itself, but presenting together, in combination (in the absence of a global confusional state), it is strongly localizing to the dominant inferior parietal lobule. These symptoms are agraphia, acalculia (for basic mathematics), left-right disorientation and finger agnosia.

Table 7.9. Regional Brain Syndromes

Frontal lobe			
Unilateral large lesion		Classic manifestations include apathy and abulia.	
Frontal eye field		Destructive lesions cause impaired gaze to the contralateral side (hence looking towards the lesion).	
		Seizures cause stimulation of the contralateral gaze center (hence looking away from the lesion).	
Olfactory groove		Foster-Kennedy syndrome	Ipsilateral Anosmia
			Ipsilateral central scotoma, optic atrophy
			Contralateral papilledema
Prefrontal lobe		Executive functions	
Parietal lobe			
Either side	Cortical sensory syndrome	Lesion of post-central gyrus, mainly in the hand region	
		Loss of position sense, inability to localize tactile stimuli	
		Astereognosis (inability to judge size and shape by touch)	
		Agraphesthesia (cannot detect no. written on hand)	
	Sensory extinction		
	Contralateral homonymous hemianopia		
	Contralateral neglect		
	Anton syndrome	Bilateral occipital lobe strokes. Caused by bilateral PCA or Top of Basilar syndrome. Manifests with visual deficit without recognition of blindness (visual agnosia)	
	Balint syndrome	Bilateral PCA artery (parietal-occipital). Manifest with loss of voluntary but not reflexive eye movements, Optic ataxia, Asimultagnosia	
Dominant	Aphasia	Wernicke's	Lesion in the auditory association cortex inferior to the angular gyrus (Refer to table 7.8).
		Conduction	Disruption to the connections between the frontal and temporal speech areas. It is similar clinically to Wernick's aphasia with the note that repetition is the only severely affected ability and the patient is aware of the deficit (Refer to table 7.8).
		Pure word blindness	Alexia without agraphia. Rare, lesion in parieto-occipital lobe interrupts connections between left angular gyrus and both occipital lobes (Refer to table 7.8).
	Gerstmann's syndrome		Agraphia without alexia, right-left confusion, digit agnosia, acalculia
	Bilateral Astereognosis		
Non-dominant		Topographic memory loss, anosognosia, dressing apraxia	
Occipital lobe			
Homonymous hemianopia			
Cerebellum			
Hemisphere		Ipsilateral appendicular Ataxia.	
Vermis		Truncal ataxia	
Pineal region			
Perinaud's syndrome		Convergence and supranuclear upward gaze palsy with normal response to vertical doll's eyes, lid retraction (together termed "setting sun sign", with fixed pupils).	
The syndrome of the Sylvian Aqueduct		When Perinaud's syndrome is combined with downgaze palsy.	

7.8.3. Apraxia

Apraxia refers to the loss of a learned motor skill. A good example is an adult patient presenting with an infant like walk, characterized by asymmetrical steps and leg movements. This type of apraxia, termed as motor apraxia, is seen in normal pressure hydrocephalus, secondary to white matter hemispheral changes mainly in the depth of the frontal lobes. Ideomotor apraxia is a term referring to the inability to carry out an action in response to verbal command. The patient may initiate motor actions, speak and understand when spoken to, but unable to follow commands. It is not a very localizing symptom, having some association to aphasia. Aphemia (verbal apraxia) refers to apraxia of the speech and articulatory apparatus, without language disturbances. It is caused by small lesions of the dominant frontal operculum, with normal written language (unlike Broca's). Speech is referred to as foreign accent syndrome.

7.8.4. Cortical Deafness

Cortical deafness may be caused by bilateral lesions of the primary auditory cortex (located at Heschl's gyrus). Patients are aware of a sound existing but are unable to interpret verbal stimuli or nonverbal stimuli. Pure word deafness (e.g., verbal auditory agnosia) is a subset of cortical deafness. In this presentation, patients can identify nonverbal sounds but cannot understand any spoken words. The lesion characteristically causing pure word deafness is an infarct in the auditory area of the dominant hemisphere, extending to the subcortical white matter, cutting off the auditory input from the contralateral hemisphere.

Chapter 8

The Meninges, the Cerebrospinal Fluid and the Lateral Ventricles

8.1. Abstract

This chapter deals with the anatomy of related non-purely speaking neurological structures, which are pivotal both clinically and for the understanding of CNS architecture. We begin our discussion with the cranial meninges, describing the layers and meningeal folding and continue with a description of the dural venous sinuses and the venous drainage of the cerebral hemispheres. The cerebral cisterns are presented followed in direct clinical correlation, with a description of the herniation syndromes and common intracranial hemorrhages. The concept of true and potential intracranial spaces is presented. Next we discuss the cerebrospinal fluid, both in its laboratory features as well as the blood brain barrier (BBB) and finally we present the circumventricular organs, those regions lacking BBB in the brain. The chapter ends with a gross anatomical description of the lateral ventricles and its relationship to other neural structures following its "C" shaped form.

8.2. The Cranial Meninges

8.2.1. Introduction

Although the meninges have been introduced in earlier chapters and discussed to certain degrees in the frame of specific CNS regions, a focused discussion is in order. The dura matter, the most external of the meninges is a tough thick layer (giving it its name). The dura receives its blood supply from external carotid artery branches (anterior, middle and posterior meningeal arteries, occipital arteries etc). It has a somatosensory innervation, mainly for pain and temperture via the trigeminal nerve. The dura is composed of two distinct layers: an outer periosteal later and an inner true dura membranous layer. The periosteal layer is rich in blood vessels and sensory nerve endings, hard to separate from the tabula interna of the skull. The membranous true dural meningeal layer is a sheath of fibrous tissue. Dural sinuses form between the two layers at specific locations, whenever the dura leaves the inner skull surface or at its free edges (i.e., where it leaves to form the flax cerebri, as well as at the falx free edge and correspondingly where it leaves to form the tentorium cerebelli and in the incisura). Refer to figure 8.1.

The meningeal membranous dura is adhered in normal cases and in health to its underlying arachnoid layer. No subdural space exists under normal conditions. The arachnoid matter is a thin layer, adjacent to the dura. It has an external membranous layer and an inner web-like layer connected to the pia by thin strands of connective tissue (the arachnoid trabeculae). The subarachnoid space (between arachnoid and pia) it a true space, through which the different blood vessels and cranial nerves course, filled with CSF. Enlargements of this volume layer form the subarachnoid cisterns (discussed later). The pia matter is a thin, delicate layer made of elastic fibers, found adjacent to the brain surface. It follows the contours of the brain and penetrating blood vessels (giving these a cuff upon exiting brain tissue).

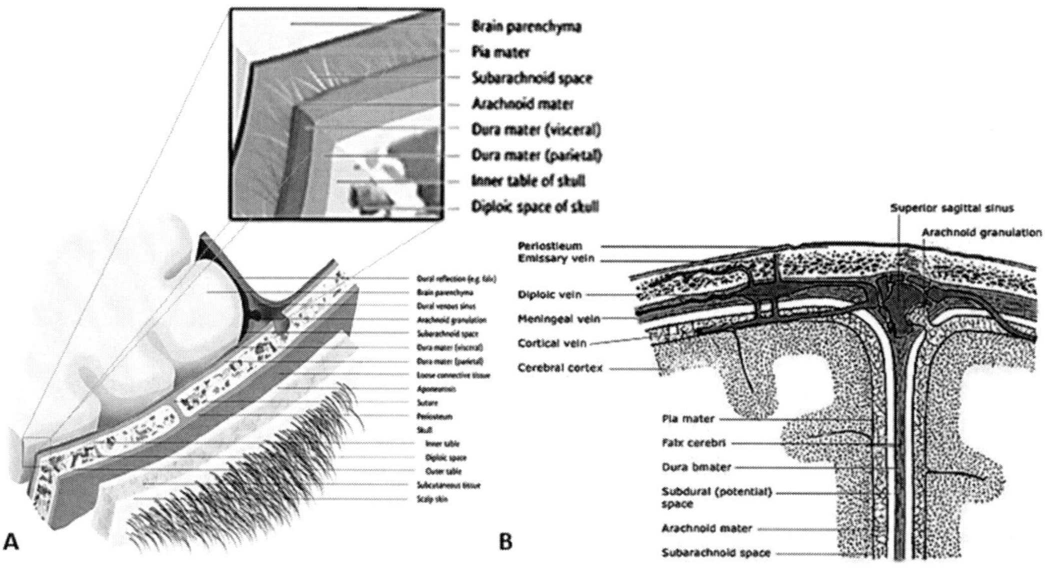

Figure 8.1. The Layers of the scalp and meninges. A, Taken with permission from www.radiopaedia.org. B, An illustration demonstrating the inner meningeal and outer endosteal (periosteal) layer. Taken from Gray's Anatomy (out of copyright and in the public domain).

8.2.2. Meningeal Foldings

The dura follows the inner table of the skull in general except in specific designated locations where folds of meningeal dura leave the skull to partition the intracranial cavity. These folds separate particular brain regions (Refer to figures 8.2-8.7). The falx cerebri separates between the two cerebral hemispheres, bordering at its lower free margin the corpus callosum. It extends the entire anterior-posterior diameter of the skull. The tentorium cerebelli separates the cerebrum from the cerebellum. It emerges from the inner occipital table (at a location marked externally usually by the nuchal lines) and the petrous temporal bone. It spans only the posterior aspect of the skull, with its free edge (The incisura) bordering the midbrain region, allowing for the midbrain to be continuous with the diencephalon. This junction between the falx cerebri and the tentorium cerebelli forms the tentorial notch (incisura) that envelopes the midbrain. Its ends are relatively tough and sharp. Structures traveling through the incisura include, except the midbrain (at the interpeduncular fossa), the oculomotor nerve (CN-III) and the basilar artery. The posterior cerebral arteries, emerging from the tip of the basilar artery course above the incisura to travel in the supratentorial plane. This point is important when discussing brain herniation syndromes (discussed later). The falx cerebelli separates the two cerebellar hemispheres. Dural sinuses form at junctions between meningeal foldings and the periosteal dura or between different meningeal folding.

8.2.3. Dural Venous Sinuses and the Cerebral Venous Drainage

As mentioned, dural sinuses form at junctions between meningeal foldings and the periosteal dura or another folding and are in fact vascular (venous) sinuses. As vascular conduits, these structures are quite unique in structure. An important histological point to remember, which at times carry a grave clinical significance is the fact that the dural sinuses are meningeal layers lined by endothelial cells. The dural sinuses do not have venous valves or smooth muscle in its walls. Thus, these venous structures are incapable of venocontriction or any type of reflex response to being breeched (unlike peripheral arteries and veins). These vascular structures thus are indifferent to any vasoactive drug as well. Venous blood emptied into the dural sinuses from different cortical and ventral veins ultimately leaves the cranium via the internal jugular vein. Venous blood then flows (via the brachiocephalic veins) into the superior vena cava.

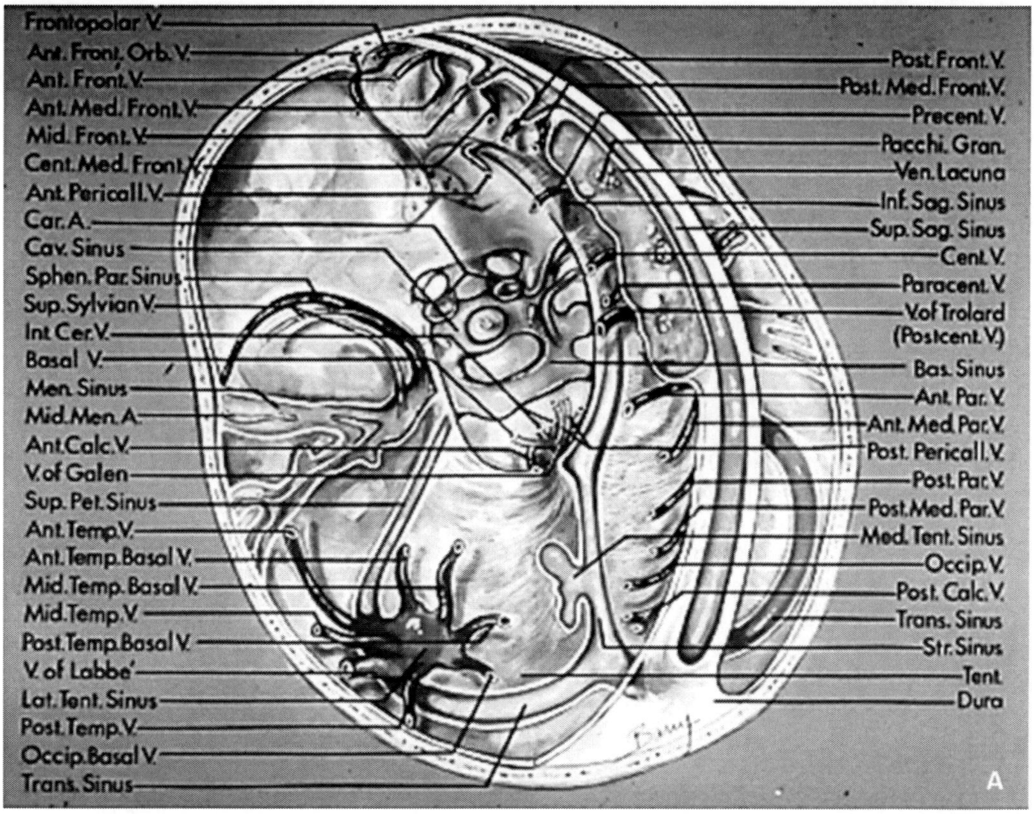

Figure 8.2. (Continued)

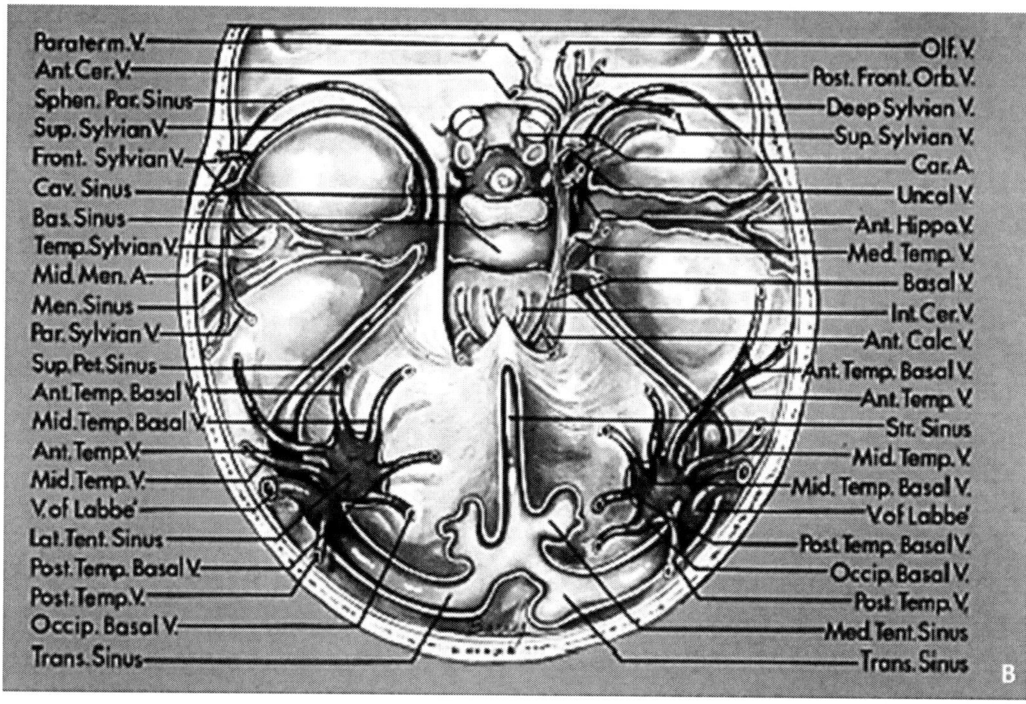

Figure 8.2. Dural sinuses and bridging veins. A, oblique superior view; B, direct superior view with the falx and superior sagittal sinus removed. A., artery; Ant., anterior; Ant.Med., anteromedial; Bas., basilar; Calc., calcarine; Car., carotid; Cav., cavernous; Cent., central; Cer., cerebral; Front., frontal; Front.Orb., fronto-orbital; Hippo., hippocampal; Inf., inferior; Int., internal; Lat., lateral; Med., medial; Men., meningeal; Mid., middle; Occip., occipital; Olf., olfactory; Pacci. Gran., Pacchionian granulations; Par., parietal; Paracent., paracentral; Paraterm., paraterminal; Pericall., pericallosal; Pet., petrosal; Post., posterior; Post.Med., posteromedial; Precent., precentral; Sag., sagittal; Sphen.Par., sphenoparietal; Str., straight; Sup., superior; Temp., temporal; Tent., tentorial, tentorium; Trans., transverse; V., vein; Ven., venous. Taken with permission from the Rhoton Collection.

In terms of terminology, whenever two sinuses join together they form another sinus. Refer to table 8.1 for the venous sinuses structure and hierarchy. The confluence of sinuses (i.e., Torcula herophili) is the occipital location where the superior sagittal sinus, the straight sinus (sinus rectus) and the occipital sinuses meet and drain to the transverse sinuses. It is often shaped in a manner that the superior sagittal sinus drains to the right transverse sinus while the straight sinus drains to the left transverse sinus.

The Cavernous sinus (discussed previously and in chapter 10) is a plexus of veins located on either sides of the sella Turcica. This plexus surrounds portions of the internal carotid artery and the oculomotor, trochlear, trigeminal and abducens cranial nerves (CN-III, IV, V, and VI).

The cavernous sinus drains via the superior petrosal sinus into the transverse sinus and via inferior petrosal sinus to the internal jugular vein.

Table 8.1. Venous drainage of the brain

<table>
<tr><td colspan="4">Miscellaneous outflow shunt</td><td colspan="4">Except the internal jugular vein (IJV), there are a few more intracranial-extracranial venous shunts. These are minimal in health, carrying no clinical significant, but seen in cases of increased intracranial pressure or venous congestion (like in sinus vein thrombosis). These are Orbital veins, vertebral venous plexus, scalp veins.</td></tr>
<tr><td rowspan="11">IJV</td><td colspan="7">The IJV are the major source of outflow, right is usually dominant. We present the venous structures draining back from the IJV (opposite to the blood flow)</td></tr>
<tr><td colspan="7">Inferior petrosal sinus</td></tr>
<tr><td rowspan="9">Sigmoid sinus</td><td colspan="6">Superior petrosal sinus</td></tr>
<tr><td rowspan="8">Transverse sinus</td><td colspan="5">Inferior anastomotic vein of Labbe</td></tr>
<tr><td rowspan="7">Torcula herophili</td><td colspan="4">Occipital sinus</td></tr>
<tr><td colspan="2">Superior sagittal sinus</td><td colspan="2">Superior anastomotic vein of Trolard (refer to text and figure 8.8 for the other veins)</td></tr>
<tr><td rowspan="5">Straight sinus</td><td colspan="3">Inferior sagittal sinus</td></tr>
<tr><td rowspan="4">Vein of Galen</td><td colspan="2">Pre-central cerebellar veins</td></tr>
<tr><td colspan="2">Basal vein of Rosenthal</td></tr>
<tr><td rowspan="2">Internal cerebral veins (joined at Monro foramen by)</td><td>Anterior septal vein.</td></tr>
<tr><td>Thalamostriate vein.</td></tr>
</table>

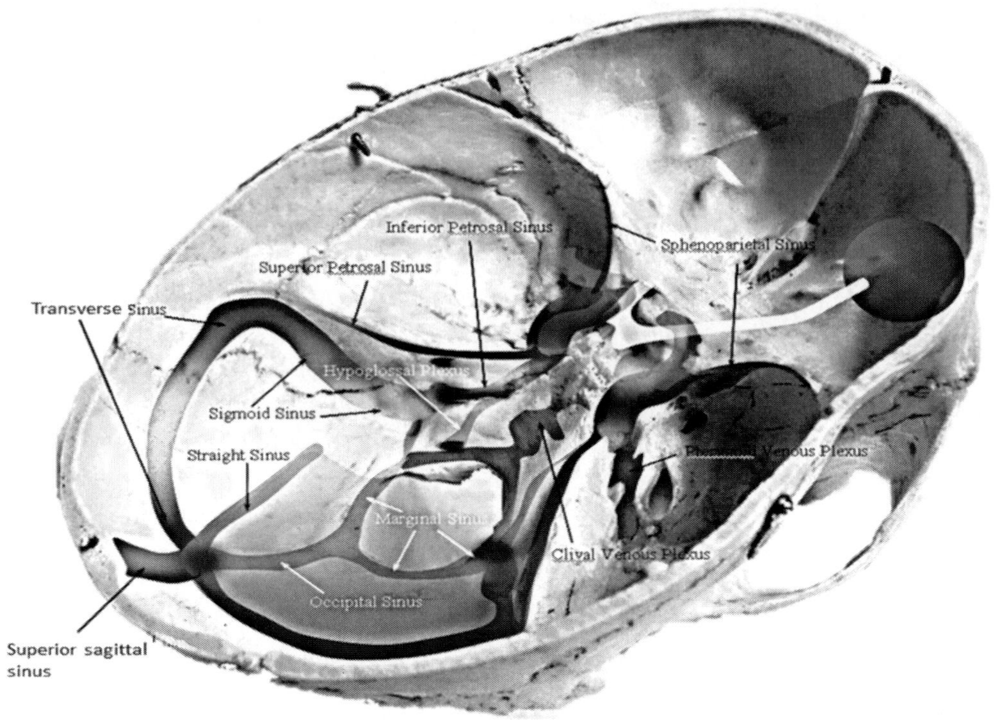

Figure 8.3. Illustration of the dural venous sinuses. Some sinuses are present less commonly than others. The more uncommon ones are labeled in white. The superior and inferior sagittal sinuses are not shown to full extent for clarity. Note how the sphenoparietal sinus runs along the edge of the lesser sphenoid wing, and superior petrosal sinus follows the petrous ridge. Most people have quite asymmetric sinuses. Taken with permission from www.neuroangio.org.

8.2.3.1. Venous Drainage of the Cerebral Hemispheres

Like the arterial system, the intracranial venous system has superficial and deep territories. As discussed next, generally speaking, the superficial veins drain mainly to the superior sagittal sinus and cavernous sinus. The cortical veins highly variable, but a few constant ones merit mentioning like the inferior anastomotic vein of Labbe (draining to the transverse sinus) and the superior anastomotic vein of Trolard (draining to the superior sagittal sinus). The superficial middle cerebral veins drain to the cavernous sinus. The deep cerebral veins drain into the internal cerebral vein, the basal vein of Rosenthal as well as the great vein of Galen (which also drain the Rosenthal vein). The great vein of Galen is joined by the inferior sagittal sinus to form the straight sinus (sinus rectus).

The veins are divided into four groups based on their site of termination: a superior sagittal group, which drains into the superior sagittal sinus; a tentorial group, which drains into the transverse or lateral tentorial sinus; a sphenoidal group, which drains into the sphenoparietal or cavernous sinus; and a falcine group, which drains into the straight or inferior sagittal sinus either directly or through the basal, great, or internal cerebral veins. The veins emptying into the superior sagittal sinus drain the upper part of the medial or lateral surfaces of the frontal, parietal, and occipital lobes and the anterior part of the orbital surface of the frontal lobe. The veins from the lateral surface that terminate in the superior sagittal sinus are the frontopolar, anterior frontal, middle frontal, posterior frontal, precentral, central, anterior parietal, posterior parietal, and occipital veins and the vein of Trolard, which, in this case, is a large postcentral vein. The veins from the medial surface that drain into the superior sagittal sinus are the anteromedial frontal, centromedial frontal, posteromedial frontal, paracentral, anteromedial parietal, posteromedial parietal, and posterior calcarine veins. The veins from the orbital surface that drain into the superior sagittal sinus are the anterior orbitofrontal veins.

The veins emptying into the sinuses in the tentorium drain the lateral and basal surfaces of the temporal lobe and the basal surface of the occipital lobe. The veins from the lateral surface that drain into the sinuses in the tentorium are the anterior temporal, middle temporal, and posterior temporal veins and the vein of Labbé. The veins from the inferior surface that drain into the sinuses in the tentorium are the anterior temporobasal, middle temporobasal, posterior temporobasal, and occipitobasal veins. The veins that empty into the cavernous or sphenoparietal sinus course along the sylvian fissure and drain the parts of the frontal, parietal, and temporal lobes adjoining the sylvian fissure. These branches are the superficial sylvian vein and its tributaries, the frontosylvian, parietosylvian, and temporosylvian veins.

The veins emptying into the straight sinus or its tributaries drain the part of the frontal and parietal lobes surrounding the corpus callosum and the medial part of the temporal lobe. The area drained by this group corresponds roughly to the limbic lobe of the brain. The veins in this group are the paraterminal, posterior fronto-orbital, olfactory, anterior pericallosal, posterior pericallosal, uncal, anterior hippocampal, medial temporal, and anterior calcarine veins. The right superficial sylvian veins are directed toward the sphenoparietal sinus and the anterior part of the cavernous sinus, and the left superficial sylvian veins are directed further posteriorly toward a lateral extension of the cavernous sinus. The deep sylvian and anterior cerebral veins also empty into the anterior end of the basal vein. The carotid arteries pass through the cavernous sinuses. The meningeal sinuses in the floor of the middle cranial fossae course with the middle meningeal arteries. The medial tentorial sinuses receive tributaries from the cerebellum and join the straight sinus. The basilar sinus sits on the clivus. Pacchionian granulations protrude into the venous lacunae.

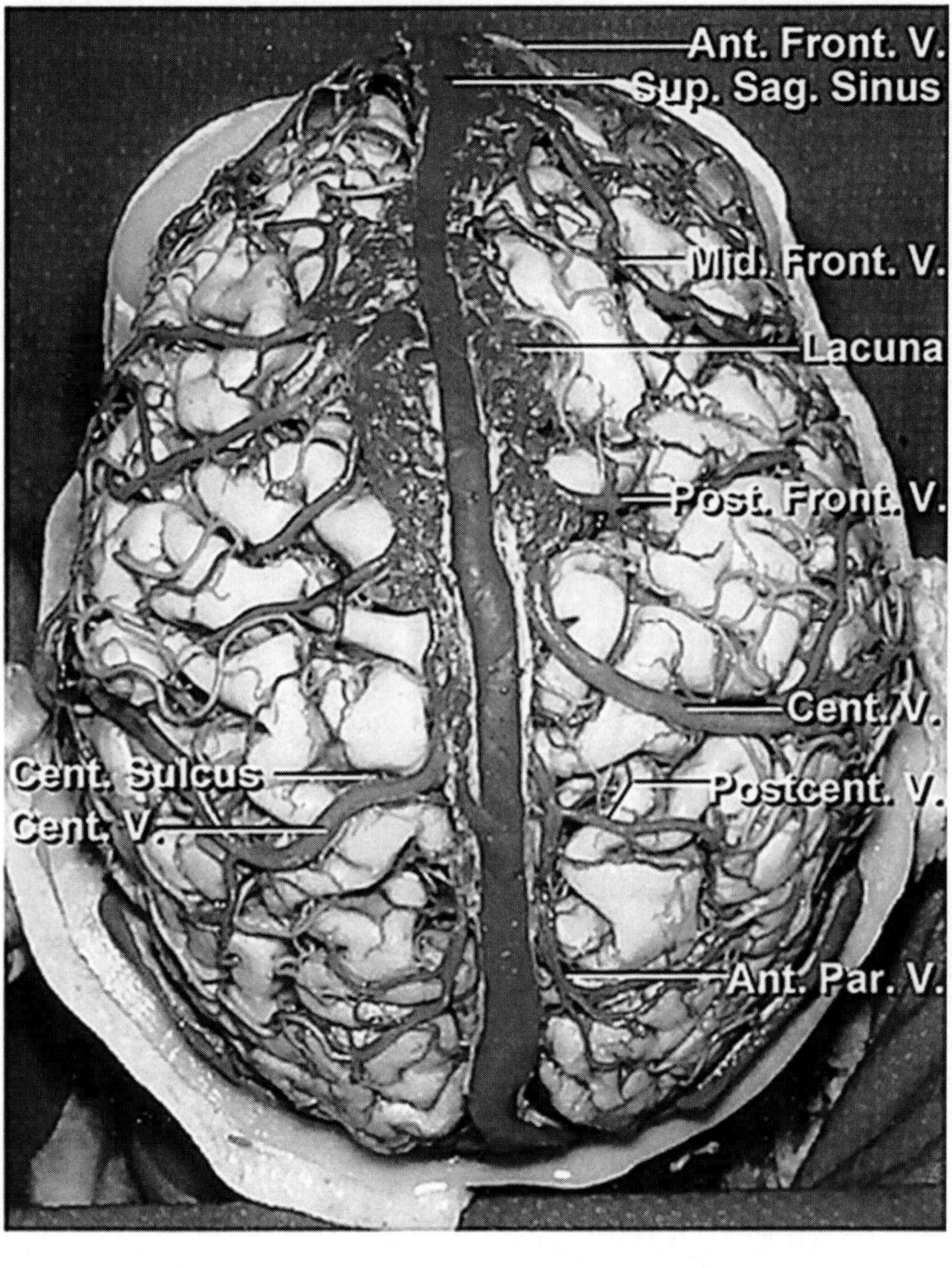

Figure 8.4. Venous lacunae and bridging veins to the superior sagittal sinus, superior view. A large venous lacuna adjoining the sagittal sinus extends above the bridging veins emptying into the superior sagittal sinus. The veins from the right hemisphere emptying into the superior sagittal sinus are the anterior, middle, and posterior frontal, central, postcentral, and anterior parietal veins. The precentral and central areas are drained by the large central vein. The veins draining the posterior part of The hemisphere are directed forward. Taken with permission from the Rhoton Collection.

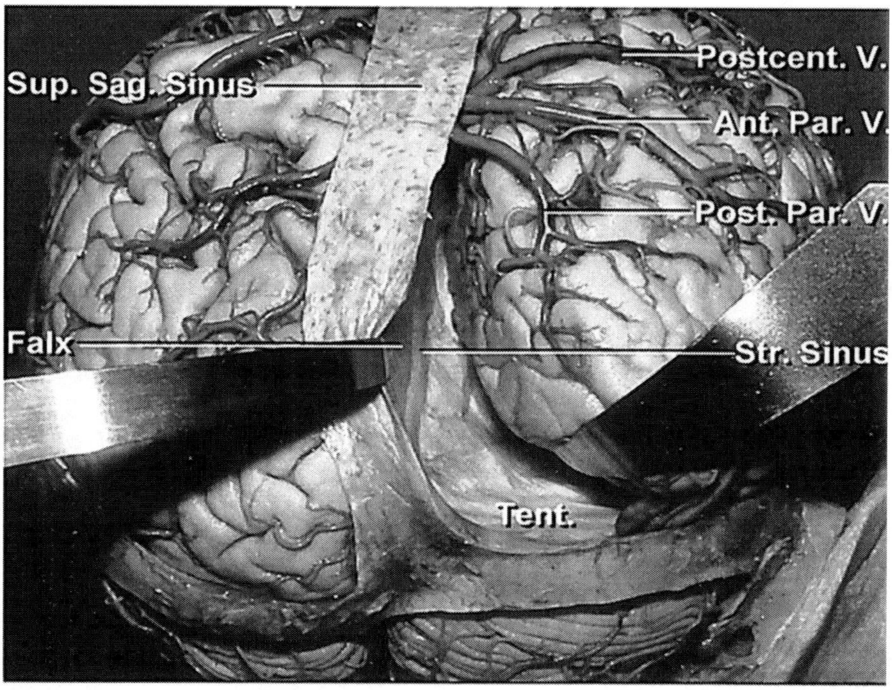

Figure 8.5. The lambdoid suture has been removed to show the absence of bridging veins entering the posterior part of the superior sagittal sinus. Right postcentral and anterior and posterior parietal veins empty into the superior sagittal sinus. The right occipital lobe has been retracted to expose the tentorium, falx, and straight sinus. There are no bridging veins between the occipital pole and the superior sagittal or straight sinus. Ant., anterior; Cent., central; Front., frontal; Mid., middle; Par., parietal; Post., posterior; Postcent., postcentral; Precent., precentral; Sag., sagittal; Squam., squamosal; Str., straight; Sup., superior; Temp., temporal; Tent., tentorium; V., vein. Taken with permission from the Rhoton Collection.

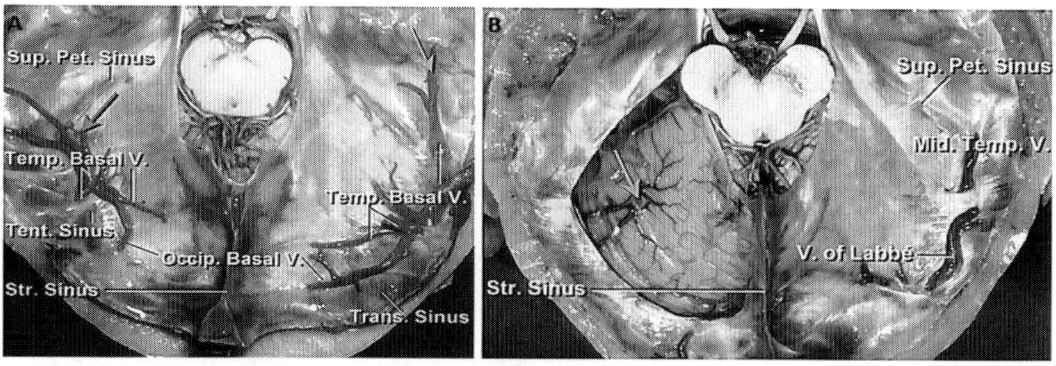

Figure 8.6. Veins of the basal surface. A, Superior view of the tentorial sinuses. The long vein on the left basal surface empties into the tributary of the left tentorial sinus shown by the dark arrow. The temporobasal veins on the right side empty into the right tentorial sinus with multiple tributaries. The tributary of right tentorial sinus shown with a light arrow. B, Tributaries of the transverse and tentorial sinuses. The left half of the tentorium has been removed. The bridging cerebellar vein, shown with an arrow, empties into the tentorial sinus. Mid., middle; Occip., occipital; Pet., petrosal; Post., posterior; Str., straight; Sup., superior; Temp., temporal; Tent., tentorial; Trans., transverse; V., vein. Taken with permission from the Rhoton Collection.

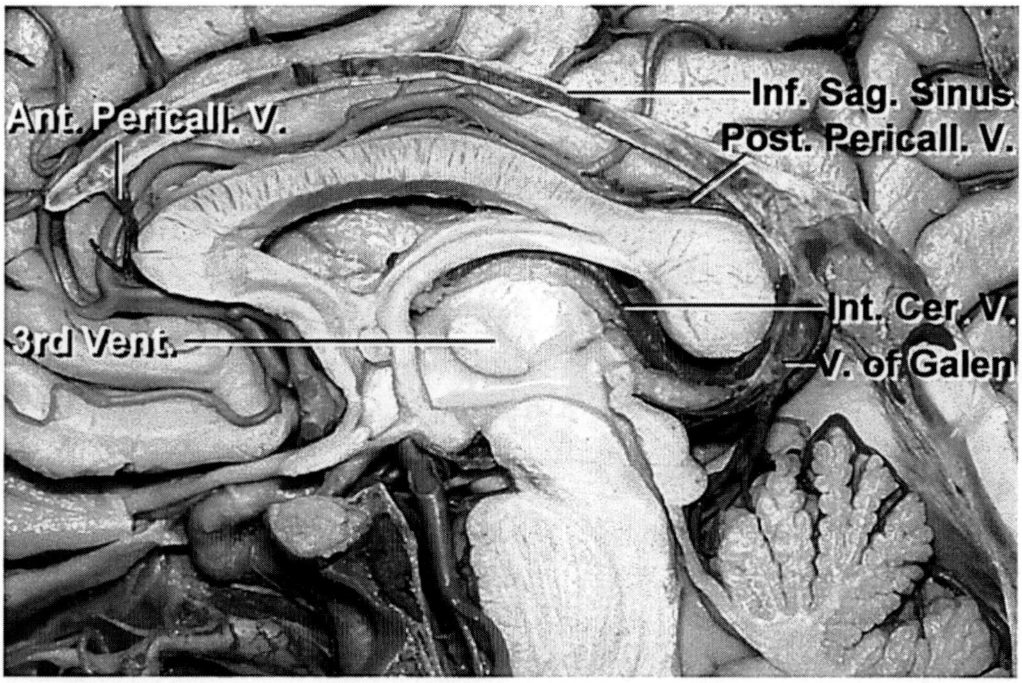

Figure 8.7. Veins of the medial surface. Enlarged view of the inferior sagittal sinus coursing in the lower edge of the falx. An anterior pericallosal vein empties into the anterior end of the inferior sagittal sinus. A small posterior pericallosal vein empties into the vein of Galen. Ant., anterior; Atr., atrial; Cer., cerebral; Cing., cingulate; Inf., inferior; Int., internal; Pericall., pericallosal; Post., posterior; Sag., sagittal; Sept., septal; V., vein; Vent., ventricle. Taken with permission from the Rhoton Collection.

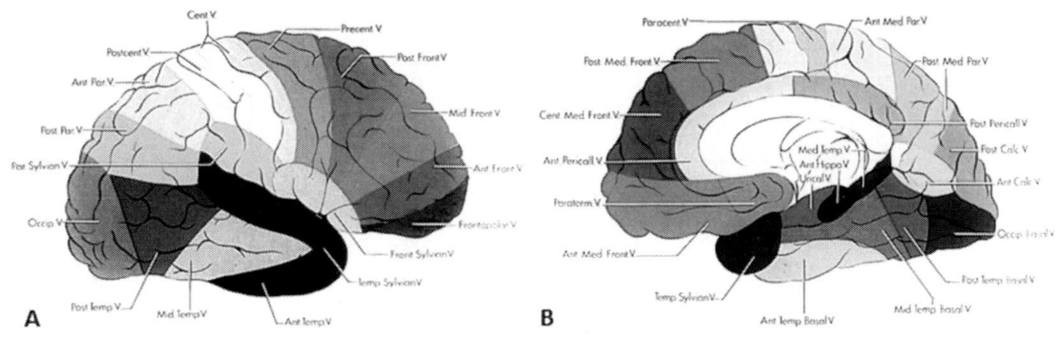

Figure 8.8. Territory and direction of drainage of the cortical veins. A, lateral surface. B, Medial surface. Taken with permission from the Rhoton Collection.

8.2.4. The Subarachnoid Cisterns

The subarachnoid cisterns are naturally occurring widening of this space, occurring in location where the arachnoid does not follow perfectly the curvatures of the CNS structures. Their importance stems from the clinical need to deduce physiological conclusions from anatomical images. A clinician looking at a CT scan (or MRI for that matter) trying to evaluate for an increased intracranial pressure is faced with the question when studying the brain structures of whether this is an anatomical variant or a new clinical finding. Detailed knowledge of the cisterns existence allows us to evaluate that patient's relative size of a certain structure. If a cistern is effaced or obliterated in imaging, than the right conclusion is that the brain region close to it is swollen (edematous). Otherwise, the absolute size of the brainstem or any other brain structure does not influence the intracranial pressure. Refer to table 8.2 for a short description of the cerebral cisterns.

Table 8.2. The Cerebral Cisterns

Cistern	Location, structures		Content
Chiasmatic	At the junction of the optic chiasm and the pituitary gland		CN-II, Ophthalmic artery
Lamina terminalis	It is the superior continuation of the chiasmatic cistern, at supraoptic crest.		
Cisterna fossae lateralis	It is located lateral to the pituitary gland, at the border of the temporal and frontal lobes, continuing as the Sylvian cistern at the Sylvian fissure.		
Perimesencephalic cisterns	Interpeduncular cistern	Located in so named fossa, bordered by the mamillary bodied and the crus cerebri.	CN-III Basilar artery
	Ambient cistern	Located lateral to crus cerebri (on midbrain sides)	CN-IV, PCA (P_2 segment)
	Quadrigeminal cistern	Located over the superior and inferior colliculi	CN-IV root
		At the junction where the inferior sagittal sinus joins the vein of Galen to form the straight sinus.	
Trigeminal cistern	Located Between the different branch fibers and the trigeminal ganglion		
Prepontine cistern	Located anteriorly at the pontomedullary junction, posterior to the clivus.		CN-VI Basilar artery
Cerebellopontine cistern	Superior	Located at the fold of Pons	CN-V, VII, VIII AICA
	Inferior	Located at the lateral cerebello-medullary junction and inferior Olivary eminence	CN-VIII-XII Vertebral artery PICA
Cisterna magna	Located between cerebellum and medulla		Distal PICA
Lumbar cistern	A large space located caudal to the conus medullaris		Cauda equine

The Liliequist's membrane (LM) is a subarachnoid membranous thickening, considered to separate the interpeduncular cistern from the chiasmatic cistern. Although a part of classical teaching, it forms a competent barrier between these cisterns in only 10 to 30%). Its superior leaflet (i.e., its diencephalic membrane) separates the interpeduncular cistern from the chiasmatic cistern medially and from the carotid cisterns laterally. Its inferior leaflet (i.e., its mesencephalic membrane) separates the interpeduncular cistern from the prepontine cistern. The diencephalic membrane is thicker and thus more often a competent barrier, effectively isolating the chiasmatic cistern. Its importance stems from the need to try isolating the source of a non-traumatic (aneurysmal) subarachnoid hemorrhage. Classic teaching states that hemorrhages anterior to LM are of the ACA, anterior communicating or MCA origin, whereas hemorrhages posterior to the LM are of basilar artery, posterior communicating or PCA origin. However, the carotid cisterns often communicate with the crural cisterns and in turn with the interpeduncular cistern (a bypass route). Still, blood in the carotid or prepontine cistern is more compatible with a low-pressure pretruncal source of bleeding and not an anterior communicating artery aneurysmal rupture.

8.3. Herniation Syndromes

8.3.1. Introduction

This term refers to shifts in brain tissue (caused by a mass effect) through rigid openings in the skull or meningeal foldings, causing compression to other structures of the CNS and producing symptoms. A herniation syndrome requires by definition a change in consciousness (either deteriorating consciousness or a comatose state). Brain structure shifts (the radiological correlation of the herniation syndrome) may not always be accompanied by the clinical syndrome, and may actually represent an epiphenomenon that occurs late in the process and is not actually the cause of the observations. Refer to figure 8.9 and to tables 8.3-8.5 for an overview.

There are many possible herniation syndromes, the most common are:

1) **Central (transtentorial) herniation** – discussed below. It refers to a central downward displacement of the brainstem. In milder cases it results in traction of the CN-VI during its long course over the clivus. Large lesions in posterior fossa may cause pressure to progress through foramen magnum, resulting in cerebellar tonsillar herniation, which is associated with compression of the medulla and respiratory arrest, blood pressure instability, death.
2) **Uncal herniation** - discussed below. It refers to the herniation of the medial temporal lobe inferiorly through the tentorial notch. The clinical triad includes a "Blown" pupil (compression of CN-III ipsilaterally), hemiplegia (compression of cerebral peduncles) and coma (distortion of midbrain ARAS).Compression of PCA's as they pass through the tentorial notch may cause infarctions.
3) **Cingulate (subflacine) herniation** - When the cingulate gyrus herniates under falx cerebri. It is usually asymptomatic unless the ACA kinks under the falx as well, causing bifrontal infarctions. This herniation type usually warns of impending transtentorial herniation.
4) **Upward cerebellar** – rare, iatrogenic. Caused when a ventricular external drain is allowed to over drain, causing a shift of cerebellum and brainstem structures through the incisura. The cerebellar vermis ascends above the tentorium, compressing the midbrain and possibly occluding the SCAs resulting in cerebellar infarction. It may compress the sylvian aqueduct resulting in hydrocephalus.
5) **Tonsillar herniation** – an extension of the central herniation.
6) **External herniation** – through an opening in the dura matter and skull. Not always accompanied by loss of consciousness. Danger of compromised blood supply or draining veins compressed against the free bone or dural edge, resulting in arterial or venous infarcts.

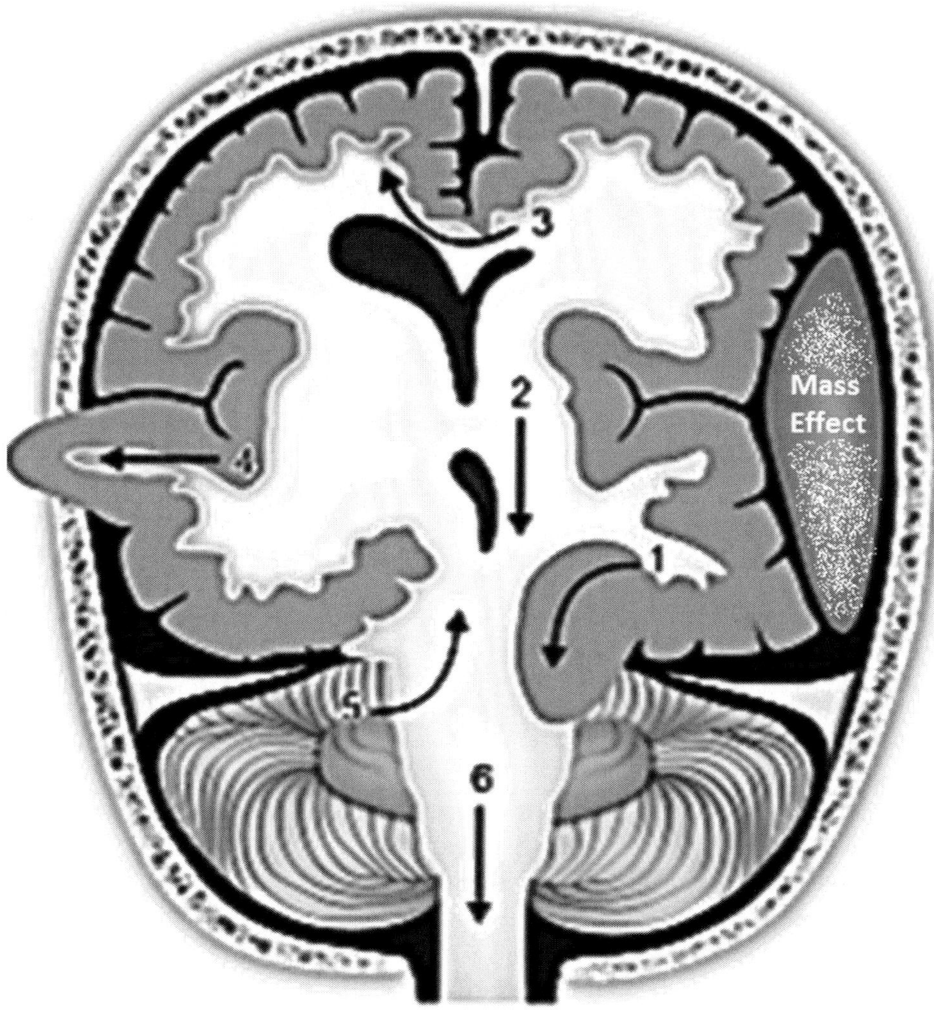

Figure 8.9. Type of brain herniation syndromes. 1-Uncal herniation. 2-Central herniation. 3-Cingulate herniation. 4-Transcalvarial (external) herniation. 5-upward herniation. 6-tonsillar herniation. Modified from Focused neurosurgery textbook, 2014.

8.3.1.1. Coma from a Supratentorial or Infratentorial Mass

Central herniation results in the sequential failure of the diencephalon, midbrain, pons, and medulla oblongata. The "Classic" signs of increased intracranial pressure (ICP) are hypertension, bradycardia and an altered respiratory pattern. These are usually seen with a posterior fossa lesion and may be absent in slowly developing supratentorial masses. An important note tough is that predicting the location of the lesion based on the herniation syndrome is unreliable. Decreased consciousness occurs early in central herniation and late in uncal herniation (also rarely gives decorticate posturing, refer to chapter 3). Etiologies range from vascular (stroke, intracerebral hemorrhage, subarachnoid hemorrhage), inflammatory (cerebral abscess, subdural empyema, herpes simplex encephalitis) neoplastic or traumatic.

Coma caused by infratentorial masses span the same etiologic spectrum. Hydrocephalus, caused by compression of the sylvian aqueduct and/or fourth ventricle is an aggravating factor.

8.3.2. Central Herniation

Central herniation, AKA transtentorial herniation, is usually more chronic than uncal herniation (due to tumor, especially of frontal, parietal or occipital lobes). The diencephalon is gradually forced through the tentorial incisura. The pituitary stalk may be sheared, resulting in diabetes insipidus. The PCAs may be trapped along the open edge of the incisura and may occlude, producing cortical blindness. The brainstem suffers ischemia from compression and shearing of the perforating arteries arising from the basilar artery. This results in hemorrhages within the brainstem parenchyma (the so called Duret's hemorrhages).

Imaging shows a downward displacement (shown more in the pineal region). The perimesencephalic cisterns are compressed. This herniation syndrome typically progresses through several stages, named according to the compromised structure at that stage (refer to table 8.3). These are successive steps, which if halted sooner carry a better prognosis. The diencephalic stage, the earliest stage, may be due to diffuse bilateral hemisphere dysfunction or (more likely) from bilateral diencephalic dysfunction due to downward displacement. This stage warns of impending (irreversible) midbrain damage but is frequently reversible if the cause is treated. The midbrain–upper pons stage occurs when midbrain signs fully develop (in adults), in which point prognosis is very poor. Fewer than 5% of cases will have a good recovery if treatment is successfully undertaken at this stage.

Table 8.3. Symptoms and signs of central herniation

Stages	Consciousness	Respiration	Pupils	Oculomotor	Motor
Diencephalic	Altered alertness is the first sign, may manifest as lethargy or agitation, later coma.	Sighs, yawns, later Cheyne-Stokes.	Small (1-3 mm).	Usually positive Doll's eyes and conjugate ipsilateral response to cold water calorics test.	Early bilateral Babinski sign, later the patients may become motionless, and then decorticate posturing.
Upper pons		Cheyne-Stokes.	Mid-position (3-5 mm)	Doll's eyes, Caloric test impaired. In MLF lesion inter-nuclear ophthalmoplegia	Initially decorticate, than bilateral decerebrate posturing.
Lower Pons - Upper Medullary		Regular. Shallow, rapid (20-40/min)			Flaccid, bilateral Babinski
Medullary (Terminal stage)		Slow, irregular rate and depth.	Widely dilated		

Outcome after central herniation varies but generally dismal. 9% of patients have good recovery, 18% have good functional outcome, 10% are severely disabled, and 60% die. Factors associated with a better result include a young age and an anisocoria (unequal pupils, indicating peripheral CN-III damage) with deteriorating Glasgow coma score and a nonflaccid motor function. Factors associated with poor outcome are bilaterally fixed pupils, indicating midbrain damage.

8.3.3. Uncal Herniation

This type of herniation usually occurs in rapidly expanding traumatic hematomas, frequently in the lateral middle-fossa or temporal lobe pushing the medial uncus and hippocampal gyrus over edge of tentorium, entrapping third nerve and directly compressing midbrain (discussed later). The PCA's may be occluded (as with central herniation). Impaired consciousness is NOT a reliable early sign. Earliest consistent sign are a unilaterally dilating pupil, caused by the compression of the CN-III nerve (not CNS compression). Deterioration may be rapid (deep coma in hours). The vasomotor fibers of the CN-III are located at its periphery, whereas its somatomotor fibers are located at its center. Thus, external compression causes a blown pupil prior to causing ophthalmoplegia. A vascular event (like secondary to diabetes) causes ophthalmoplegia with pupil sparing.

Table 8.4. Symptoms and signs of central herniation

Stages	Respiration	Pupils	Oculomotor	Motor
Early CN-III	Normal	Unilateral dilated, 85% ipsilateral to lesion	Doll's eye are normal or dysconjugate	Contralateral Babinski
Late CN-III	Sustained hyper-ventilation	Blown pupil	After blown pupil external ophthalmoplegia	Contralateral or ipsilateral weakness (Kernohan's), bilateral decerebration
Midbrain–upper Pons	Sustained hyperpnea	Blown and fixed, finally bilateral	Absent movement	Rigidity, bilateral decerebration

Table 8.5. Cerebral Herniation Syndromes Overview

Herniation	Anatomical structures involved	Clinical symptoms
Subfalcine / Cingulate	Cingulate gyrus	Leg weakness
	Pericallosal arteries	
Transtentorial / Uncal	CN-III palsy	Ipsilateral ptosis and mydriasis
	Cerebral peduncle	Contralateral / Ipsilateral (Kernohan's) hemiparesis
	PCA	Cortical blindness
	Brainstem reticular formation compression	Decreased consciousness
Posterior (Tectal)	Superior colliculi	Bilateral ptosis
	Brainstem compression	Vertical gaze paralysis
Central (axial)	Basilar artery perforators (brainstem damage)	Depressed consciousness, impaired eye movements (MLF)
		Respiratory irregularity, apnea.
		Hypertension, bradycardia
Tonsillar	Medulla oblongata	Apnea, respiratory depression

In terms of radiological appearance, the tentorial incisura surrounds the interpeduncular and pre-pontine cisterns and brainstem. There is great interpersonal variability in the amount of space in the incisura. Impending uncal or hippocampal herniation may be indicated by encroachment on the lateral aspect of the suprasellar cistern with flattening of normal pentagonal shape. Once herniation occurs imaging may show brainstem displacement and flattening, compression of the contralateral cerebral peduncle or midbrain rotation with slight increase of ipsilateral subarachnoid space. Obliteration of the parasellar and interpeduncular cisterns occurs as the uncus and / or hippocampus are forced through the hiatus. This type of herniation is also segregated into stages (refer to table 8.4). The early CN-III stage is not a brainstem finding, caused by CN-III compression. The late CN-III stage manifests with midbrain dysfunction.

8.3.4. Intracranial True and Potential Spaces and Related Hemorrhages

The epidural space is located between the periosteal and membranous dural layers of the skull. Within the spinal column, it is a real space filled with fat and the Batson's venous plexus. This space may be developed by a hemorrhage caused by rupture of the middle meningeal artery mostly, secondary to a fracture of the temporal bone. It is a lens shaped biconvex hematoma, not spreading across suture lines (refer to figure 8.10). Clinically, it manifests with a lucid interval, and in hours elevated ICP.

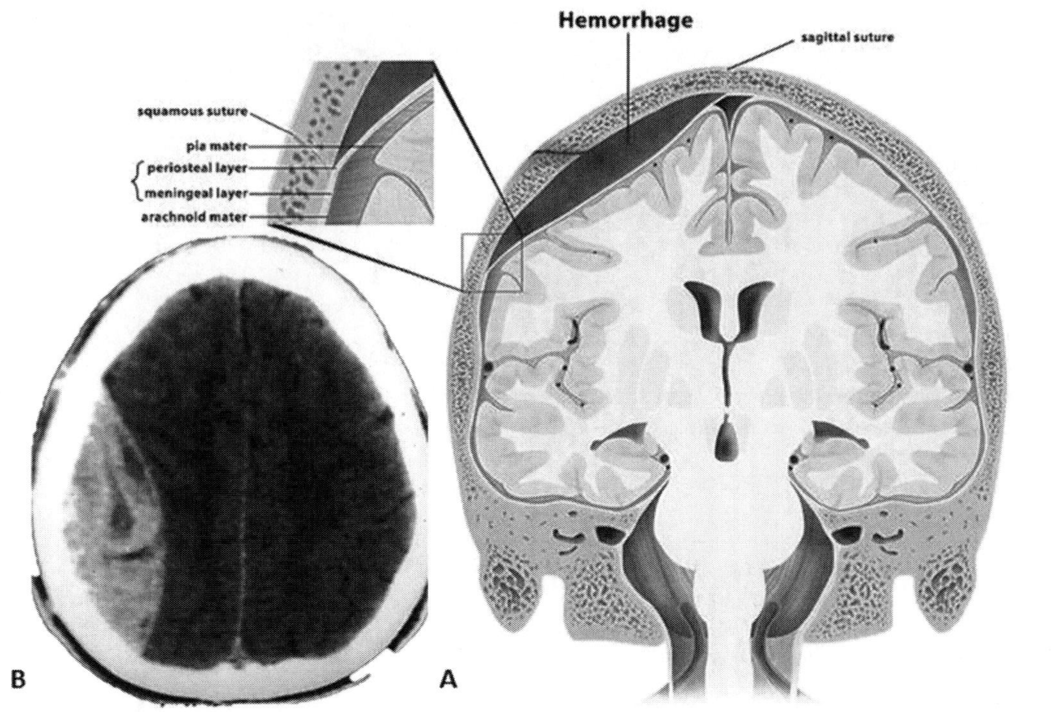

Figure 8.10. An extradural (Epidural) Hemorrhage. A, illustration. B, Non-contrast enhanced CAT scan showing the lens shape of an acute subdural hematoma. Taken with permission from www.radiopaedia.org.

The subdural space is located between the membranous dura and the membranous arachnoid layers. This space may be developed by a hemorrhage caused due to rupture of the bridging veins, vulnerable to shear injury particularly as they cross the arachnoid into the dura. It results in a crescent (lenticular) shaped hematoma (refer to figure 8.11). The subarachnoid space is a true space, span by blood vessels and cranial nerves and bathes by CSF. A non-traumatic hemorrhage is caused in 80% due to an arterial aneurysm and in 4% due to an AVM (arteriovenous malformation).

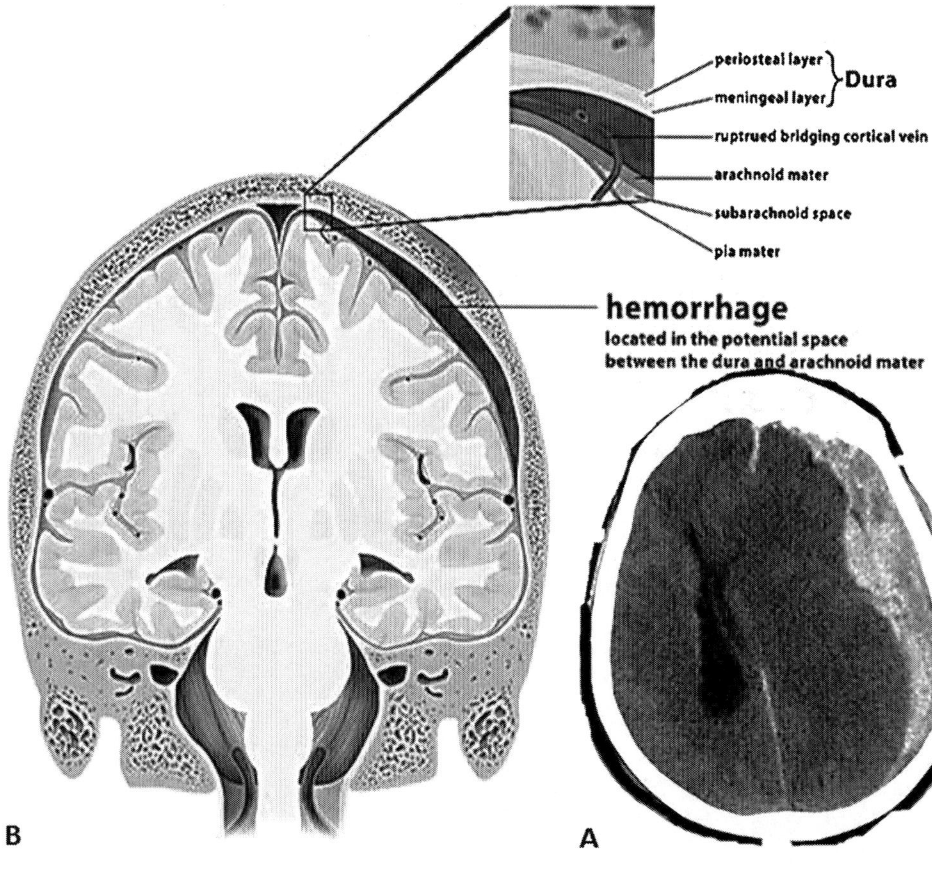

Figure 8.11. A subdural hemorrhage. A, A Non-contrast enhanced CAT scan showing the lenticular shape of an acute subdural hematoma. B, illustration. Taken with permission from www.radiopaedia.org.

8.4. The Cerebrospinal Fluid (CSF)

8.4.1. General Information

The CSF surrounds the brain and spinal cord, and may function as a shock absorber for the CNS. It may also serve an immunological function analogous to the lymphatic system (no lymphatics in the brain). The CSF normally is a clear colorless fluid with a specific gravity of 1.007 and a pH of 7.33~7.35. About 80% of the CSF is produced by the choroid plexus of the ventricles, located in both lateral ventricles (accounts for - 95% of CSF produced in the choroid plexuses) and in the third and fourth ventricles. Most of the reminder of the CSF production occurs in the interstitial space. A small amount may also be produced by the ependymal lining of the ventricles. Refer o table 8.6 for normal CSF production, volume and pressure.

In the adult, the CSF is produced at a rate of 0.3 ml/min. about 450 ml are produced in a 24hrs which means that in a normal adult, the CSF is "turned over" or recycled about three times every day. The rate of CSF formation is independent of the intracranial pressure.

The CSF is absorbed by the arachnoid villi (or arachnoid granulations) that extend into the dural venous sinuses. The rate of absorption is intracranial-pressure dependent.

Table 8.6. Normal CSF production, volume and pressure

Property	Pediatrics		Adult
	Newborn	1-10 years	
Total volume	5		150
Formation rate	25 ml/day		0.3 ml/min (450 ml/day)
Pressure (cm)	9-12	Mean 10, normal <15	7-16

8.4.2. CSF Constituents

In normal adult CSF, there are 0~5 lymphocytes or mononuclear cells/ mm^3, and no polymorphinuclear cells (PMN's) or red blood cells (RBC). In the absence of RBCs, 5-10 WBCs per mm^3 is suspicious of an infectious or pathological condition, with over 10 white blood cells (WBCs) per mm^3 is defined as abnormal. Refer to tables 8.7.

Table 8.7. Variations in CSF Content With Age

Age group		WBC	RBC	Protein (mg/dl)	Glucose (mg/dl)	Glucose ratio (CSF:Plasma)
Newborn	Preemie	10	Many	150	20-65	0.5-1.6
	Term	7-8	Moderate	80	30-120	0.4-2.5
Infants	1-12 mos	5-6	0	15-80		
	1-2 yrs	2-3	0	15		
Young child		2-3	0	20		
Children 5-15 years		2-3	0	25		
Adults		3	0	30	40-80	0.5
Senile		5	0	40		

Table 8.8. CSF solutes

Constituent	Units	CSF	Plasma	CSF:Plasma
Osmolarity	mOsm/L	295	295	1.0
Water content		99%	93%	
Na	mEq/L	138	138	1.0
K	mEq/L	2.8	4.5	0.6

Table 8.8. (Continued)

Constituent	Units	CSF	Plasma	CSF:Plasma
Cl	mEq/L	119	102	1.2
Ca	mEq/L	2.1	4.8	0.4
pCO_2	mm Hg	47	41	1.1
pH		7.33	7.41	
pO_2	mm Hg	43	104	0.4
Glucose	Mg/dl	60	90	0.67
Lactate	mEq/L	1.6	1	1.6
Pyruvate	mEq/L	0.08	0.11	0.73
Total protein	Mg/dl	35	7000	0.005
Albumin	Mg/L	155	36600	0.004
IgG	Mg/L	12.3	9870	0.001

Table 8.9. CSF findings in various pathologic conditions (Adult values)

Condition	OP*	Appearance	Cells (per mm^3)	Protein (mg%)	Glucose (%serum)	Comments
Normal	7-18	Clear	0 PMN, 0 RBC, 0-5 mono	15-45	50	
Bacterial meningitis	↑	Turbid	↑↑↑ (mostly PMN)	100-1000	< 20	PMN's early
Viral meningitis / encephalitis	nl**	nl	↑ (mostly monocytes)	40-100	nl	
Guillain – Barre syndrome	nl	nl	nl	50-1000	nl	Protein ↑, IgG
Tuberculus meningitis	↑	Opalescent fibrin clot on standing	50-500 (lymphocytes, monocytes)	60-700	20-40	PMN's, acid fast(+), Ziel-Neelson stain
Multiple sclerosis	nl	nl	5-50 monocytes	0-800	nl	↑ IgG

*Opening pressure (cm H_2O), ** normal

Table 8.10. SF Features in Subarachnoid Hemorrhage and in a Traumatic Spinal Tap

	Traumatic LP tap	SAH
RBC count	Gradually decreasing	Constant
Clotting	Clots	Do not clot
Xantochromia	None	Present
RBC / WBC ratio	Normal	May be decreased
Protein content	Normal or increased	May be increased
Hemosiderin laden macrophages	absent	Present within days
CSF opening pressure	Normal	Increased
Repeated LP tap	Normal	Consistent with SAH

8.4.3. The Blood Brain Barrier

The blood–brain barrier (BBB) is a highly selective permeability barrier that separates the circulating blood from the brain extracellular fluid (BECF) in the CNS. The BBB is formed by the capillary endothelial cells, which are connected by tight junctions with an extremely high electrical resistance. The BBB allows the passage of water, some gases, and lipid soluble molecules by passive diffusion, as well as the selective transport of molecules such as glucose and amino acids that are crucial to neural function. On the other hand, the BBB may prevent the entry of lipophilic, potential neurotoxins by way of an active transport mechanism mediated by P-glycoprotein. Astrocytes are necessary to create the blood–brain barrier. A small number of regions in the brain, including the circumventricular organs (CVOs), do not have a BBB (discussed later).

The BBB occurs along all capillaries and consists of tight junctions around the capillaries that do not exist in normal circulation. Endothelial cells restrict the diffusion of microscopic objects (e.g., bacteria) and large or hydrophilic molecules into the CSF, while allowing the diffusion of small hydrophobic molecules (O_2, CO_2, hormones). Cells of the barrier actively transport metabolic products such as glucose across the barrier with specific proteins. This barrier also includes a thick basement membrane and astrocytic end-feet. The CSF is an ultra-filtrate of the blood, low in immune and toxic constituents. The BBB is in actuality the sum of filtering capabilities of four layers: the capillary endothelium, the endothelial basement membrane, the astrocytic foot processes and the astrocytes (refer to figure 8.12).

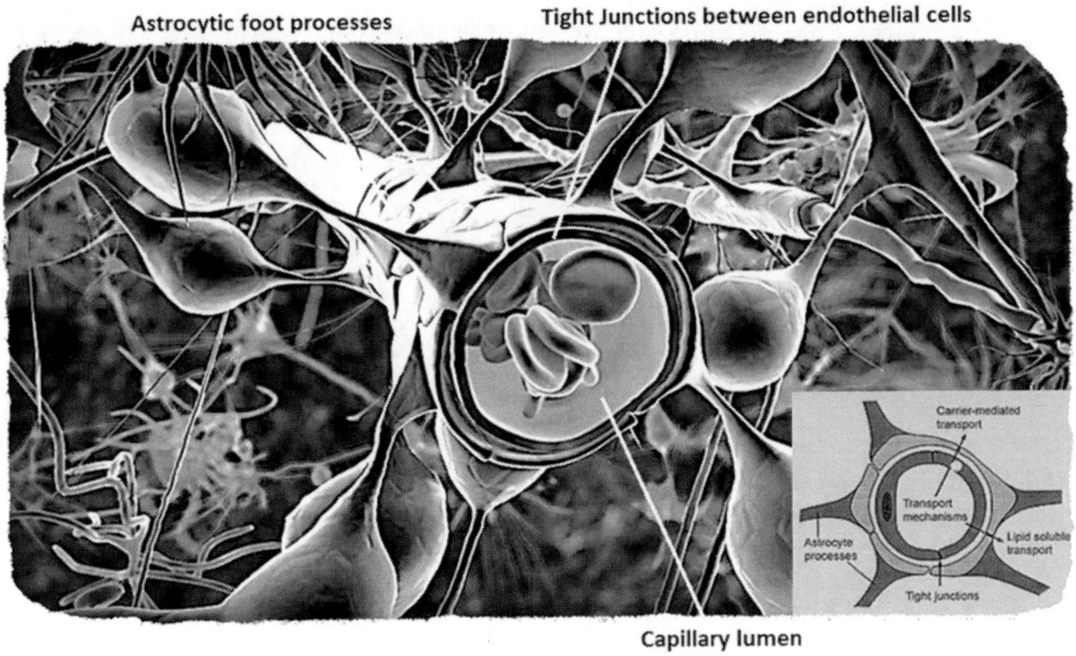

Figure 8.12. The blood brain barrier (BBB) in 3-Dimensions. Refer to the text.

8.4.4. The Circumventricular Organs

The Circumventricular organs (CVOs) are structures in the brain that are characterized by their extensive vasculature and lack of a normal BBB. These CVOs allow for the linkage between the CNS and the peripheral blood flow; additionally they are an integral part of neuroendocrine function. The lack of a blood brain barrier allows the CVOs to act as an alternative route for peptides and hormones in the neural tissue to the peripheral blood stream, while still protecting it from toxic substances. CVOs can be classified into sensory and secretory organs. The sensory organs include area postrema (AP), the subfornical organ (SFO) and the organum vasculosum of lamina terminalis (OVLT). These have the ability to sense plasma molecules and then pass that information into other regions of the brain. Through this, they provide direct information to the autonomic nervous system from systemic circulation. The secretory organs include the subcommissural organ(SCO), the posterior pituitary (i.e., the neurohypophysis), the pineal gland, the median eminence and the intermediate lobe of the pituitary. These organs are responsible for secreting hormones and glycoproteins into the peripheral vascular system using feedback from both the brain environment and external stimuli.

All of the circumventricular organs, besides the SCO, contain extensive vasculature and fenestrated capillaries which leads to a 'leaky' BBB at the site of the organs. Furthermore, all CVOs contain neural tissue, allowing them to play a role in the neuroendocrine system (refer to figure 8.13).

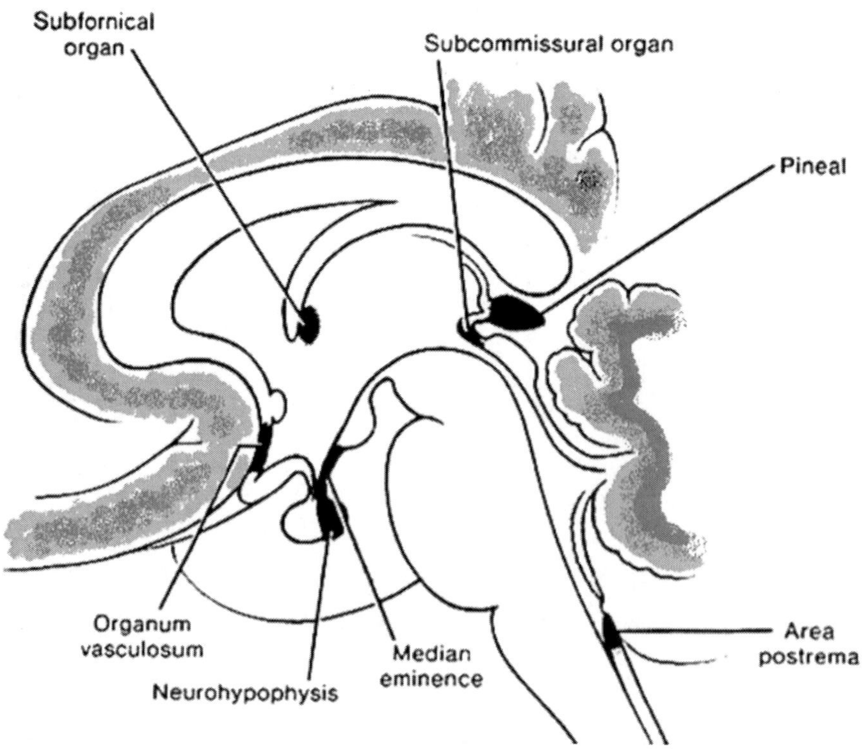

Figure 8.13. The Circumventricular organs. Refer to text. Taken from Gray's Anatomy (out of copyright and in the public domain).

8.4.4.1. Area Postrema

Its bilateral structure makes it lie on either side of the medullary midline, at the junction between the medulla and the spinal cord. It is the chemoreceptor trigger zone for vomiting.

8.4.4.2. Organum Vasculosum of the Lamina Terminalis (OVLT)

Classified as a sensory CVO, the OVLT is situated in the anterior wall of the third cerebral ventricle. It receives afferent inputs from the subfornical organ (SFO), the median pre-optic nucleus region, the brainstem, and even the hypothalamus. Conversely, the organum vasculosum maintains efferent projections to the stria medullaris and basal ganglia. It is an important component of the body's system of maintaining fluid homeostasis and thus it features the primary neurons responsible for osmosensory balance. The OVLT may also play a role in the regulation of LH secretion via a negative feedback mechanism. It is also hypothesized that the OVLT may be the mechanism through which pyrogens function to initiate a febrile response in the CNS. Finally, OVLT neurons have been observed to respond to temperature changes indicating that the organum vasculosum of the lamina terminalis is subject to different climates.

8.4.4.3. The Subfornical Organ (SFO)

The subfornical organ is a sensory CVO situated in the lamina terminalis and lacking the BBB, the absence of which characterizes the circumventricular organs. Protruding into the third ventricle of the brain, the highly vascularized SFO can be divided into three anatomical zones. Its central zone is composed exclusively of the glial cells and neuronal cell bodies. Conversely, it's rostral and caudal areas are mostly made of nerve fibers while very few neurons and glial cells can be seen in this area. Functionally, however, the SFO may be viewed in two portions, the dorsolateral peripheral (pSFO) division and the ventromedial core segment. As an important mechanism of both energy and osmotic homeostasis, the SFO has many efferent projections. It seems that the most essential of all these connections is the SFO's projections to the paraventricular hypothalamic nucleus. The subfornical organ is a circumventricular organ active in many bodily processes including, but not limited to, osmoregulation, cardiovascular regulation, and energy homeostasis.

8.4.4.4. The Subcommissural Organ

The subcommissural organ (SCO) is a small secretory organ located near the anterior entrance of the sylvian aqueduct and at the midline roof of the third ventricle. The SCO also covers and penetrates the posterior commissure. It is aberrant from other CVOs in that lacks a high concentration of fenestrated capillaries, making its BBB less permeable. On the other hand, its large role in the neuroendocrine system awards it the CVO classification. The main function of the SCO is the secretion of the glycoprotein SCO-spondin. When SCO-spondin is released, it travels into the third ventricle, where it aggregates to create Reissner's fibers (RF). Reissner's fibers are long fibrous projections that travel caudally through the sylvian aqueduct and can terminate as far as the spinal cord. These fibers contribute to the maintenance of the patency of the sylvian aqueduct. If the SCO were to malfunction, causing a loss of the Reissner's fibers, a medical condition known as Congenital Hydrocephalus (CH) can develop. The SCO is innervated by many systems, the most common of which is associated with the serotonergic system.

8.4.4.5. The Neurohypophysis

The pituitary is subdivided into two principal lobes, anterior and posterior, the latter of which is also known as the neurohypophysis (refer to chapter 4). The posterior pituitary is made up by a stalk, the infundibulum, which consists of axonal projections that extend from the hypothalamus. The posterior lobe stores and releases oxytocin and vasopressin, also known as antidiuretic hormone (ADH), which are produced in the hypothalamus.

8.4.4.6. The Median Eminence

The median eminence (ME) is located in the inferior portion of the hypothalamus and is ventral to the third ventricle. The median eminence is rich in fenestrated capillaries, allowing for the passage of proteins and neurohormones. Specifically, the median eminence allows for the transport of neurohormones between the CSF and the peripheral blood supply. The major cell type that makes up the median eminence is specialized ependymal cells known as tanycytes. These contribute to the organ's ability to selectively allow macromolecules to pass from the central to the peripheral neuroendocrine systems.

8.4.4.7. The Pineal Gland

The pineal gland rests proximally to the posterior section of the diencephalon. It is located within 1-2mm of the midline of the brain. In the average adult, the dimensions are 5-9mm in length, 1-5mm in width and 3-5mm in thickness. Its average weight is 100–180 mg. The pineal gland is considered a secretory organ and its activity shows circadian oscillations. Its main function, secretion of the hormone melatonin, dies out when there is no input from the primary circadian pacemaker in the suprachiasmatic nuclei (SCN). Other peptides aside from melatonin have been detected in the pineal. They are most likely associated with a type of innervation deemed "pineal peptidergic innervation." These include vasopressin, oxytocin, VIP, NPY, peptide histidine isoleucine, calcitonin gene-related peptide, substance P and somatostatin.

8.5. The Lateral Ventricles

The fourth ventricle was discussed in details in the chapter focused on the brainstem (chapter 3), the third ventricle was described in details in the chapter focused on the diencephalon (chapter 4). The lateral ventricles, formerly termed as the first and second ventricles are the superior remnants of the lumen in the original neural tube. The two bilaterally symmetric lateral ventricles lie in close apposition to the caudate nucleus in certain locations. Other C-shaped structures that follow the curve of the ventricles include the caudate nucleus, the corpus callosum, the fornix and the stria terminalis. The third ventricle (along midline) is located between the two thalami. Refer to figure 8.14 for the neural relationships.

Each lateral ventricle wraps around the thalamus (figure 8.14-8.15). The frontal horn is anterior to the thalamus, the body is above the thalamus, the atrium and occipital horn are behind the thalamus, and the temporal horns is below and lateral to the thalamus. The septum pellucidum is in the medial wall of the frontal horn and body of the lateral ventricle. The hippocampal formation is in the floor of the temporal horn. The fornix arises in the hippocampal formation and wraps around the thalamus in the medial part of the temporal horn, atrium, and body. The fimbria of the fornix arises on the surface of the hippocampal formation in the temporal horn. The crus of the fornix are posterior to the thalamus in the wall of the atrium. The body of the fornix passes above the thalamus in the lower part of the medial wall of the body. The columns of the fornix are formed at the level of the foramen of Monro and pass inferior to the mamillary bodies. The crura of the fornix are connected across the midline in the roof of the third ventricle by the hippocampal commissure. The septum pellucidum, which separates the frontal horns in the midline, does not extend to the anterior tip of the frontal horn in the lateral view because the frontal horn is directed forward and laterally from the anterior margin of the septum pellucidum.

The head and body of the caudate nucleus form the lateral wall of the frontal horn and body of the lateral ventricle. The tail of the caudate nucleus extends into the anterior part of the lateral wall of the atrium and into the medial part of the roof of the temporal horn to the level of the amygdaloid nucleus, which is in the anterior wall of the temporal horn. The corpus callosum is made up of the rostrum (which is in the floor of the frontal horn), the genu (which forms the anterior wall and roof of the frontal horn), the body (which forms the roof of the body of the lateral ventricle), and the splenium (which gives rise to the fiber bundles making up the forceps major, which forms a prominence in the medial wall of the atrium called the bulb of the corpus callosum). The genu of the corpus callosum gives rise to a fiber bundle called the forceps minor, which forms the anterior wall of the frontal horn. The body and splenium give rise to a fiber bundle called the tapetum, which sweeps downward to form the roof and lateral wall of the atrium and temporal horn. The relationship of the hippocampal formation, fornix, and mamillary bodies to these structures is shown in the middle figure. A prominence in the medial wall of the atrium, called the calcar avis, overlies the calcarine sulcus.

Looking at the structures forming the walls of the lateral ventricles (refer to figure 8.16), in the frontal horn, the genu of the corpus callosum is in the roof, the caudate nucleus is in the lateral wall, the rostrum of the corpus callosum is in the floor, and the septum pellucidum is in the medial wall. In the body of the lateral ventricle, the body of the corpus callosum is in the roof, the caudate nucleus is in the lateral wall, the thalamus is in the floor, and the septum pellucidum and fornix are in the medial wall. The choroidal fissure, the site of the attachment of the choroid plexus in the lateral ventricle, is situated between the fornix and the thalamus. At the atrium, the lateral wall and roof are formed by the tapetum of the corpus callosum, and the floor is formed by the collateral trigone, which overlies the collateral sulcus. The inferior part of the medial wall is formed by the calcar avis, the prominence that overlies the deep end of the calcarine sulcus, and the superior part of the medial wall is formed by the bulb of the corpus callosum, which overlies the forceps major. At the temporal horn, the medial part of the floor of the temporal horn is formed by the prominence overlying the hippocampal formation, and the lateral part of the floor is formed by the prominence called the collateral eminence, which overlies the deep end of the collateral sulcus. The roof is formed by the caudate nucleus and the tapetum of the corpus callosum, the lateral wall is formed by the tapetum of the corpus callosum, and the medial wall of the temporal horn is little more than the cleft between the fimbria of the fornix and the inferolateral aspect of the thalamus.

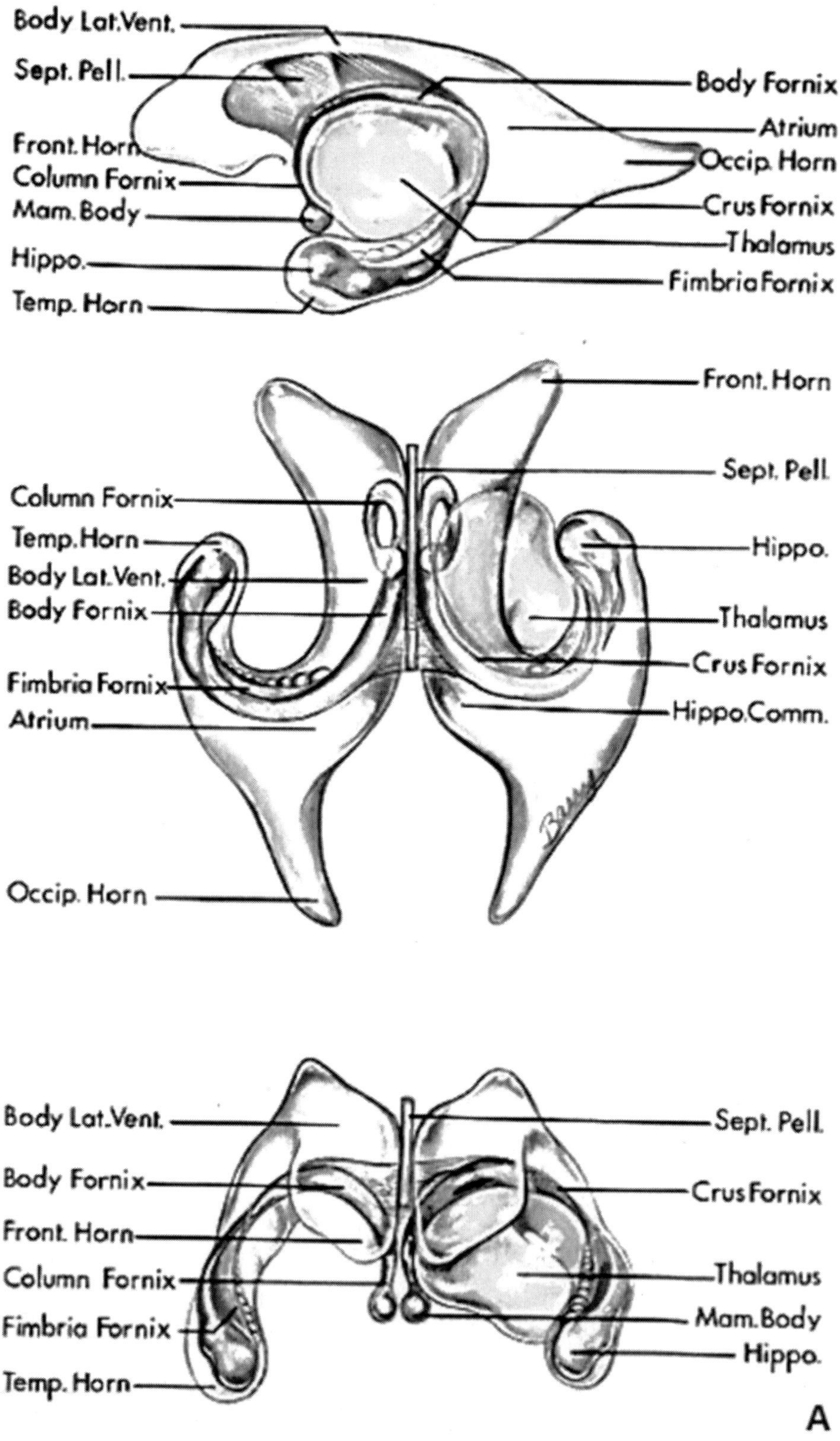

Body Lat.Vent.
Sept. Pell.
Front. Horn
Column Fornix
Mam. Body
Hippo.
Temp. Horn
Body Fornix
Atrium
Occip. Horn
Crus Fornix
Thalamus
Fimbria Fornix
Front. Horn
Sept. Pell.
Column Fornix
Temp. Horn
Body Lat. Vent.
Body Fornix
Hippo.
Thalamus
Crus Fornix
Fimbria Fornix
Atrium
Hippo. Comm.
Occip. Horn
Body Lat. Vent.
Sept. Pell.
Body Fornix
Crus Fornix
Front. Horn
Column Fornix
Thalamus
Mam. Body
Fimbria Fornix
Hippo.
Temp. Horn
A

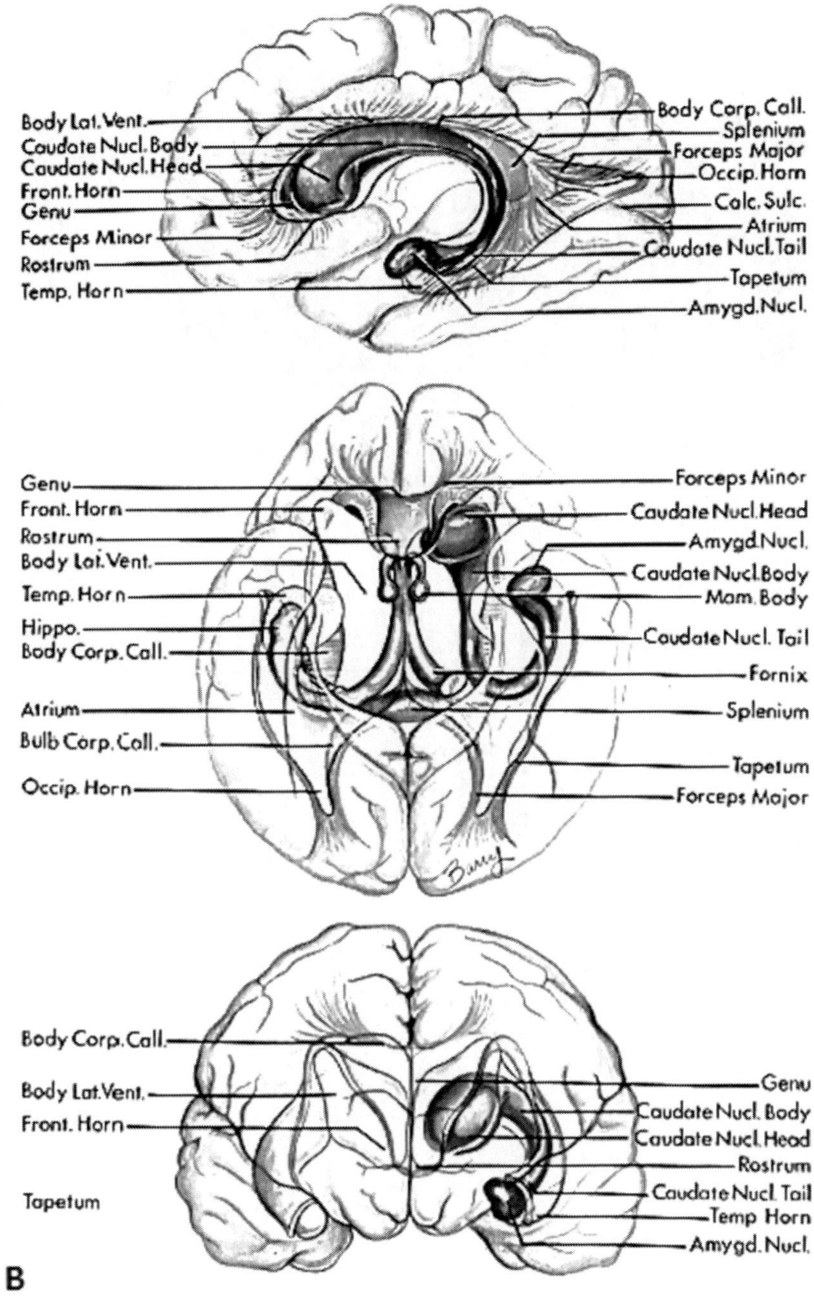

Figure 8.14. Neural relationships. A, relationship of the septum pellucidum, thalamus and hippocampal formation and fornix to the lateral ventricles. Top, lateral view; middle, superior view; bottom, anterior view. B, relationship of the corpus callosum, caudate nucleus, and fornix and hippocampal formation to the lateral ventricles. Top, view through medial surface of the hemisphere; middle, view through inferior surface of the hemisphere; bottom, view through the anterior surface of the hemisphere. Amygd., amygdaloid; Calc., calcarine; Comm., commissure; Corp., corpus; Front., frontal; Hippo., hippocampal, hippocampus; Lat., lateral; Mam., mamillary; Nucl., nucleus; Occip., occipital; Pell., pellucidum; Sept., septum; Sulc., sulcus; Temp., temporal; Vent., ventricle. Taken with permission from the Rhoton Collection.

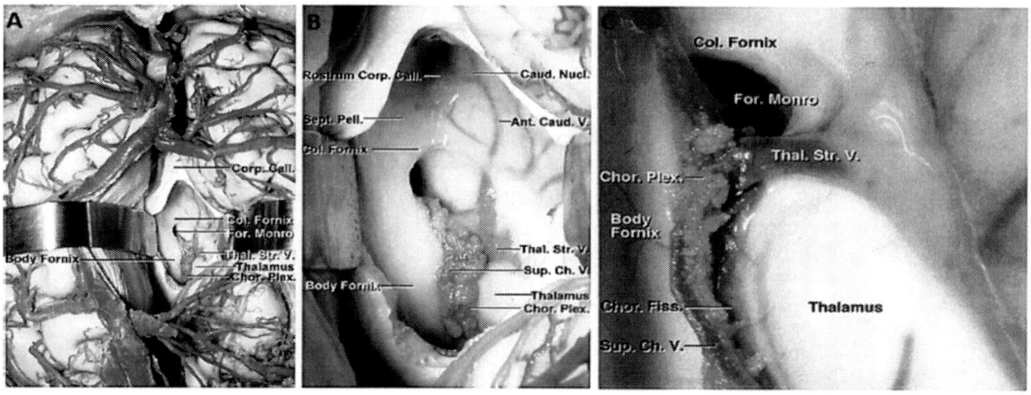

Figure 8.15. Stepwise dissection into the lateral and third ventricle via an interhemispheric approach. A, The corpus callosum has been opened to expose the fornix coursing anterior and superior to the foramen of Monro. B, enlarged view. The anterior caudate and superior choroidal veins join the anterior end of the thalamostriate vein. The column of the fornix passes anterior and superior to the foramen of Monro. The floor of the frontal horn is formed by the rostrum of the corpus callosum, the medial wall by the septum pellucidum, and the lateral wall by the caudate nucleus. C, Enlarged view of the foramen of Monro. The columns of the fornix pass around the superior and anterior margins of the foramen of Monro. The anterior nucleus of the thalamus sits in the posterior margin of the foramen of Monro. The thalamostriate vein passes forward between the caudate nucleus and thalamus and through the posterior margin of the foramen of Monro. The choroidal fissure in the body of the lateral ventricle is located between the body of the fornix and the thalamus. Taken with permission from the Rhoton Collection.

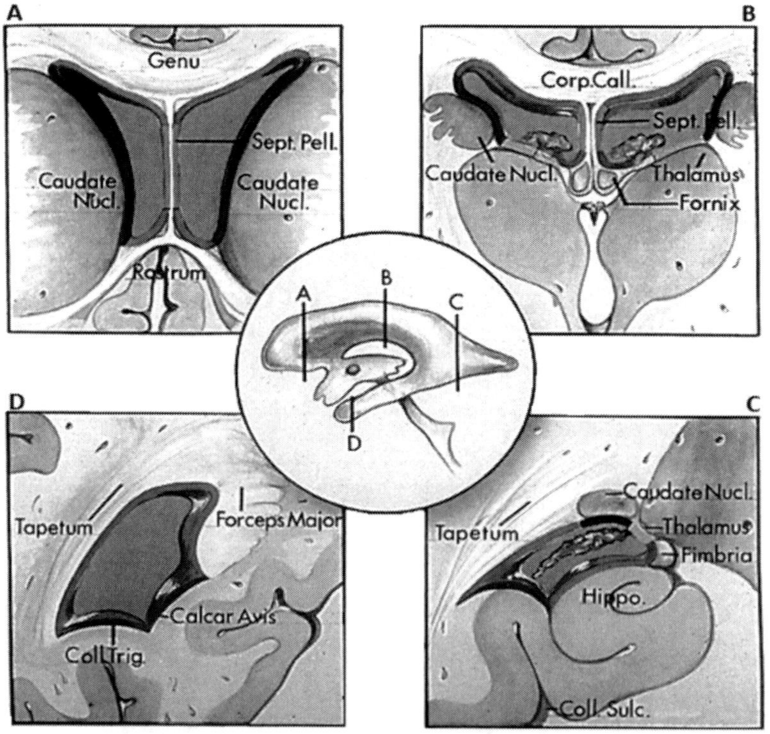

Figure 8.16. Structures in the walls of the lateral ventricles. The central diagram shows the level of the cross sections through the frontal horn (A), body (B), atrium (C), and temporal horn (D). Call., callosum; Coll., collateral; Corp., corpus; Hippo., hippocampus; Nucl., nucleus; Pell., pellucidum; Sept., septum; Sulc., sulcus; Trig., trigone. Taken with permission from the Rhoton Collection.

Chapter 9

Cerebral Blood Supply

9.1. Abstract

This chapter reviews many of the anatomical landmarks discussed previously, with a focused look at the arterial supply to the brain. The development of the arterial brain vasculature, initially with the internal carotid system and next with the joining of the vertebrobasilar system is reviewed, along with a short description of the anastomoses between these systems. The internal carotid artery and the vertebrobasilar system are described next, focusing on clinically relevant details and a concise, table based description. The circle of Willis is described next, followed by a description of the three main cerebral arteries using dissection images, angiographic studies and illustrations. After a discussion on the vascular territories, a short description of the Basal Cisterns Vascular Architecture follows, based on dissections from the timeless Rhoton Collection. The chapter ends with a short overview of ischemic clinical syndromes, not repeating those taught in the brainstem (chapter 3) and cerebral cortex (chapter 7) discussions.

9.2. Introduction

Arterial blood reaches the brain mainly via two arterial systems (pairs of arteries), the vertebral arteries (VA) which fuse to form the single basilar artery and the internal carotid arteries (ICA) coming off the common carotid artery. Arteries penetrate the dura and arachnoid to form a complex network that covers the brain surface in the subarachnoid space (and cisterns). Arterial branches penetrate the surface, (taking a pia "cuff" with them) and irrigate deeper regions. Arteries give rise to smaller and smaller arteries that form capillary beds. Blood is drained into veins and dural sinuses and ultimately into the internal jugular vein. The dura is irrigated by the meningeal arteries that are branches of the external carotid arteries. The vertebrobasilar system has been discussed in details in the chapters dealing with brainstem and cerebellar anatomy, and will be mentioned here for completeness. The external carotid artery (ECA) and possible ECA-ICA anastomoses will be presented as well.

9.3. Development of the Blood Supply to the Brain

During the closure of the neural tube, primordial endothelial blood-containing channels are established. From these all other vessels, arteries, veins and capillaries are derived. At stage 12, capital venous plexuses, the capital vein and three aortic arches are present. The internal carotids develop early (at stages 11–13), followed by the posterior communicating artery, the caudal branch of the internal carotid at stage 14, the basilar and vertebral arteries (stage 16), the main cerebral arteries (stage 17) and finally the anterior communicating artery, thereby completing the circle of Willis.

Bilaterally, longitudinal arteries are established at stage 13 and are connected with the internal carotids by temporary trigeminal, otic and hypoglossal arteries. At first, the posterior communicating artery provides the major blood supply of the brainstem. Anastomotic channels unite the two longitudinal arteries, thereby initiating the formation of the basilar artery. The temporary arteries are gradually eliminated, but each of them may persist. The primitive trigeminal artery is the most common of the primitive carotid–basilar anastomoses that persists into adulthood, with an incidence of 0.1–1.0%.

Capillaries at the level of the cerebral hemispheres begin to appear at 5 weeks, probably earlier in the brainstem. By 5 weeks (stage 16), many of the definitive arteries are present and are being transformed into the definitive pattern. At the end of the embryonic period, an annular network of leptomeningeal arteries arises from each middle cerebral artery and extends over each developing hemisphere. Similar meningeal branches, originating from the vertebral and basilar arteries, embrace the brain stem and cerebellum. From these gradually muscularizing leptomeningeal arterial branches grow into the brain. Both supratentorially and infratentorially, paramedian, short circumferential and long circumferential arteries can be distinguished. The first vessels penetrate the telencephalon in the seventh week of gestation, form a subventricular plexus at about 12 weeks of gestation and also gradually muscularize. At 16 weeks of gestation, the anterior, middle and posterior cerebral arteries, contributing to the formation of the circle of Willis, are well established.

9.4. External Carotid Artery (ECA) Branches and Major Extracranial-Intracranial (EC-IC) Anastomoses

The External carotid artery branches include (in correct order from proximal to distal):

1) Superior thyroid - It is the first branch, supplies the larynx and upper thyroid gland. In 20%, it arises above the carotid bifurcation and in 10% it arises from the common carotid artery (CCA).
2) Ascending pharyngeal artery- APA, it is the posterior branch. It anastomoses with the vertebral artery (VA) at the C3 vertebra level. It supplies the nasopharynx, oropharynx, middle ear, cranial nerves IX-XI, meninges.
3) Lingual artery – It is the major blood supply to the tongue and floor of the oral cavity.

4) Facial artery - It crosses the mandible, supplying the face, palate and lips.
5) Occipital artery – It runs posterior superior between the C1 vertebra and the occipital bone. It supplies the posterior scalp, upper cervical muscles and posterior fossa meninges. It anastomoses with VA at the C1-C2 level.
6) Posterior auricular artery - It supplies the pinna, external auditory canal and scalp.
7) Superficial temporal artery - It supplies the scalp and anterior ear.
8) Internal maxillary (IMA) – it is a terminal branch, coursing within the parotid gland, behind the mandible, to terminate in the pterygopalatine fossa. The middle meningeal artery (MMA) branches from it.

Different intracranial-intracranial (IC-IC) and extracranial-intracranial (EC-IC) arterial anastomoses exist, all having potential significance in different pathological situations, some manifest as a bypass route once a conventional route is narrowed or blocked. One such IC-IC anastomoses group is the ICA anastomoses with the basilar artery (BA) system via persistent trigeminal arteries, proatlantal, otic or hypoglossal arteries. At the C6 segment (ophthalmic), the ICA anastomoses with the lingual artery, the recurrent meningeal artery, the MMA, or the facial artery. The ECA has several anastomoses as well. It's APA anastomoses with the with C2-4 segments (caroticotympanic artery, vidian artery, and inferolateral trunk respectively). The ECA may anastomose with the vertebral artery via muscular branches, with the occipital artery via musculospinal branches or the IMA may anastomose with the ophthalmic artery and the vidian artery.

9.5. The Internal Carotid Artery

The two internal carotid arteries enter the skull via the carotid canal in the temporal bone. The arteries than course forward in the cavernous sinus, turns upward and pierces the dura to join the Circle of Willis. These twist in turn to form the carotid siphon. Just before joining the circle of Willis the ophthalmic arteries branch off (these have anastomotic connections with the external carotid artery and the anterior choroidal artery). The internal carotid arteries are segmented to seven different segments, according to the anatomical structure they traverse. Refer to table 9.1 and figures 9.1-9.3.

Table 9.1. The Internal carotid artery (ICA) – branches and segments

C1	Cervical. It travels in the carotid sheath with the internal jugular vein and the vagus nerve, surrounded by sympathetic postganglionic nerves. It has no branches.	
C2	Petrous. It ends at the posterior aspect of foramen lacerum, infero-medially to the edges of the Gasserian ganglion in Meckle's cave.	
	Segments	Vertical
		Posterior loop
		Horizontal
C3	Lacerum. It passes over, not through the foramen lacerum	
	Branches	Caroticotympanic (inconsistent)
		Pterygoid (Vidian)

Table 9.1. (Continued)

C4	Cavernous. It ends at the proximal dural ring, has many branches	
	Meningo-hypophyseal trunk (the largest and most proximal branch)	Artery of Bernasconi & Cassinari (to tentorium)
		Dorsal meningeal artery
		Inferior Hypophyseal artery (to neurohypophysis)
	Anterior Meningeal artery	
	Artery to the inferior portion of the cavernous sinus (Present in 80%)	
	McConnell Capsular artery (to pituitary capsule, present in 30%)	
C5	Clinoid. Ends in the distal dural ring, where ICA becomes intradural	
C6	Ophthalmic. Ends proximal to Posterior communicating artery (Pcomm.)	
	Ophthalmic artery	Origin is distal to cavernous sinus in 89%, passing through the optic canal into the orbit.
	Superior hypophyseal artery	To anterior pituitary and stalk
	Posterior communicating artery (Pcomm.)	Thalamo-perforators (supplies the optic tract, chiasm, post. Hypothalamus).
	Anterior Choroidal	It supplies the optic tract, globus pallidus, genu of internal capsule, uncus, optic radiation, LGN.
		Its plexal segment enters the supracornual recess of the temporal horn. Its cisternal segment passes through the crural cistern.
C7	Communicating. Begins proximal to Pcomm, travels between CN-II and III, terminates below the anterior perforated substance where it bifurcates to the MCA and ACA.	

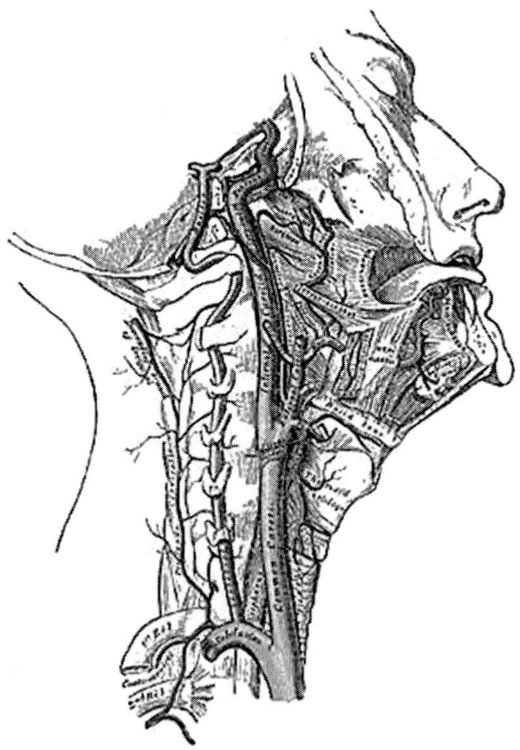

Figure 9.1. The Carotid arterial system. Taken from Gray's Anatomy (out of copyright and in the public domain).

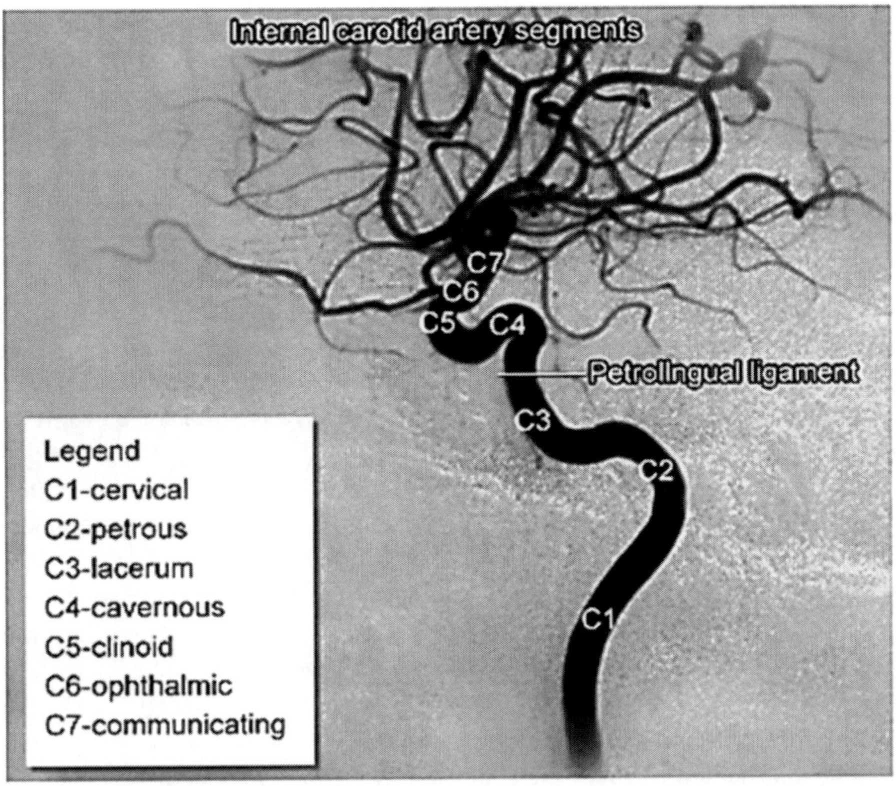

Figure 9.2. The internal carotid artery segments. Taken with permission from www.radiopaedia.org.

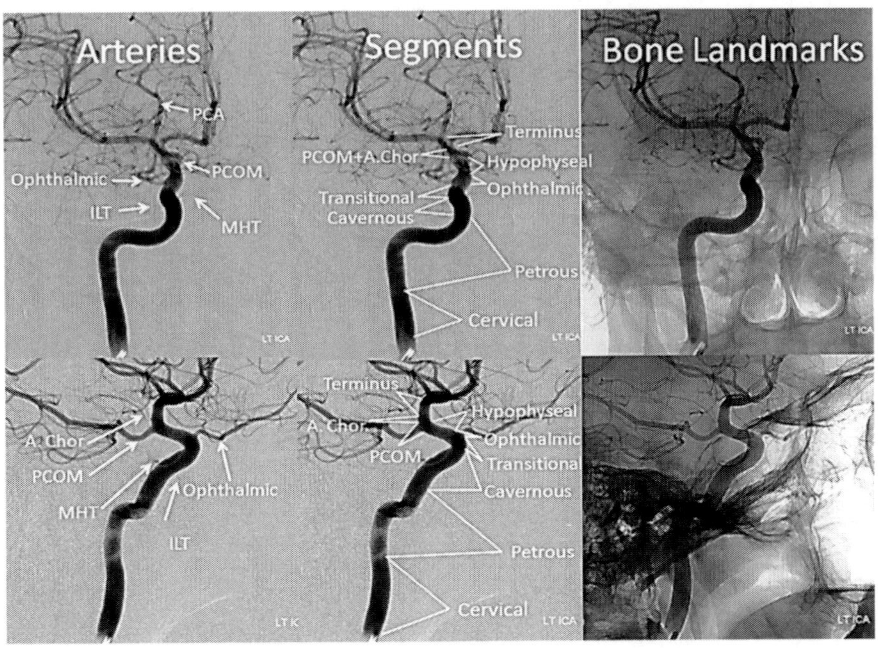

Figure 9.3. The internal carotid artery. Arteries, segments and bone landmarks. Taken with permission from www.neuroangio.org.

The internal carotid artery gives rise to the ophthalmic, posterior communicating, anterior choroidal, anterior cerebral, and the middle cerebral arteries. The supraclinoid portion of the ICA is divided into three segments based on the origin of these branches: an ophthalmic segment (C4-Op.) that extends from the origin of the ophthalmic artery to the origin of the PComA; a communicating segment (C4-Co.) that extends from the origin of the PComA to the origin of the AChA; and a choroidal segment (C4-Ch.) that extends from the origin of the AChA to the bifurcation of the ICA into the anterior and middle cerebral arteries. The perforating branches arising from the ophthalmic segment extend to the optic nerve, optic chiasm and the optic tracts, and the floor of the third ventricle around the infundibulum and tuber cinereum (refer to figure 9.4). The superior hypophyseal arteries arise from the ophthalmic segment and extend to the infundibulum of the pituitary gland. The branches arising from the communicating segment reach the optic tracts, floor of the third ventricle, and the area around the mamillary bodies. The perforating branches of the choroidal segment pass upward and enter the anterior perforated substance. The posterior cerebral arteries arise from the basilar artery and pass backward below the optic tracts. The ACA and AComA course above the optic chiasm and pass between the frontal lobes. The olfactory nerves are lateral to the gyrus rectus. The ophthalmic artery (Figure 9.4B) arises above the cavernous sinus. The carotid artery courses through the cavernous sinus and then laterally and produces a prominence in the wall of the sphenoid sinus before giving rise to the ophthalmic artery. The oculomotor, trochlear, abducens, and the ophthalmic, maxillary, and mandibular divisions of the trigeminal nerve pass lateral to the sphenoid sinus in the walls of the cavernous sinus. The superior hypophyseal arteries arise from the ophthalmic segment.

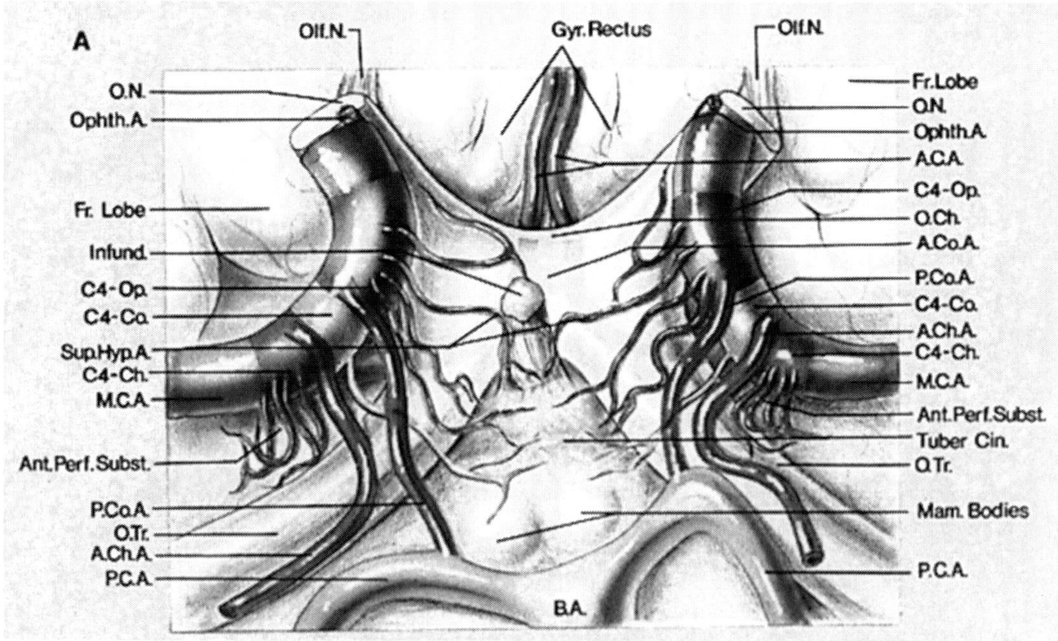

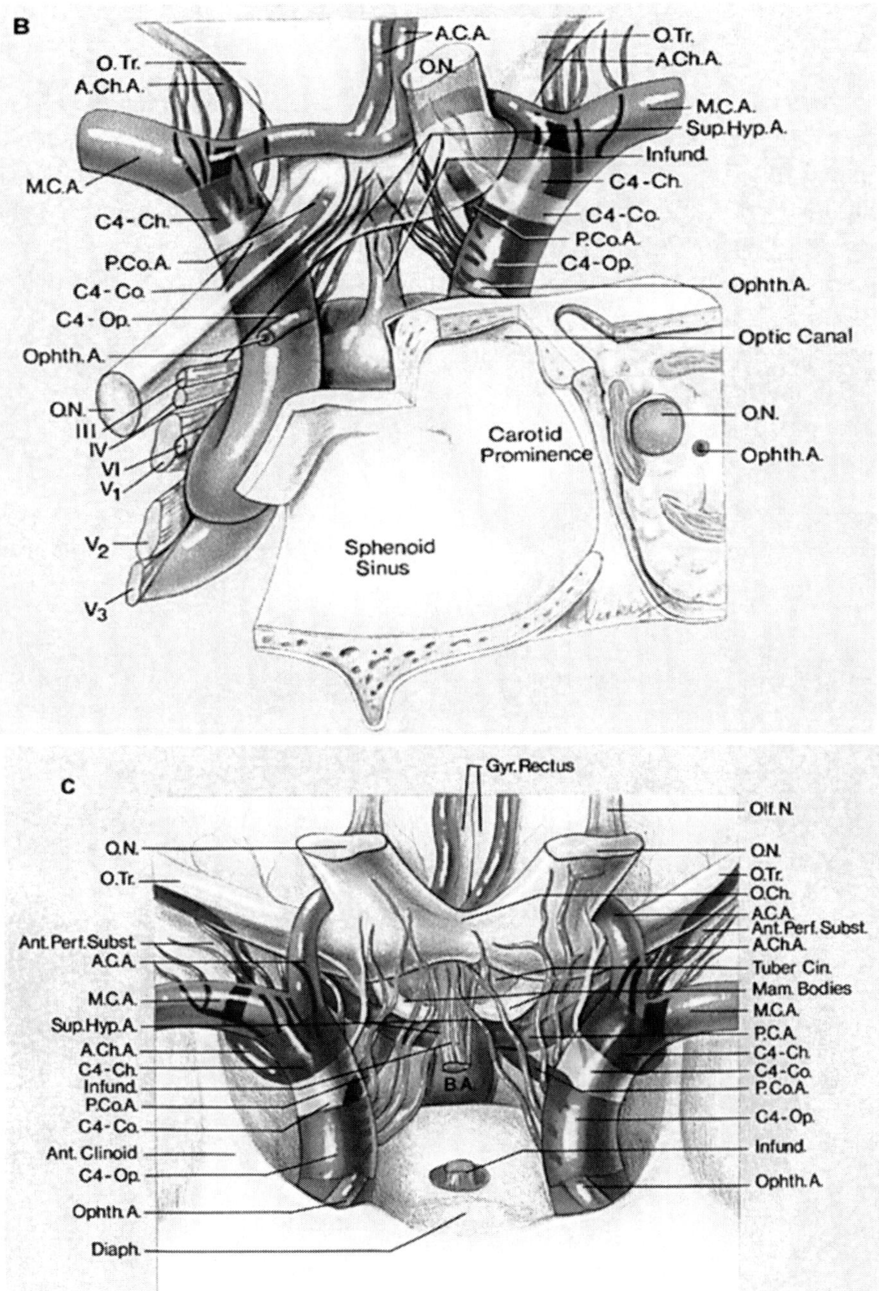

Figure 9.4. Perforating branches of the ICA. A, inferior view. B, anterior view. The left optic nerve has been divided near its entrance into the optic canal and elevated to give a clearer view of the perforating branches. C, anterior view with both optic nerves divided and elevated to show the lower surface of the floor of the third ventricle and the perforating branches passing to it. The infundibulum has been divided above the diaphragma sellae. A., artery; A.C.A., anterior cerebral artery; A.Ch.A., anterior choroidal artery; A.Co.A., anterior communicating artery; Ant., anterior; Ch., choroidal; Cin., cinereum; Co., communicating; Diaph., diaphragm; Fr., frontal; Gyr., gyrus; Hyp., hypophyseal; Infund., infundibulum; M.C.A., middle cerebral artery; Mam., mamillary; N., nerve; O., optic; Olf., olfactory; Op., ophthalmic; Ophth., ophthalmic; P.C.A., posterior cerebral artery; P.Co.A., posterior communicating artery; Perf., perforated; Subst., substance; Sup., superior; Tr., tract. Taken with permission from the Rhoton Collection.

9.6. The Vertebrobasilar System

The intracranial vertebrobasilar system develops after the internal carotid system is already well established, probably as demand for nourishment by the enlarging telencephalon begins to exhaust the reserve of the internal carotid system. A number of segmental vessels arising from the dorsal aortae supply endo-, ecto-, and mesodermal elements and support the developing neural tube. Subsequently, longitudinal anastomoses between these vessels give rise to the vertebral artery, which eventually assumes a role in cerebral supply (refer to figures 9.5-9.6). Because of its segmental nature, the vertebral artery is prone to many variations, including fenestrations and duplications. Adjacent longitudinal systems include ascending and deep cervical arteries.

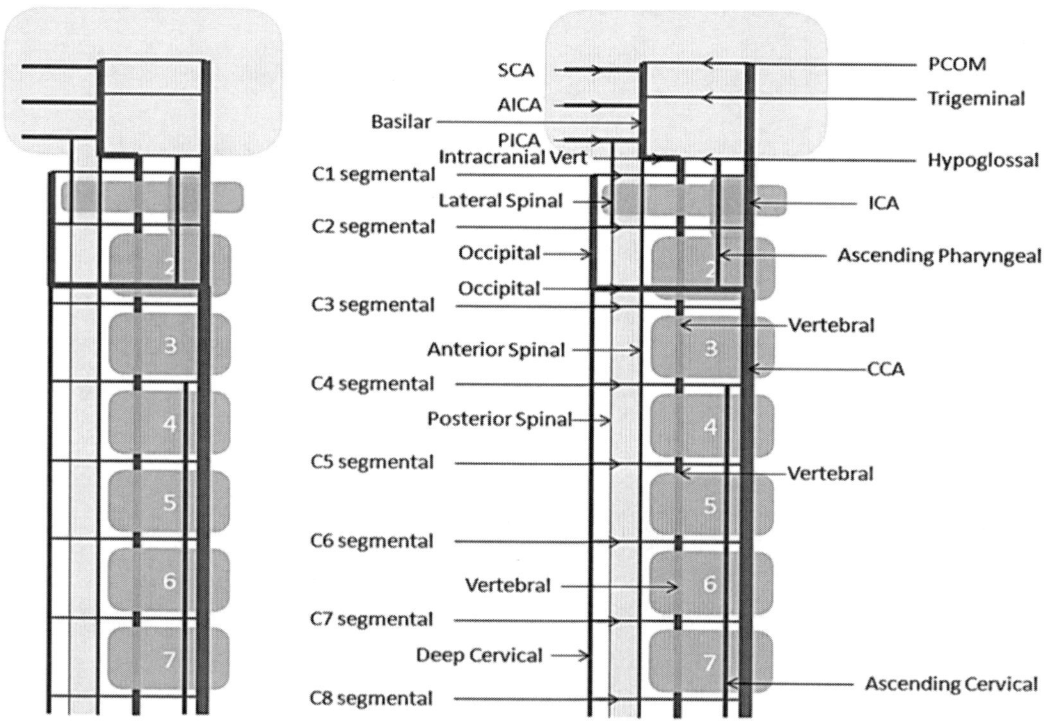

Figure 9.5. A scheme of the vertebrobasilar system. Taken with permission from www.neuroangio.org.

The two vertebral arteries penetrate the dura near the Foramen magnum. At the lower border of the Pons they fuse to form the single basilar artery. Along the brain stem, they supply blood to the medulla, pons, midbrain, and cerebellum, and end in the circle of Willis. The vertebral artery is divided into four segments giving off different branches (refer to figure 9.7 and table 9.2). Basilar artery features and branches are presented in table 9.3 and figure 9.8.

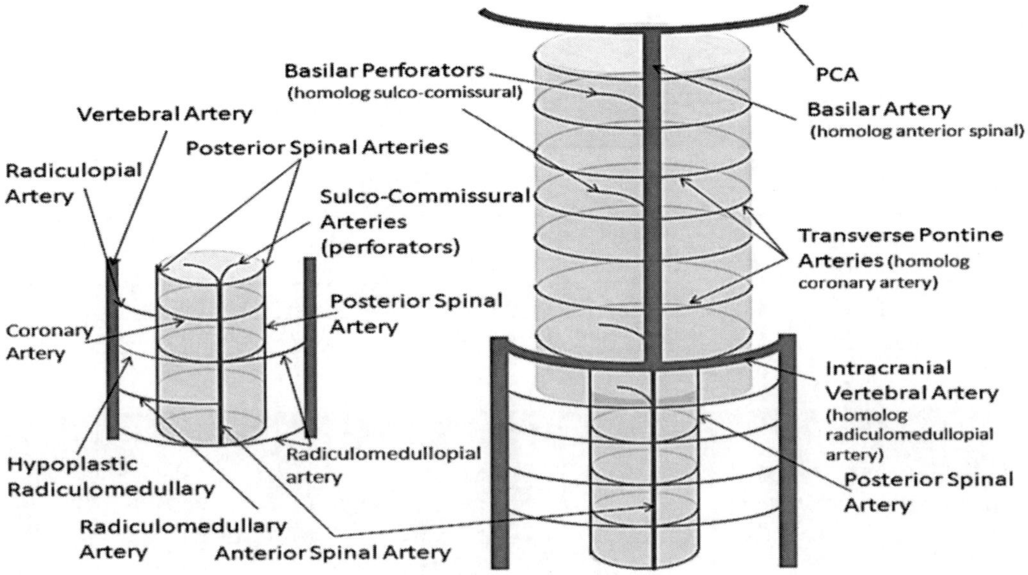

Figure 9.6. A diagram of cervical spinal vasculature (left), and brainstem vasculature (right), without the cerebellum. The image on the LEFT represents cervical spinal cord arterial supply, consisting of anterior spinal artery and a loose network of posterolateral vessels known as the posterior spinal arteries. The anterior and posterior spinal systems are connected by anastomoses running along the circumference of the cord, although known as "**coronary**" arteries, are conceptually quite clear. A number of perforating arteries into the substance of the cord exist; when arising from the anterior spinal artery and penetrating through the ventral cord sulcus, they are named "**sulco-comissural**" arteries. The entire spinal cord is supplied via segmental radiculomedullary arteries, connecting VA to anterior spinal artery. Taken with permission from www.neuroangio.org.

Table 9.2. The Vertebral Arteries

Segments	V_1	Enters the C6 transverse foramen.		
	V_2	Ascends within the vertebral foramina with a sympathetic fibers and venous plexus		
	V_3	Exits and curves posteromedially.		
	V_4	Pierces the dura, enter the subarachnoid space.		
Branches	Anterior meningeal artery			
	Posterior meningeal artery			
	Medullary (bulbar) artery			
	Posterior spinal artery			
	PICA (largest branch)	Arises 15mm proximal to the vertebrobasilar junction.		
		Segments	Anterior Medullary (from PICA origin to inferior olivary prominence).	
			Lateral medullary (to the origin of CN-IX-XI)	
			Tonsillo-medullary	
			Telovelotonsillar (supratonsillar, ascends in the tonsillomedullary fissure).	
			Cortical segments	
		Branches	Choroidal artery (to choroid plexus of the fourth ventricle)	
			Terminal branches	Tonsillohemispheric
				Inf. vermian
	Anterior spinal			

Table 9.3. The Basilar Artery

AICA	Runs posterolateral, anteriorly to CN-VI-VIII giving a loop that runs into the internal acoustic meatus. It gives off the labyrinthine artery.
	Supplies the anterior-lateral-inferior cerebellum and anastomoses with PICA
Internal auditory (labyrinthine)	
Pontine branches	Short circumferential arteries
	Long circumferential arteries
SCA	The superior cerebellar artery, having a superior vermian branch.
PCA	In 15% arises from Pcomm (termed as "fetal circulation"). Refer to table 9.6.

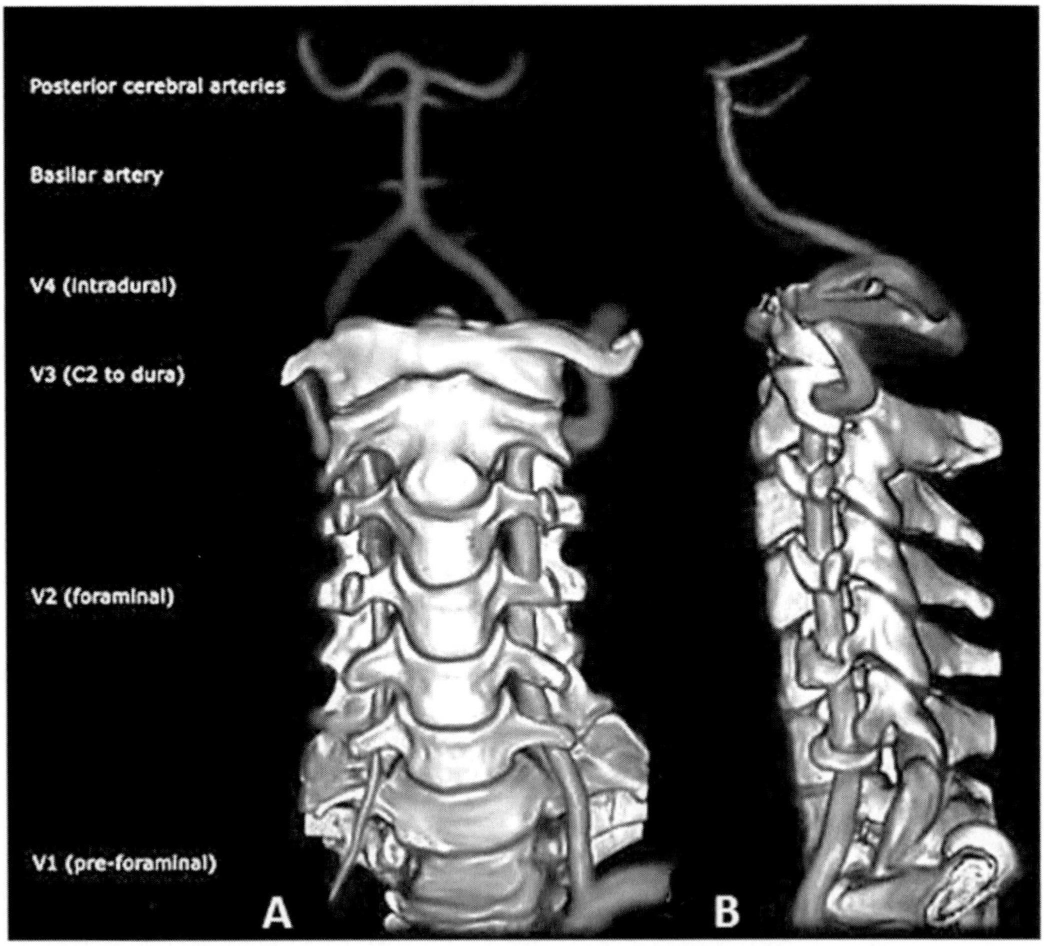

Figure 9.7. Segments of the vertebral artery. A, anterior-posterior. B, Lateral. Taken with permission from www.radiopaedia.org.

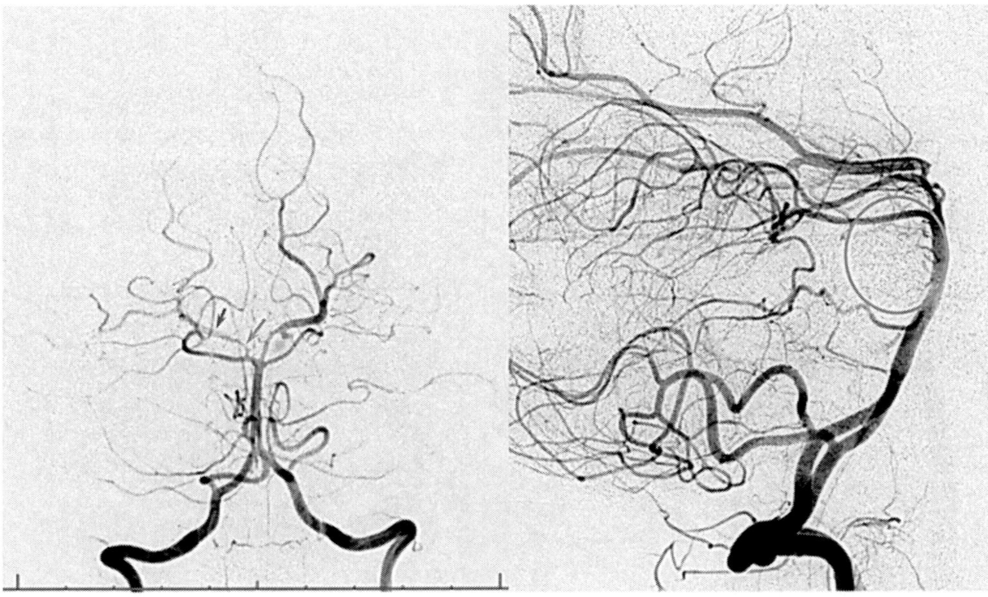

Figure 9.8. Basilar artery perforators. Classical dispostion depicts AICA and SCA arising from the basilar artery, in addition to multiple short basilar perforators whose supply is limited to the brainstem. Almost always, one or more "large" perforator is present between the AICA and the SCA. Taken with permission from www.neuroangio.org.

9.7. The Circle of Willis

Thomas Willis (1621-1675) was one of the most influential 17th century physicians. He was not the first to describe the circle, rather the first to describe it so extensively, having produced his pivotal drawing (figure 9.9). Gabriel Fallopius (after whom the uterine tubes are named, 1523-1563) gave an incomplete description in 1561. Giulio Gasserio (of the Gasserian ganglion, 1561-1616) was the first to draw the circle. Johann Vesling (1598-1649) described it in treatise in 1653, as did a Swiss physician Johann Jakob Wepfer (1620-1695) in 1658.

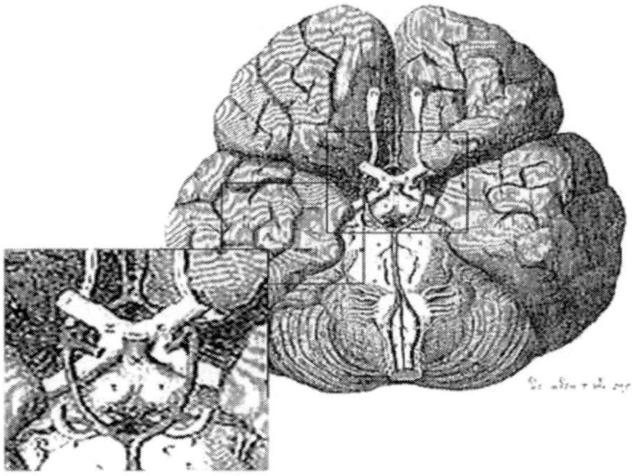

Figure 9.9. Willis. Thomas. The anatomy of the brain and nerves. McGill University press. 1965.

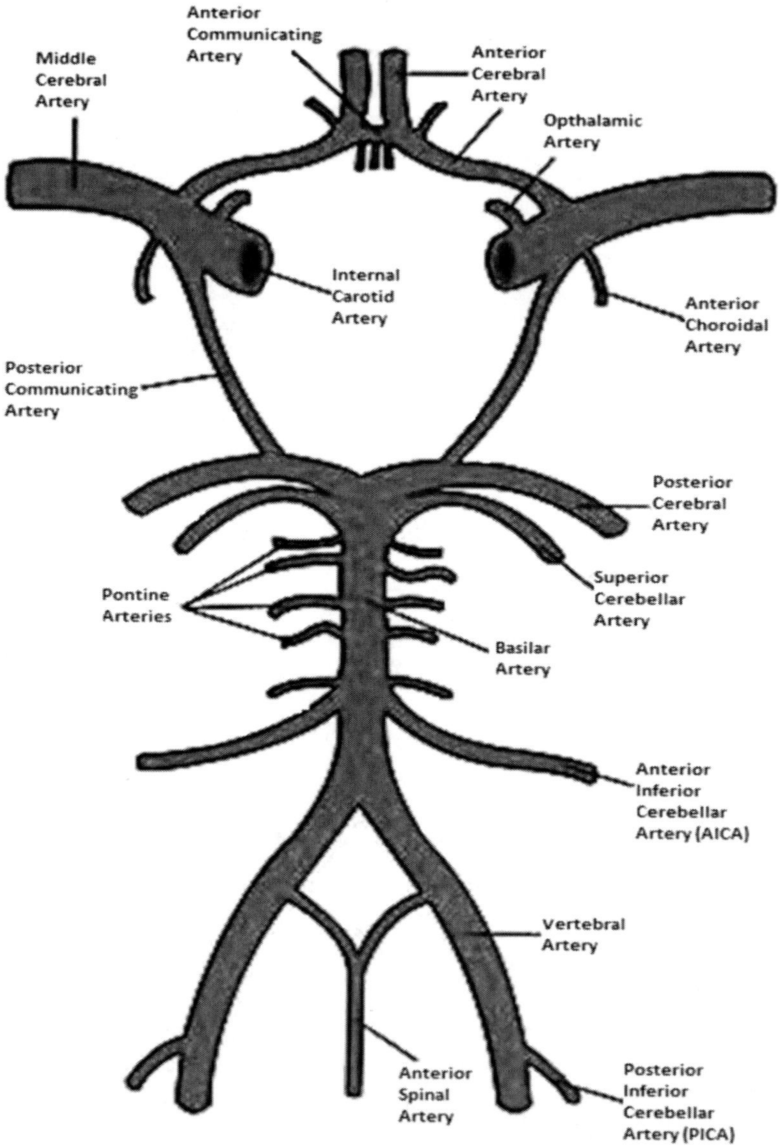

Figure 9.10. Diagram of the basilar artery and circle of Willis. This diagram has been reproduced from Gray's Anatomy (out of copyright and in the public domain).

The vertebral arteries and the internal carotid arteries meet in a circular arterial arrangement known as the circle of Willis. This circular structure is found at the base of the brain, encircling the hypophysis (pituitary) gland. The circle of Willis allows arterial blood from one system to compensate for the other in case it is partially occluded. It is composed of the following arteries: Basilar artery, PCA's, posterior communicating arteries, ICA's, ACA's and the anterior communicating arteries (refer to figure 9.10). As shown in figure 9.11, there are several common anatomical variants to the circle of Willis. A balanced configuration is present in only 18%. Hypoplasia of the posterior communicating arteries occurs in 22-32% of cases.

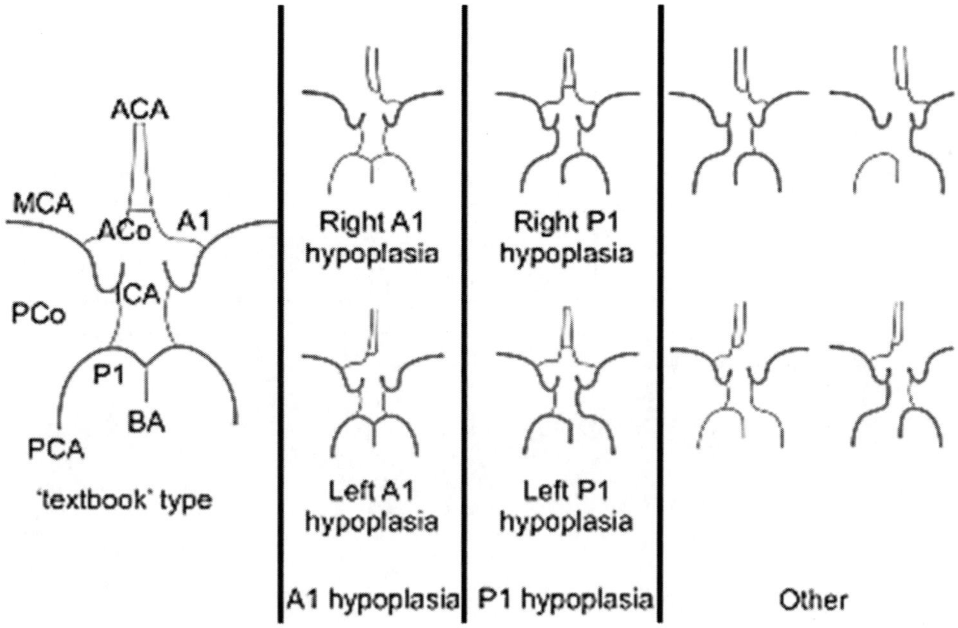

Figure 9.11. Circle of Willis Variants.

9.8. Anatomy of the Three Main Cerebral Arteries

9.8.1. The Anterior Cerebral Artery (ACA)

The ACA travels in the interhemispheric fissure, sweeping over corpus callosum. Table 9.4 presents the segments and branches of the ACA. The callosomarginal artery arises anterior to the genu of the corpus callosum. The cortical branches pass around the superior margin to reach the lateral cortical surface. The A2 segment courses below the corpus callosum, the A3 segment courses around the callosal genu, and the A4 and A5 segments course above the corpus callosum. Refer to figures 9.12-9.14 for dissection and angiographic presentation of the ACA. The ACA supplies the medial regions of the frontal and parietal lobes, Frontal regions of basal nuclei septal area, corpus callosum, anterior limb of internal capsule. Refer to figure 9.15 for the different ACA cortical branches.

Table 9.4. The Anterior Cerebral Artery (ACA) – Branches and segments

Segments	A1	From ACA origin to the anterior communicating artery (AComA.)
	A2	From AComA. to the branching of the callosomarginal artery
	A3	From callosomarginal artery to the superior surface of corpus callosum 3cm posterior to the genu of corpus callosum.
	A4	Pericallosal branches
	A5	Terminal branches

Table 9.4. (Continued)

Branches	Recurrent artery of Heubner	80% from A1, to head of caudate, putamen, anterior internal capsule. Often looks like a small artery running alongside and above the much bigger A1.
	Medial Orbitofrontal	
	Frontopolar	
	Callosomarginal	Internal frontal (anterior, middle, posterior)
		Paracentral arteries
	Pericallosal	Superior, internal parietal, precuneate arteries.
		Inferior internal parietal arteries

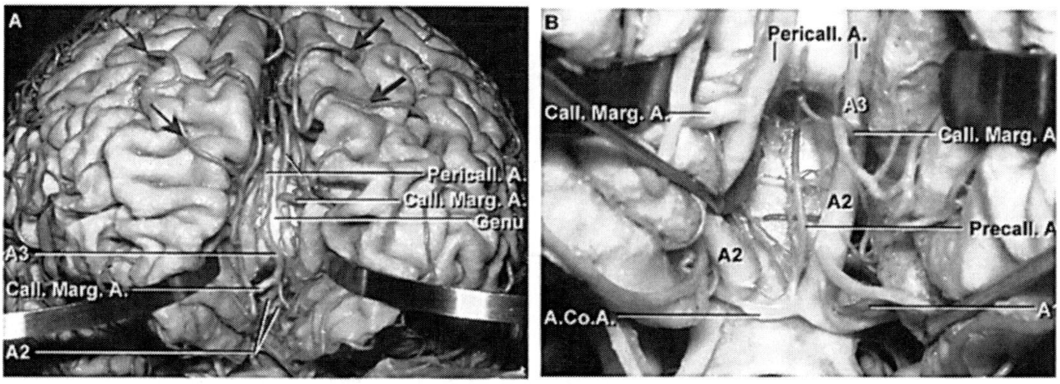

Figure 9.12. The Anterior cerebral artery. A, the lips of the anterior part of the interhemispheric fissure have been retracted to expose the branches of the pericallosal and callosomarginal arteries coursing around the genu of the corpus callosum. B, enlarged view. A precallosal artery arises from the AComA adjacent to the left ACA and passes upward in front of the lamina terminalis and rostrum of the corpus callosum, sending branches to the diencephalon and corpus callosum along its course. A., artery; A.Co.A., anterior communicating artery; Bas., basilar; Call. Marg., callosomarginal; Mam., mamillary; Pericall., pericallosal; Precall., precallosal. Taken with permission from the Rhoton Collection.

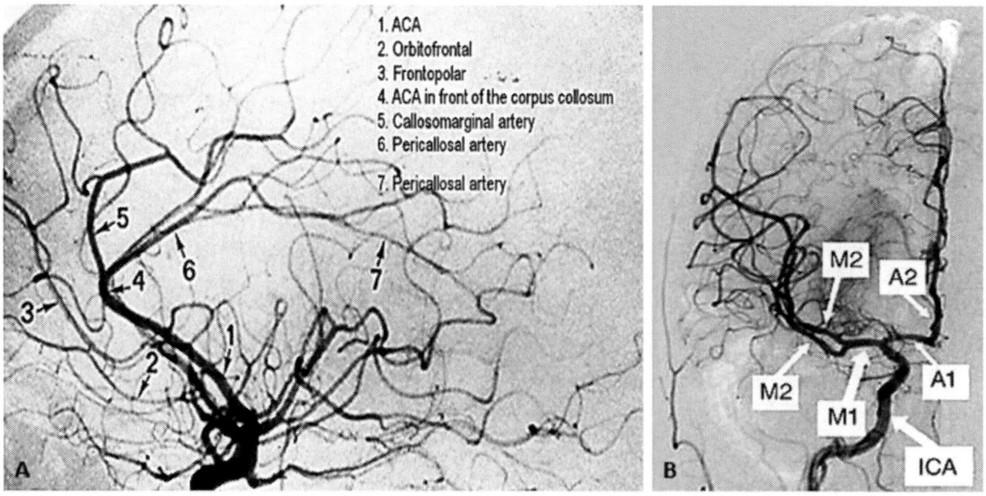

Figure 9.13. Angiographic representation of the anterior cerebral artery. A, Lateral View, annotated. B, anterior-posterior view, annotated. Taken with permission from www.radiopaedia.org.

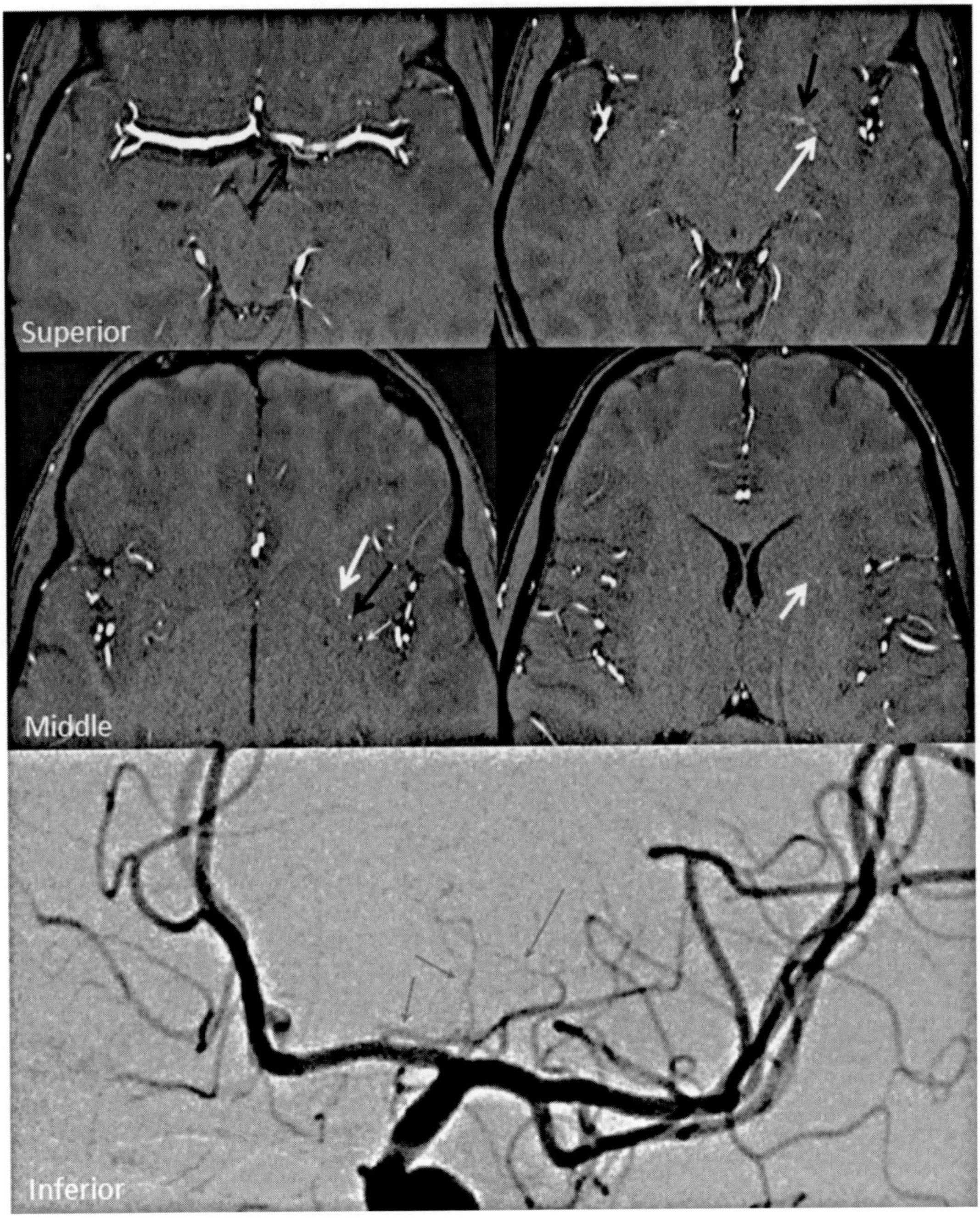

Figure 9.14. The recurrent artery of Heuber and MCA-M1 perforators. Superior image. Axial MRI (MRA) showing the artery of Heubner. In this patient, a large Heubner on the left serves the same function as the medial M1 perforators on the right, supplying the putamen, caudate, and parts of the anterior limb of the internal capsule. Taken with permission from www.neuroangio.org.

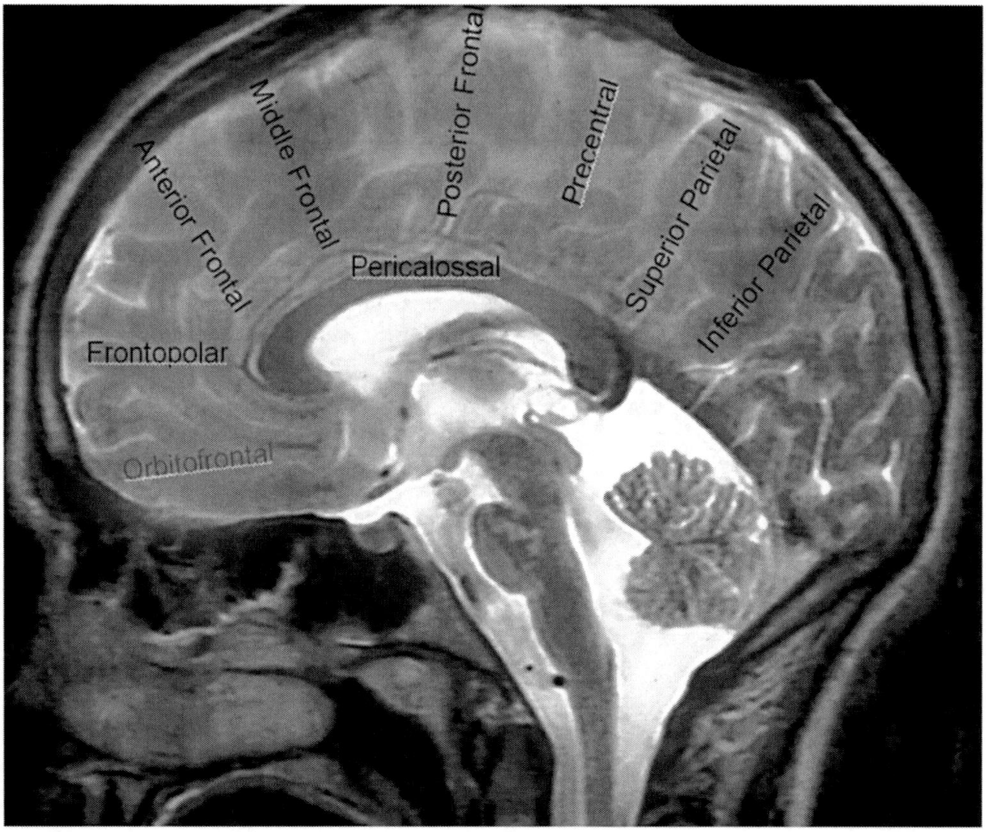

Figure 9.15. Cortical branches and variations of the ACA. Extreme variability is the rule. As long as there is understanding of where the artery is going to, naming is a matter of semantics. Taken with permission from www.neuroangio.org.

Table 9.5. The Middle Cerebral Artery (MCA) – Branches and segments

Segments	M1	From origin to bifurcation.
	M2	From bifurcation to the emergence from the sylvian fissure.
	M3-4	Distal branches.
	M5	Terminal branches.
Branches		Medial lenticulostriate
		Lateral lenticulostriate
		Anterior temporal
		Posterior temporal
		Lateral orbitofrontal
		Ascending frontal
		Precentral (pre-rolandic)
		Central (rolandic)
		Anterior parietal
		Posterior parietal
		Angular

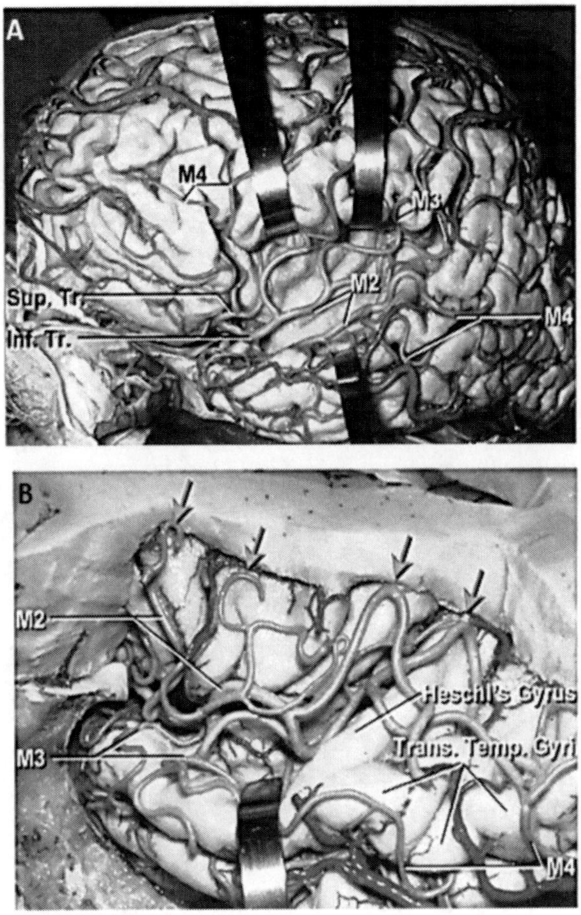

Figure 9.16. The insula and middle cerebral arteries. A, The lips of the sylvian fissure are retracted to expose the branches forming the M2, M3, and M4 crossing the insula and passing around the opercular lips to reach the cortical surface. B, The upper part of the hemisphere and the frontal and parietal operculum has been removed to expose the M2 branches crossing the insula. The posterior M3 branches cross the transverse temporal gyri, the most anterior of which forms Heschl's gyrus, to reach the cortical surface. Cent., central; Fiss., fissure; Inf., inferior; Sup., superior; Temp., temporal; Tr., trunk; Trans., transverse. Taken with permission from the Rhoton Collection.

9.8.2. The Middle Cerebral Artery (MCA)

The MCA turns laterally from the ICA to travels in the depths of the sylvian fissure. Within the depth of the Sylvian fissure, at the insular surface (refer to figure 9.16) it bifurcates to a superior division, supplying the cortex above the Sylvian fissure, including the peri-rolandic cortex. Its inferior division is destined to supply the cortex below the Sylvian fissure. The MCA branches form loops as they pass over the insula and operculum to exit the Sylvian fissure. Table 9.5 presents the segments and branches of the MCA. Refer to figure 9.17 for the angiographic presentation of the MCA branches. The MCA supplies the lateral regions of all lobes, the insular lobe, the basal nuclei, and the posterior limb of internal capsule. Refer to figure 9.18 for the different cortical MCA branches nomenclature.

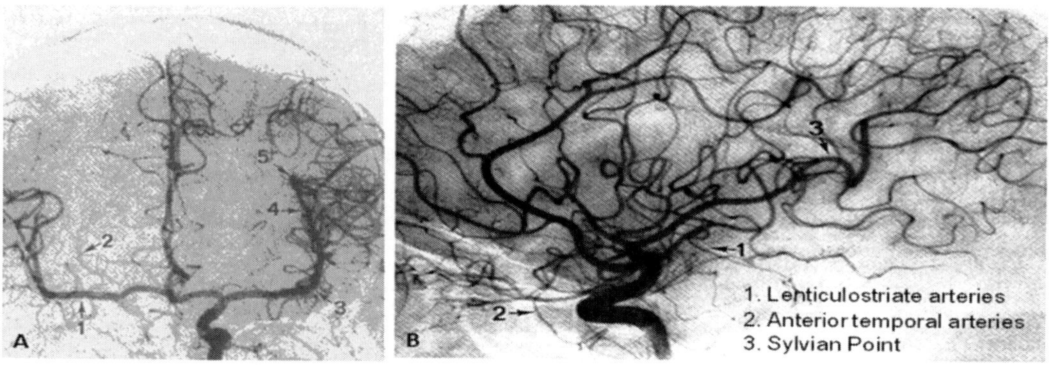

Figure 9.17. Middle cerebral artery segments. A, Anterior-posterior view. 1-M1 segment of right MCA, 2-lateral lenticulostriate arteries, 3+4-left MCA, 5-Sylvian point, located at the top of the insula. B, lateral view, annotated. Taken with permission from www.Radiopaedia.org.

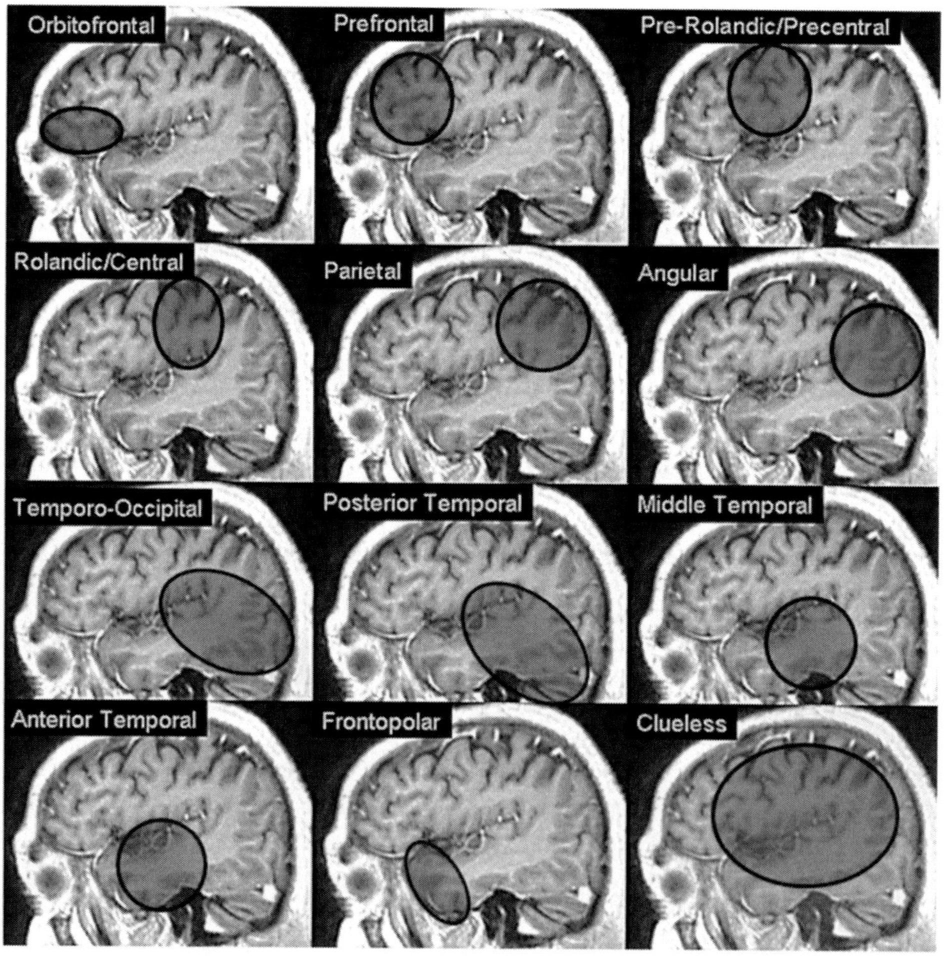

Figure 9.18. MCA branches nomenclature. Vessels are named for the cortical territory they supply, regardless of divisional origin. This nomenclature is adopted from P. Lasjaunias and A. Berenstein, Surgical Neuro-angiography, in turn referencing a series of dissection by Michotey. Taken with permission from www.neuroangio.org.

9.8.3. The Posterior Cerebral Artery (PCA)

The PCA's curve back after rising from the tip of the basilar artery, sending branches to the inferior and medial temporal lobes and over the medial occipital lobe (refer to figure 9.19). Table 9.6 presents the segments and branches of the PCA. Refer to figure 9.20 for the angiographic presentation of the PCA branches. The PCA's supply the midbrain, thalamus, choroid plexus, hippocampus, basal cortex and medial aspects of occipital lobe (calcarine and pariatooccipital sulci).

Table 9.6. The Posterior Cerebral artery – Segments and Branches

Segments	P_1	**Peduncular.** From origin to the edge of the cerebral peduncles
	P_2	**Ambient.** In so named cistern.
	P_3	**Quadrigeminal**
	P_4	**Cortical**.
Branches	P_1	Mesencephalic perforating arteries
		Interpeduncular (Thalamoperforators)
		Medial and posterior choroidal arteries
	P_2	Lateral posterior choroidal
		Thalamogeniculate
		Anterior temporal
		Posterior temporal
		Parieto-occipital
		Calcarine
	P_3	Quadrigeminal and Geniculate branches
		Posterior Pericallosal (splenial)

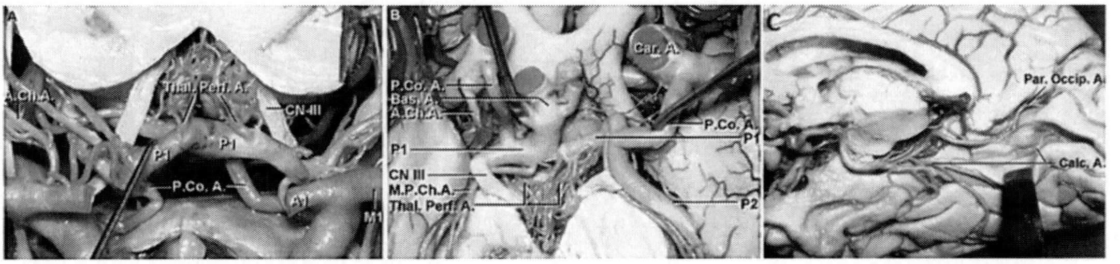

Figure 9.19. Perforating branches of the P1 and the PComA. A, superior view of the thalamoperforating arteries arising from the P1 segment. The left thalamoperforating artery is larger than the right one. The medial part of the A1s was removed to provide this view of the basilar apex. B, inferior view of another basilar bifurcation. Both P1s contribute to the tuft of thalamoperforating arteries entering the interpeduncular fossa. The right AChA courses above and lateral to the PComA and turns laterally above the uncus. An MPChA arises from the right P1. C, the lips of the parieto-occipital and calcarine sulci have been retracted. The parieto-occipital artery courses within its sulcus. The calcarine artery courses just below the calcarine sulcus and gives rise to several small branches that course along the depths of the sulcus. A., artery; A.Ch.A., anterior choroidal artery; Bas., basilar; Calc., calcarine; Car., carotid; CN, cranial nerve; Dup., duplicate; M.P.Ch.A., medial posterior choroidal artery; Par. Occip., parieto-occipital; P.Co.A., posterior communicating artery; Perf., perforating; Pit., pituitary; S.C.A., superior cerebellar artery; Thal. Perf., thalamoperforating; Tr., tract. Taken with permission from the Rhoton Collection.

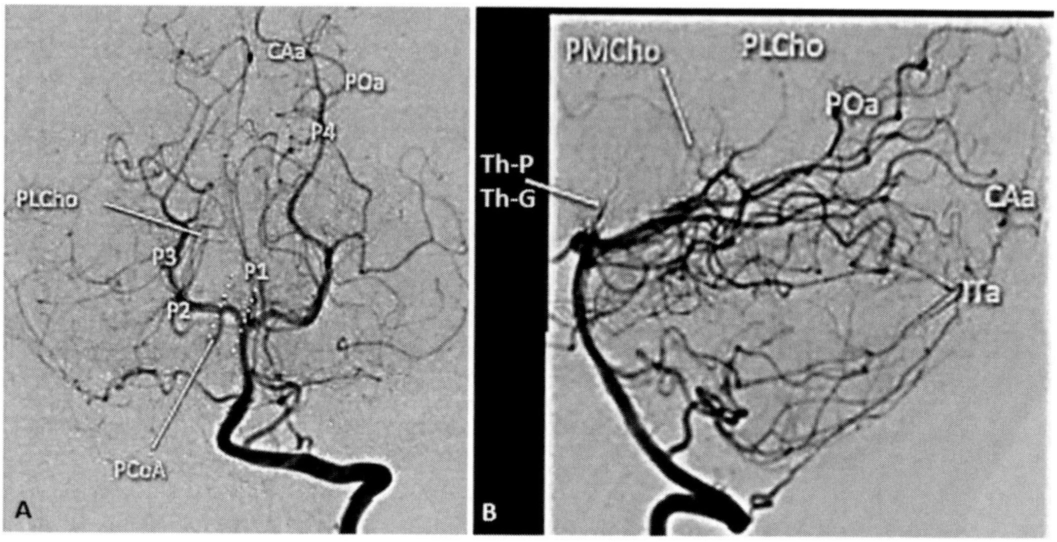

Figure 9.20. The Posterior cerebral artery. A, AP view. Segments are marked. PCOa – posterior communicating artery, PLCho – posterolateral choroidal. Caa – calcarine artery, POa – posterior occipital. B, Lateral view. Th-P thalamoperforate artery, Th-G thalamogeniculate artery. Taken with permission from www.neuroangio.org.

9.8.4. Vascular Territories

The vascular arterial territories are graphically presented in figure 9.21-9.23. In Brief, the posterior inferior cerebellar artery (PICA) territory is on the inferior occipital surface of the cerebellum and is in equilibrium with the territory of the AICA, (on the lateral side). The superior cerebellar artery (SCA) territory is in the superior and tentorial surface of the cerebellum. Branches from the vertebral and basilar arteries supply the medulla oblongata and pons. The anterior choroidal artery (AchA) supplies part of the hippocampus, the posterior limb of the internal capsule and extends upwards to an area lateral to the posterior part of the cella media. The lenticulostriate arteries (LSA's), deep penetrating arteries of MCA, supply most of the basal ganglia. The medial LSA's arise from the anterior cerebral artery (usually the A1-segment), termed as the recurrent artery of Heubner' s. This artery is the largest of the medial lenticulostriate arteries and supplies the anteromedial part of head of caudate and anteroinferior internal capsule.

The anterior cerebral artery (ACA) supplies the medial part of the frontal and the parietal lobe and the anterior portion of the corpus callosum, basal ganglia and internal capsule. The middle cerebral artery (MCA) cortical branches supply the lateral surface of the hemisphere, except for the medial part of the frontal and the parietal lobe (anterior cerebral artery), and the inferior part of the temporal lobe (posterior cerebral artery). The deep penetrating LSA-branches are discussed above. The posterior cerebral artery (PCA) P1 segment extends from origin of the PCA to the posterior communicating artery, contributing to the circle of Willis. Posterior thalamoperforating arteries branch off the P1 segment and supply blood to the midbrain and thalamus. Cortical branches of the PCA supply the inferomedial part of the temporal lobe, occipital pole, visual cortex, and splenium of the corpus callosum.

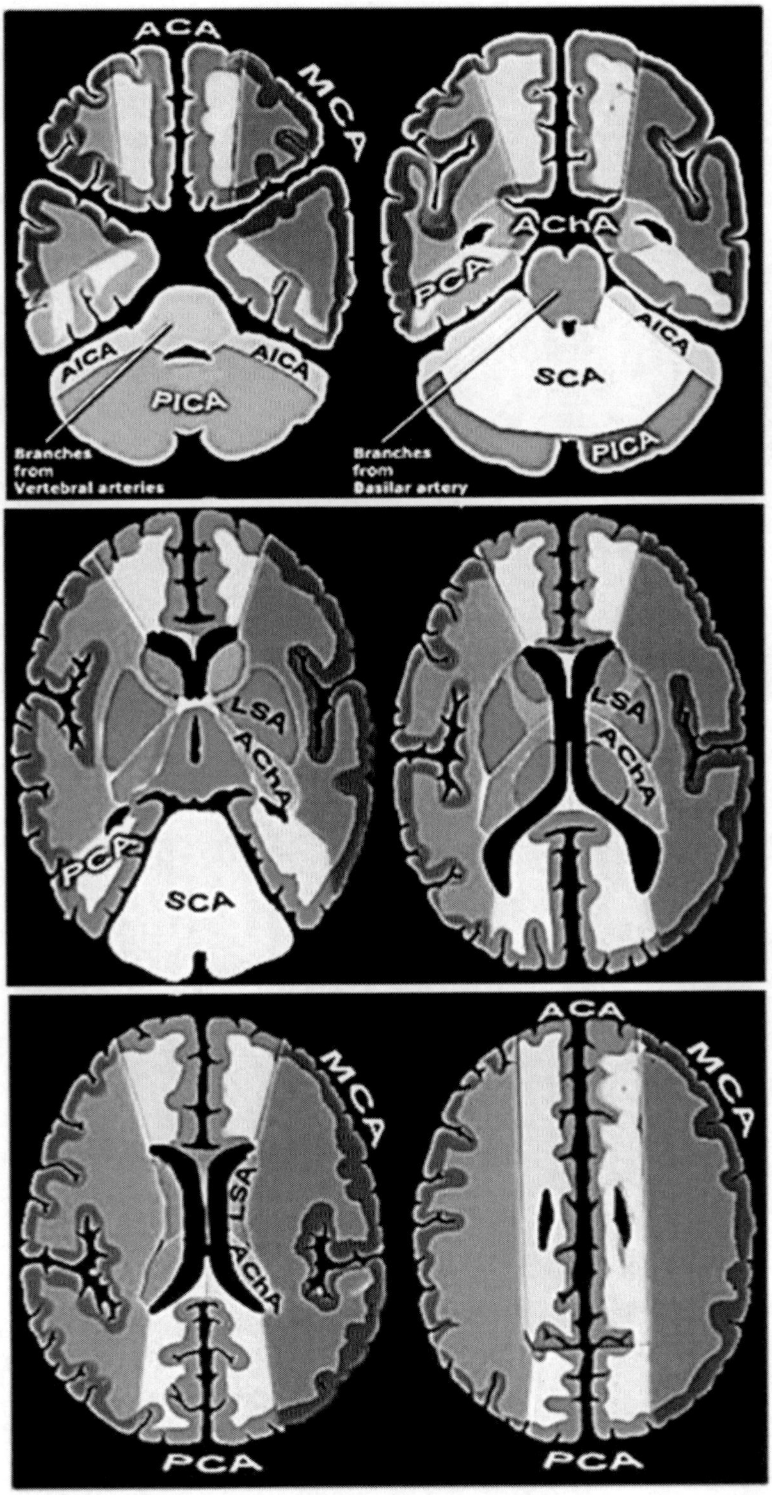

Figure 9.21. The cerebral arterial territory. Superior image is at the pons (left) and midbrain (right) levels. The middle image is at the third ventricle (left) and foramen of Monro (right) levels. The inferior image is at the lateral ventricles (left) and hemispheres (right) level. Taken with permission from http://www.radiologyassistant.nl.

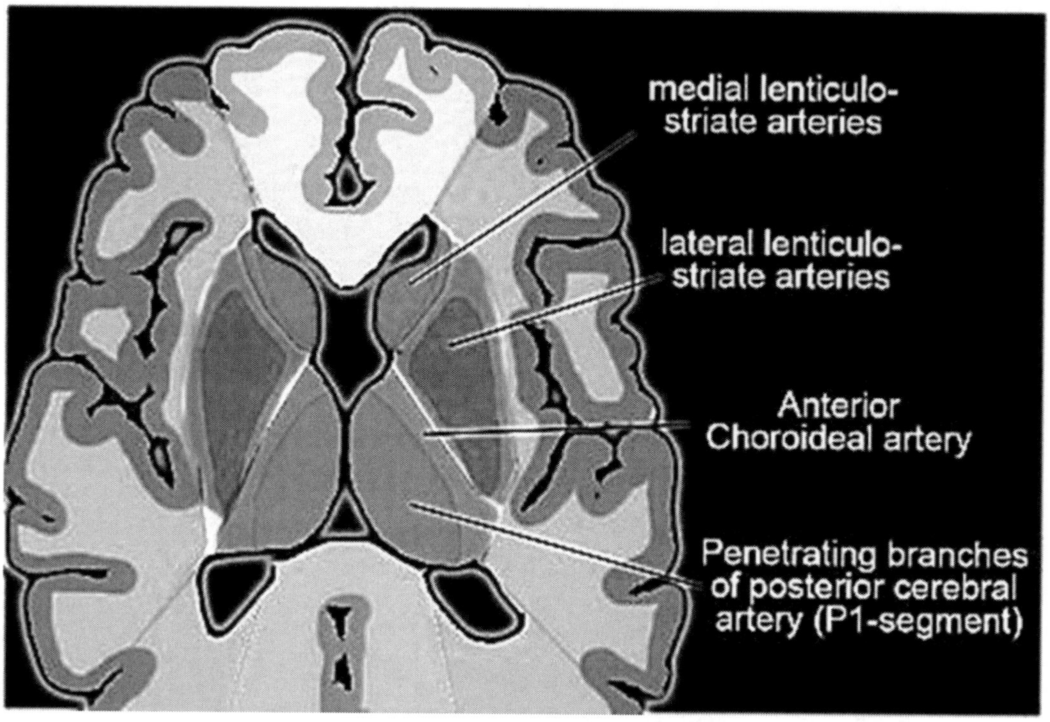

Figure 9.22. Vascular supply to the basal ganglia. Taken with permission from www.radiologyassistant.nl.

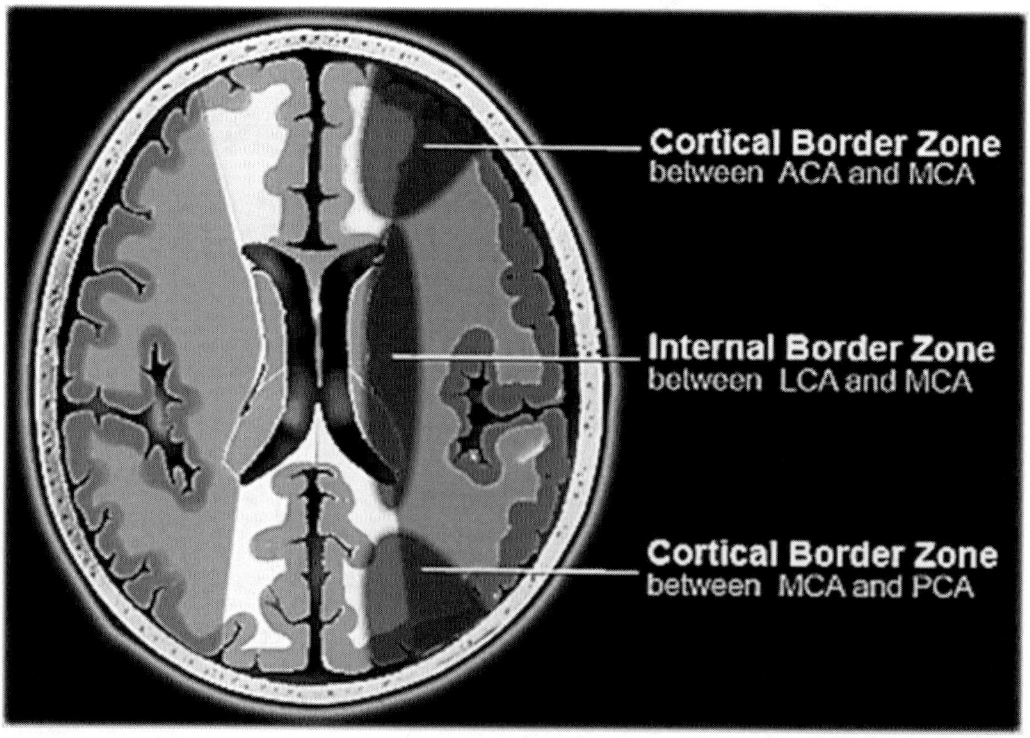

Figure 9.23. Watershed infarcts. Taken with permission from www.radiologyassistant.nl.

The watershed areas are those cortical or deep brain regions found at the edge of two neighboring vascular territories. General hypoperfusion (caused often due to cardiac failure, resuscitation or other causes of hypotension) results in ischemia of these border zones, already found at the edges of the diffusion distance. There are two patterns of border zone infarcts: Cortical and internal border zone infarctions. Cortical border zone infarctions are infarctions of cortex and adjacent subcortical white matter located at the border zone. These cortical zones exist at the junction of the ACA-MCA, ACA-PCA and MCA-PCA territories. Internal border zone infarctions are infarctions of the deep white matter of the centrum semiovale and corona radiata at the border zone between lenticulostriate perforators and deep penetrating cortical branches of MCA or at the border zone of deep white matter branches of MCA and ACA. Refer to figure 9.23 for a schematic representation.

9.9. Basal Cisterns Vascular Architecture

Dissecting through the basal cisterns around the circle of Willis in vivo unveils a complex architectural relationship the different vascular structures have with other cranial nerves and neural structures. A stepwise dissection of the basal cisterns is presented in figure 9.24. A lateral (so called pterional) exposure of the circle of Willis from the Sylvian fissure is presented in figure 9.25. A shown in figure 9.24A, the two A1 segments of nearly equal size cross the front of the lamina terminalis. The right A2 segment enters the interhemispheric fissure in front of the left A2 segment. The left recurrent artery arises near the level of the anterior communicating artery (AComA) and passes laterally below the anterior perforated substance. In Figure 9.24B, a perforating artery arises from the AComA. The recurrent artery passes laterally above the A1 segment and intermingles with the lenticulostriate branches of the M1 segment. The posterior communicating artery (PComA) is directed medially and is seen through the optico-carotid triangle located between the carotid artery, optic nerve, and the A1 segment. In figure 9.24C, the PComA is seen through the optico-carotid triangle (refer to chapter 10).

The M1 segment bifurcates into superior and inferior trunks at the limen insula. A shown in figure 9.24D, the PComA is directed backward above and medial to the oculomotor nerve. The superior cerebellar artery courses below the oculomotor nerve. In figure 9.24E the anterior choroidal artery (AChA) is shown to ascend on the medial side of the uncus. The PComA and the P1 segment join to form the P2 segment, which continues backward on the medial side of the posterior part of the uncus. A medial posterior choroidal artery (MPChA) passes backward around the brainstem. The superior cerebellar artery passes below the oculomotor and trochlear nerves. The branches forming the P3 segment course through the quadrigeminal cistern. The P2 segment courses through the ambient and crural cisterns. A MPChA encircles the brainstem. Figure 9.24F shows the trigeminal nerve in the lateral margin of the tentorial opening. The posterior cerebral artery (PCA) courses above and the superior cerebellar artery courses below the oculomotor nerve. Figure 9.24G shows the oculomotor nerve passing forward between the PCA and the superior cerebellar arteries. Figure 9.24H shows how the PCA and superior cerebellar artery encircle the brainstem to reach the quadrigeminal cistern. The P2 segment is divided into a P2A that courses in the crural cistern between the uncus and cerebral peduncle, and a P2P that courses in the ambient cisterns between the parahippocampal gyrus on the midbrain. The P3 segment courses in the quadrigeminal cistern. The trochlear nerve arises below the inferior colliculus and crosses above the branches of the superior cerebellar artery.

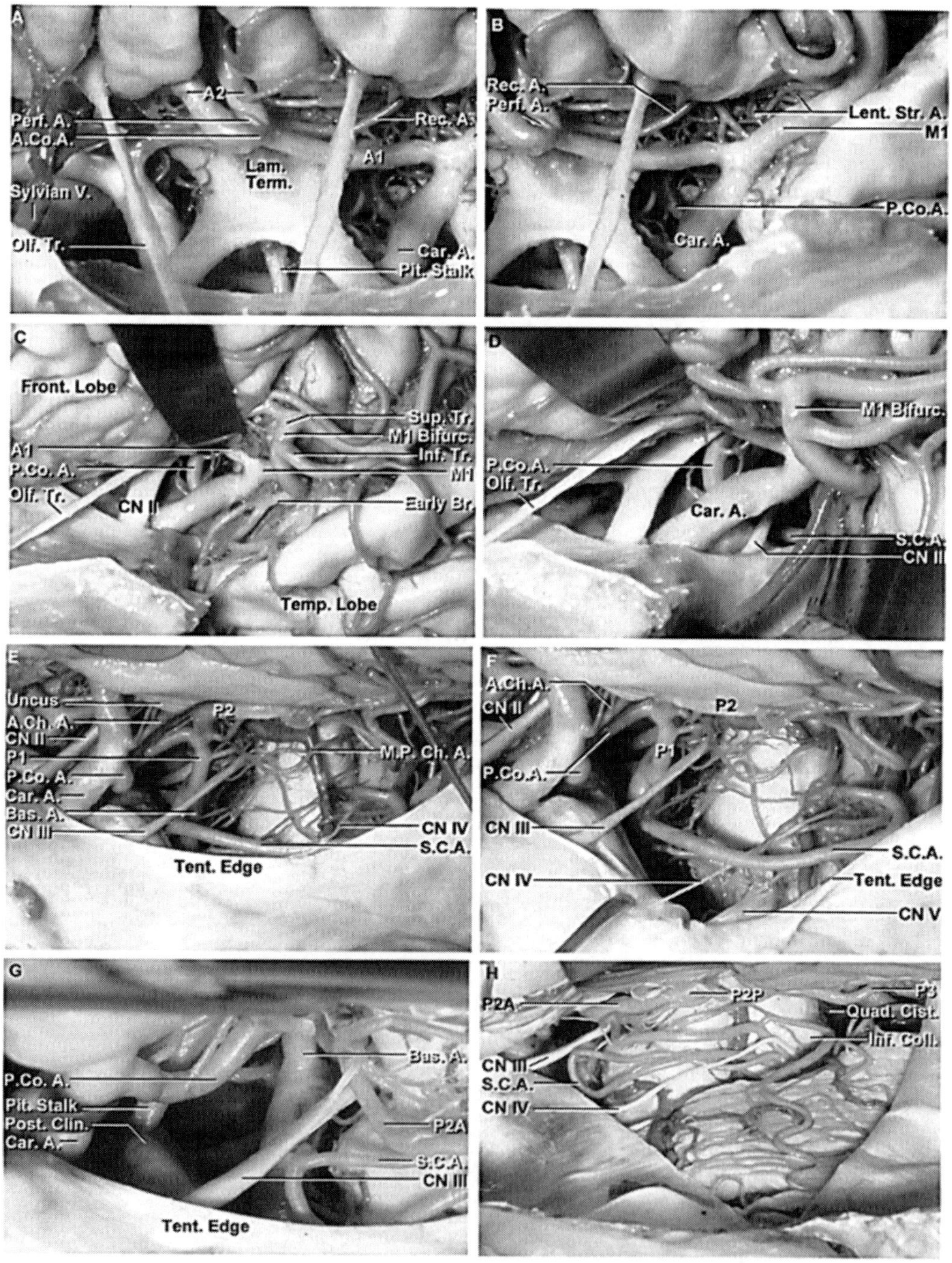

Figure 9.24. Arteries in the basal cisterns. A, anterior view. B, the view has shifted laterally above the carotid bifurcation. C, anterolateral view. D, the basal cisterns have been opened and the temporal pole retracted to expose the oculomotor nerve. E, the temporal lobe has been elevated. F, the tentorium has been divided to expose the upper part of the basilar artery. G, subtemporal exposure in another

specimen. The PComA is larger than shown in D and E. H, the exposure has been extended further posteriorly along the side of the brainstem to the quadrigeminal cistern. The tentorium has been divided to expose the upper part of the cerebellum. A., artery, arteries; A.Co.A., anterior communicating artery; Bas., basilar; Bifurc., bifurcation; Br., branch; Car., carotid; Cer., cerebral; Cist., cistern; Clin., clinoid; CN, cranial nerve; Coll., colliculus; Front., frontal; Gl., gland; Inf., inferior; Int., internal; Lam., lamina; Lent. Str., lenticulostriate; M.P.Ch.A., medial posterior choroidal artery; Olf., olfactory; P.Co.A., posterior communicating artery; Perf., perforating; Pit., pituitary; Post., posterior; Quad., quadrigeminal; Rec., recurrent; S.C.A., superior cerebellar artery; Str., straight; Sup., superior; Temp., temporal; Tent., tentorial; Term., terminalis; Tr., tract, trunk; V., vein. Taken with permission from the Rhoton Collection.

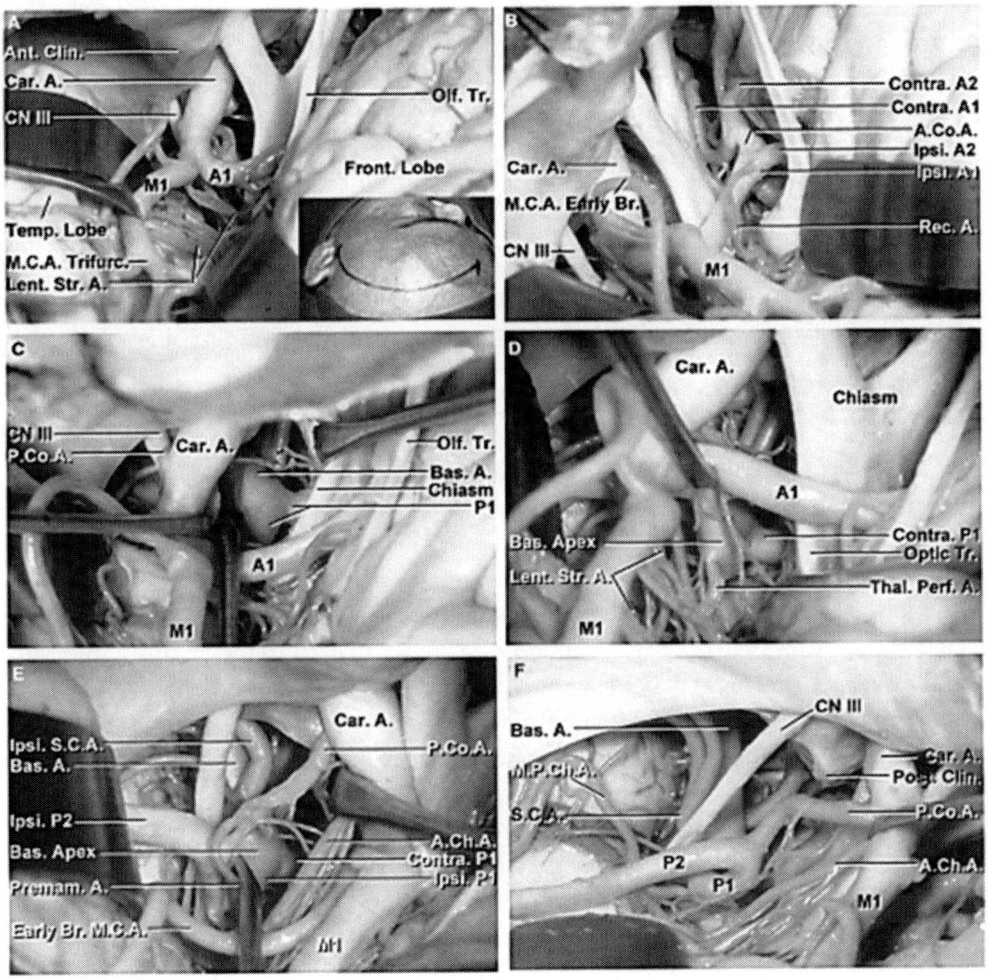

Figure 9.25. Pterional exposure of the circle of Willis. A., arteries, artery; A.Ch.A., anterior choroidal artery; A.Co.A., anterior communicating artery; A.I.C.A., anteroinferior cerebellar artery; Ant., anterior; Bas., basilar; Br., branch; Car., carotid; Clin., clinoid; CN, cranial nerve; Contra., contralateral; Front., frontal; Gr., greater; Ipsi., ipsilateral; Lent. Str., lenticulostriate; M.C.A., middle cerebral artery; M.P.Ch.A., medial posterior choroidal artery; N., nerve; Olf., olfactory; P.Co.A., posterior communicating artery; Pet., petrosal; Post., posterior; Premam., premamillary; Rec., recurrent; S.C.A., superior cerebellar artery; Seg., segment; Semicirc., semicircular; Temp., temporal; Tent., tentorial; Thal. Perf., thalamoperforating; Tr., tract; Trifurc., trifurcation. Taken with permission from the Rhoton Collection.

As show in figure 9.25-A, the left frontal and temporal lobes have been retracted to expose the carotid artery entering the dura medial to the anterior clinoid process. The carotid bifurcation has been exposed. Lenticulostriate arteries arise from the M1 segment. The M1 segment splits in a trifurcation pattern. In figure 9.25-B, the exposure has been extended between the chiasm and frontal lobe to the AComA and the contralateral A1 and A2 segments. A recurrent artery arising near the AComA passes laterally above the carotid bifurcation. In figure 9.25-C, the basilar bifurcation has been exposed through the optico-carotid triangle located between the internal carotid artery, A1 segment, and optic nerve. In figure 9.25-D, the carotid bifurcation has been depressed to expose the basilar apex in the interval between the carotid bifurcation and the lower margin of the optic tract. A thalamoperforating artery arises from the ipsilateral P1. In figure 9.25-E, the temporal pole has been retracted posteriorly. The carotid and anterior choroidal arteries have been elevated to expose the PComA, which gives rise to a large perforating branch referred to as a premamillary artery. The M1 segment gives rise to an early branch proximal to the trifurcation. The P2 segment extends above and the superior cerebellar artery (SCA) extends below the oculomotor nerve. Figure 9.25-F given an anterior subtemporal view. The temporal pole and the carotid artery have been elevated to the expose the origin of the normal-sized PComA. The AChA passes backward along the medial edge of the uncus. A large MPChA arises from the P1 and loops downward as it passes to the quadrigeminal cistern.

9.10. Clinical Syndromes of Ischemic Events

The specific clinical syndromes were discussed in the chapters detailing brainstem and cerebral cortex anatomy. Generally speaking, when considering the three arterial branches supplying the hemispheres, there are common general lines in describing the clinical manifestation of every stroke. MCA infarcts occur in one of three regions: the superior division, the inferior division or the deep territory. Infarcts affecting all regions are termed as MCA stem infarcts. Large infarcts often have a gaze preference towards the side of the lesion. ACA infarcts produce contralateral lower extremity cortical type sensory loss and weakness. These manifest as a frontal lobe dysfunction, with frontal release signs (flat affect, apraxia, abulia etc.). Alien hand syndrome occurs with damage to supplementary motor area (presents with semiautomatic movements of contralateral arm). PCA infarcts usually manifest with contralateral homonymous hemianopia. When the deep vessels are affected, infarcts in thalamus or posterior limb of internal capsule manifest. Watershed infarcts have also characteristic features. MCA-ACA watershed infarcts manifest with proximal arm and leg weakness (the so called "man in the barrel" syndrome). MCA-PCA infarcts manifest with higher order visual processing disturbances.

Chapter 10

Skull Base Synopsis

10.1. Abstract

This chapter turns the focus to a few complex unique intracranial structures, namely the cavernous sinus, the jugular foramen region and the sphenoid sinus. These regions are detailed here to a level beyond that required for the medical student, but are extremely user-friendly for the young neurology/neurosurgical resident or medical students aspiring to deepen their understanding. These structures are becoming more and more important in current neurology and neurosurgery with the evolution of surgical techniques and equipment and our growing ability to treat pathologies in these safely. The chapter begins with a discussion about the cavernous sinus, first with a detailed anatomical description and then a review of the ten triangles defined in the cavernous sinus and middle fossa and their important features. Next, the jugular foramen is tackled, describing the detailed anatomy with relevant osseous and dural architectural features and stepwise dissection, followed by the different jugular foramen clinical syndromes. Last, the sphenoid sinus, as viewed surgically via an endoscope (the so called trans-sphenoidal approach) is described.

10.2. The Cavernous Sinus

10.2.1. Introduction

The cavernous sinus was discussed previously, in the frame of the cranial nerves and brainstem discussion (chapter 3) and in chapter 8. Please refer to the text and figures presented in chapters 3, 8. The paired cavernous sinuses are located near the center of the head on each side of the sella, pituitary gland, and sphenoid sinus. Each sinus has dural walls that surround a venous space through which the fourth segment of the internal carotid artery courses. The sinus extends from the superior orbital fissure anteriorly to the area lateral to the dorsum sellae posteriorly (refer to figure 10.1). Although previously described as a tetrahedron or a pentahedron, some view it as a hexahedron-shaped space on either side of the sella turcica at the convergence of the floors of the anterior and middle cranial fossae, the sphenoid wing, and petroclival ridge (figure 10.1). The anterior edge of the cavernous sinus is attached to the margins of the superior orbital fissure and its posterior wall is located between the dorsum sellae medially and the ostium of Meckel's cave laterally.

The floor and medial wall of the cavernous sinus are formed by a periosteal layer of dura. As it continues upward along the lateral surface of the pituitary gland and clinoid processes, this thin layer is joined by another layer of dura that covers the floor of the sella turcica. The double-layered dura of the clivus extends anteriorly to form part of the posterior wall. The double-layered dura of the floor of the middle fossa extends medially at the superior border of the second division of the fifth cranial nerve to become the lateral wall of the cavernous sinus. The roof of the cavernous sinus is formed by the upward extension of the lateral wall as it joins with the thickened tentorial edge attached to both the posterior and the anterior clinoid processes. Medially, the roof is continuous with the diaphragm sella. Anteriorly, the cavernous sinus tapers and twists to terminate at the superior orbital fissure. Posterosuperiorly, it ends at the tentorium. Posteromedially, the compartment is continuous with the lateral edge of the clivus, and inferolaterally it extends into a funnel-shaped space around the internal carotid artery (ICA) through the foramen lacerum.

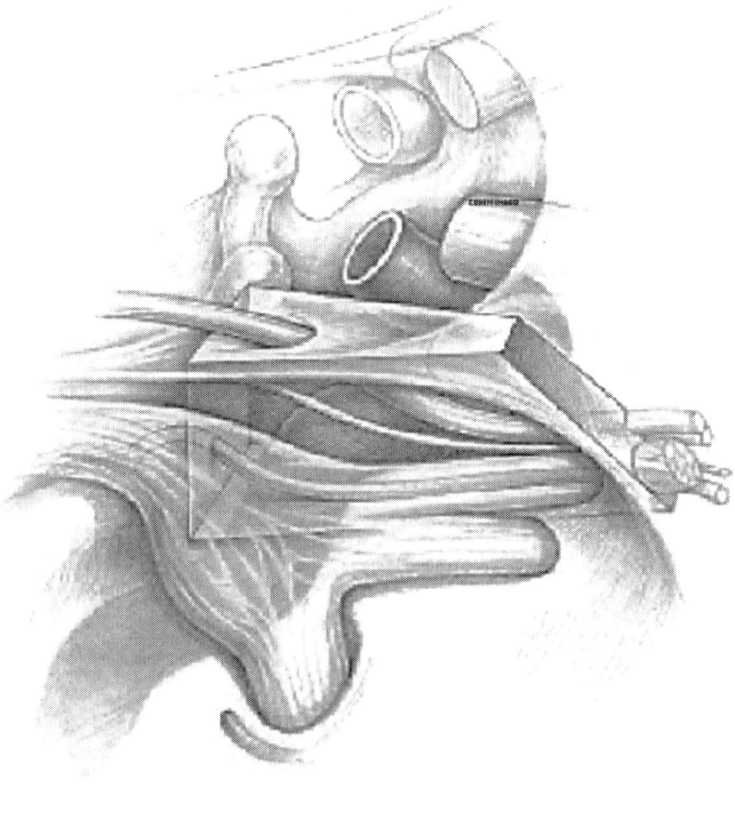

Figure 10.1. Schematic diagram of the cavernous sinus, which is defined by six surfaces: the roof, the floor, and the medial, lateral, anterior, and posterior walls. Modified from Gray's anatomy (out of copyright and in the public domain).

The oculomotor, trochlear, and ophthalmic nerves course in the lateral wall (refer to figures 3.35-3.36). The abducens nerve courses on the medial side of the ophthalmic nerve between it and the internal carotid artery. The lateral wall faces the temporal lobe, the roof faces the basal cisterns, the medial wall faces the sella, pituitary gland, and body of the sphenoid bone and the lower edge is located below the horizontal portion of the intracavernous segment of the internal carotid artery. The cavernous sinus has venous connections with the cerebrum, cerebellum, brainstem, face, eye, orbit, nasopharynx, mastoid, and middle ear (discussed later). These connections and the relationships of the cavernous sinus to the carotid artery, extraocular nerves, and pituitary gland make the sinus of special interest to neurologists, ophthalmologists, otolaryngologists, and endocrinologists, in addition to neurosurgeons.

10.2.2. Superior View of the Cavernous Sinus

The cavernous sinus extends from the superior orbital fissure anteriorly to the petrous apex posteriorly, and it is bordered by the sella medially and the middle fossa laterally. It fills the posterior margin of the superior orbital fissure, which is located below the anterior clinoid process and its posterior wall, extends from the lateral edge of the dorsum sellae to the medial margin of the trigeminal impression and Meckel's cave. Numerous venous channels open into the cavernous sinus. These include the basilar, anterior and posterior intercavernous, and the superior and inferior petrosal sinuses; the sylvian and ophthalmic veins, and the veins exiting the foramen ovale, rotundum, and spinosum; and the carotid canal and the sphenoidal emissary foramen. Each structure is shown by arrows in figure 10.2a. The basilar sinus is the largest communicating channel between the cavernous sinuses.

The oculomotor triangle (discussed later), through which the oculomotor enters the roof of the cavernous sinus, is located between the anterior and posterior petroclinoid and the interclinoid dural folds. The interclinoid fold extends from the anterior to the posterior clinoid process. The anterior petroclinoid fold extends from the petrous apex to the anterior clinoid process and the posterior petroclinoid fold extends from the petrous apex to the posterior clinoid process (figure 10.2b). The internal carotid artery has been divided at the point it exits the roof of the cavernous sinus by the dural rings. As shown in figure 10.2c, the abducens nerve passes around the lateral surface of the internal carotid artery. The oculomotor and ophthalmic nerves have been divided to expose the floor of the cavernous sinus, which is located at the level of the lower edge of the carotid sulcus on the sphenoid body below the intracavernous carotid.

The roof of the sinus extends backward from the area below the anterior clinoid process into the area between the middle fossa and sella and posteriorly, to the area lateral to the dorsum sellae (figure 10.2d). Looking at the lower margin of the sinus from inside, numerous ostia of veins drain the surrounding areas, which open into the cavernous sinus.

The lower edge of the sinus is located medial to the upper third of Meckel's cave and trigeminal ganglion and extends forward below the ophthalmic nerve, but does not include the area of the maxillary nerve. The cavernous sinus does not extend laterally to the mandibular and maxillary nerves, but extends down to just below the carotid sulcus on the body of the sphenoid bone (figure 10.2e).

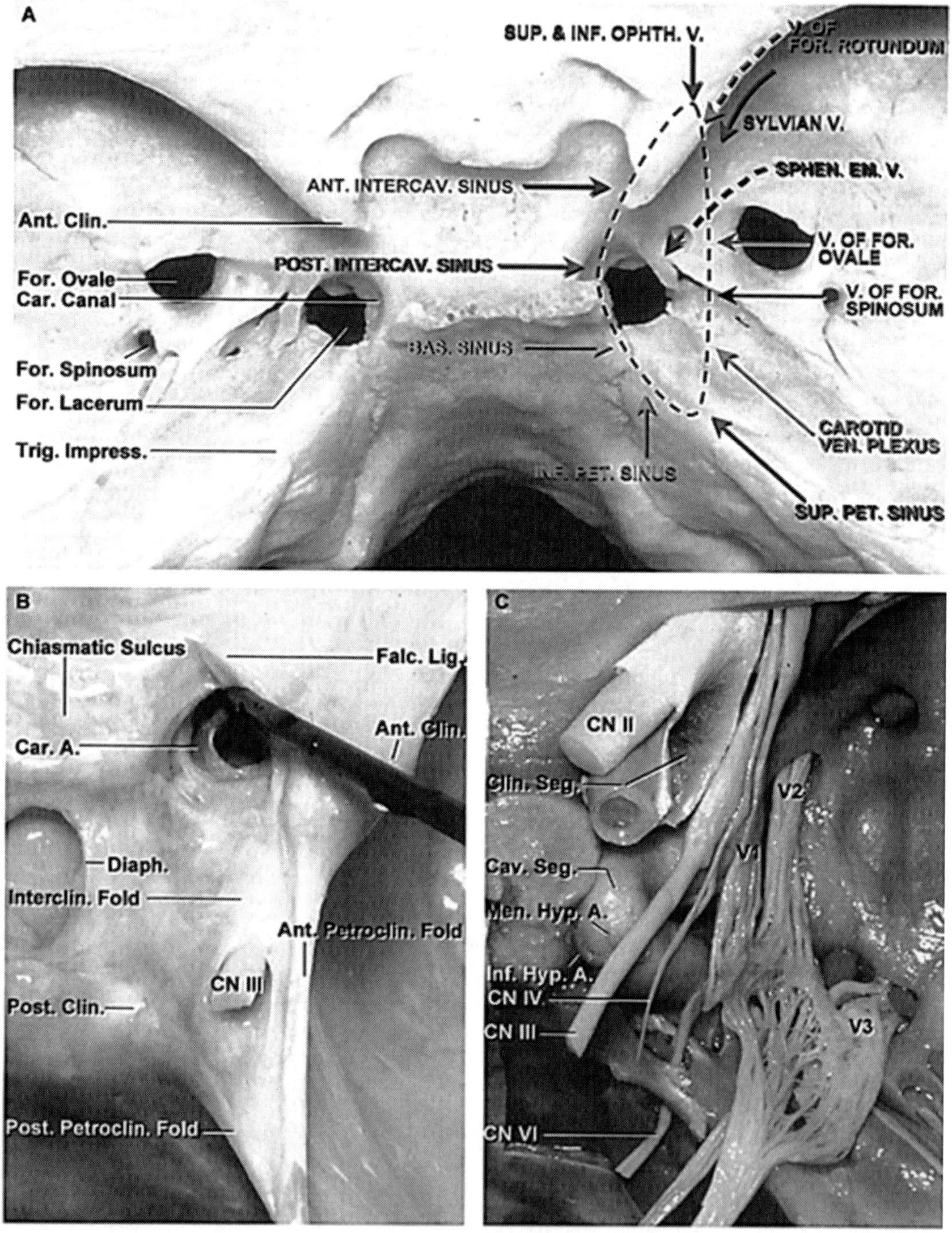
A
SUP. & INF. OPHTH. V.
V. OF FOR. ROTUNDUM
SYLVIAN V.
SPHEN. EM. V.
ANT. INTERCAV. SINUS
Ant. Clin.
V. OF FOR. OVALE
For. Ovale
POST. INTERCAV. SINUS
Car. Canal
V. OF FOR. SPINOSUM
For. Spinosum
BAS. SINUS
For. Lacerum
CAROTID VEN. PLEXUS
Trig. Impress.
INF. PET. SINUS
SUP. PET. SINUS
B
Chiasmatic Sulcus
Falc. Lig.
Car. A.
Ant. Clin.
Diaph.
Interclin. Fold
Ant. Petroclin. Fold
CN III
Post. Clin.
Post. Petroclin. Fold
C
CN II
Clin. Seg.
V2
V1
Cav. Seg.
Men. Hyp. A.
Inf. Hyp. A.
CN IV
CN III
V3
CN VI

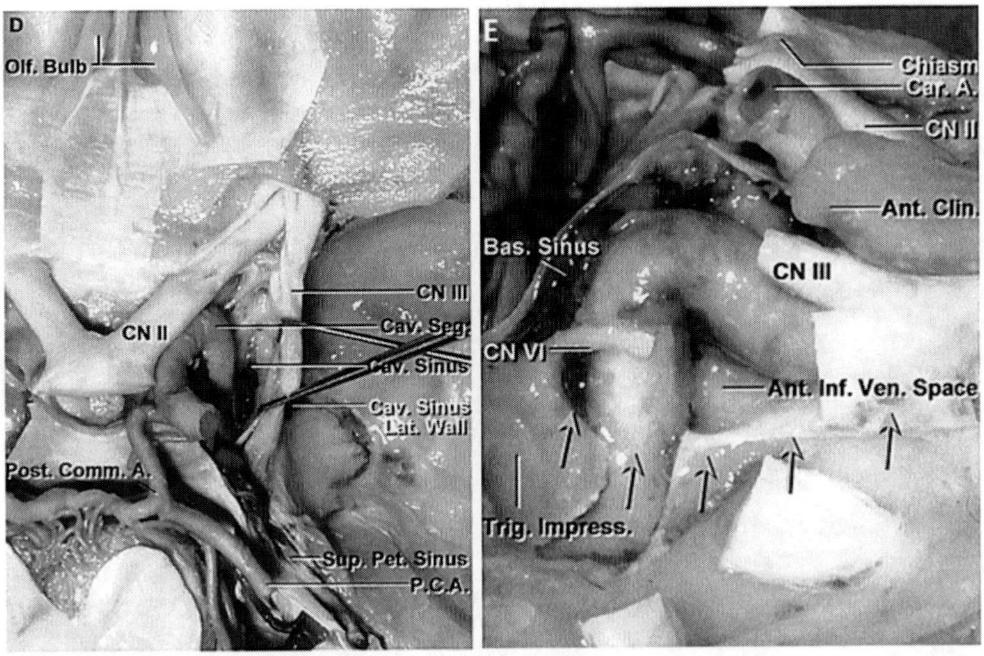

Figure 10.2. A, superior view of the cranial base in the region of the cavernous sinus. B, superior view of the roof of the cavernous sinus. A probe has been inserted under the falciform dura fold, which extends medially from the anterior clinoid process and above the optic canal to the chiasmatic sulcus. C, the dura has been removed from the roof and lateral wall of another cavernous sinus. The anterior clinoid process has been preserved. D, superior view of the cavernous sinus with the anterior clinoid process and roof removed. E, lateral view of the specimen shown in C. A segment of the oculomotor, trigeminal, trochlear, and abducens nerves has been removed. The arrows have been placed along the lower margin of the dural envelope forming the lower margin of the cavernous sinus. A., artery; Ant., anterior; Bas., basal; Car., carotid; Cav., Cavernous; Clin., clinoid; CN, cranial nerve; Comm., communicating; Diaph., diaphragm; Em., emissary; Falc., falciform; For., foramen; Hyp., hypophyseal; Impress., impression; Inf., inferior; Intercav., intercavernous; Interclin., interclinoid; Lat., lateral; Lig., ligament; Med., medial; Men., meningeal; Men. Hyp., meningohypophyseal; Olf., olfactory; Ophth., ophthalmic; P.C.A., posterior cerebral artery; Pet., petrosal; Petroclin., petroclinoid; Post., posterior; Seg., segment; Sphen., sphenoid; Sup., superior; Trig., trigeminal; V., vein; Ven., venous. Taken with permission from the Rhoton Collection.

10.2.3. Lateral View of the Cavernous Sinus

The lateral wall of the cavernous sinus extends downward from the tentorial edge and blends into the dura covering Meckel's cave and the middle fossa. The oculomotor and trochlear nerves enter the roof of the cavernous sinus. The carotid artery exits the cavernous sinus on the medial side of the anterior clinoid process. Removing the outer layer of dura from the lateral wall of the cavernous sinus and Meckel's cave (figure 10.3a) exposes the oculomotor and trochlear nerves entering the roof of the cavernous sinus and passing forward through the superior orbital fissure. The thin layer covering Meckel's cave consists in part of the arachnoid membrane extending forward from the posterior fossa and surrounding trigeminal nerve to the level of the trigeminal ganglion. The superior petrosal sinus passes above the ostium of Meckel's cave and joins the posterior part of the cavernous sinus.

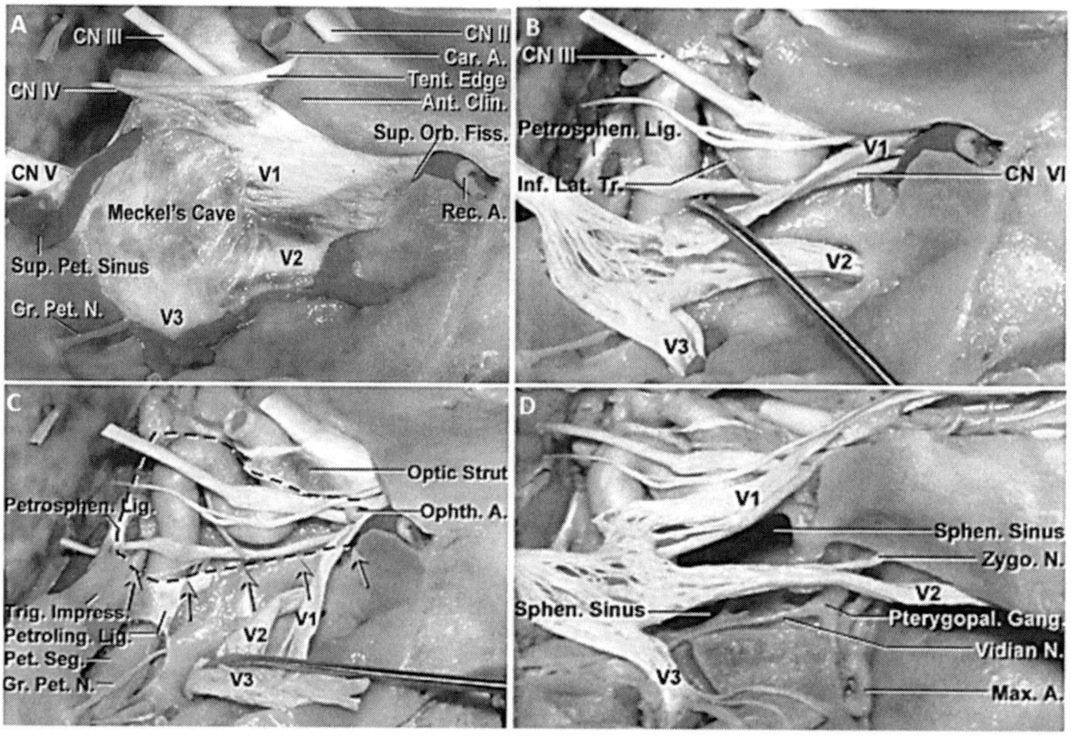

Figure 10.3. A Stepwise dissection of the right cavernous sinus lateral wall. A, the outer layer of dura has been peeled away from the lateral wall of the cavernous sinus and Meckel's cave. This exposes the oculomotor and trochlear nerves entering the roof of the cavernous sinus and passing forward through the superior orbital fissure. B, the ophthalmic nerve has been depressed to expose the abducens nerve, which passes under the petrosphenoid ligament roofing Dorello's canal, and courses medial to the ophthalmic nerve. C, the trigeminal nerve has been folded downward to expose the petrolingual ligament, which extends above the internal carotid artery, just proximal to where the artery enters the cavernous sinus. The margins of the cavernous sinus are shown with a broken line. D, the bone between the first and second and the second and third trigeminal divisions has been drilled to expose the lateral wing of the sphenoid sinus. The vidian nerve, which passes forward to enter the sphenopalatine ganglion in the pterygopalatine fossa, is exposed between the second and third trigeminal divisions. A., artery; Alv., alveolar; Ant., anterior; Bas., basilar; Brs., branches; Car., carotid; Cav., cavernous; Cist., cistern; Clin., clinoid; CN, cranial nerve; Cond., condyle; Div., division; Fiss., fissure; For., foramen; Gang., ganglion; Gen., geniculate; Gr., greater; Impress., impression; Inf., inferior; Inf. Lat., inferolateral; Infraorb., infraorbital; Infratemp., infratemporal; Lat., lateral; Less., lesser; Lig., ligament; M., muscle; Mandib., mandibular; Max., maxillary; Men., meningeal; Mid., middle; N., nerve; Oculom., oculomotor; Ophth., ophthalmic; Orb., orbital; Pericav., pericavernous; Pet., petrosal, petrous; Petroling., petrolingual; Petrosphen., petrosphenoid; Plex., plexus; Post., posterior; Proc., process; Pteryg., pterygoid; Pterygopal., pterygopalatine; Rec., recurrent; Seg., segment; Sphen., sphenoid; Sup., superior; Tent., tentorial; Tr., trunk; Trig., trigeminal; Troch., trochlear; V., vein; Ven., venous; Zygo., zygomatic. Taken with permission from the Rhoton Collection.

The cavernous sinus extends from the superior orbital fissure to the petrous apex. It is located medial to the upper third of the gasserian ganglion. The pericavernous venous plexus surrounds the maxillary and mandibular nerves in the region of the foramen rotundum and foramen ovale. The venous spaces in the cavernous sinus communicate posteriorly with the inferior and superior petrosal and basilar sinuses. In addition, the cavernous sinus communicates with the superior ophthalmic veins and the venous plexus around the maxillary and mandibular nerves and pituitary gland. As shown in figure 10.3b, the abducens nerve passes under the petrosphenoid ligament roofing Dorello's canal, coursing medial to the ophthalmic nerve. The abducens nerve crosses laterally below the ophthalmic nerve as it passes through the superior orbital fissure.

The optic strut separates the optic canal and superior orbital fissure (refer to figures 10.3c+d). The dura extending medially off the upper surface of the anterior clinoid forms the upper dural ring around the internal carotid artery, and the dura lining the lower margin of the clinoid extends medially to form the lower dural ring. The clinoid segment of the carotid artery, located between the upper and lower ring, is enclosed in the dura sheath, referred to as the carotid collar.

10.2.4. Cavernous Sinus and Middle Fossa Triangles

Parkinson described a triangle within the lateral wall of the cavernous sinus through which the intracavernous portion of the carotid artery and its branches might be exposed. Since his pioneering work, a number of significant triangular relationships formed by the convergence and divergence of the cranial nerves in the region of the cavernous sinus and middle fossa have been defined. Refer to table 10.1 for a summary. This triangular arrangement is helpful in understanding and planning approaches to the cavernous sinus.

The cavernous sinus triangles are formed by the optic, oculomotor, trochlear, and ophthalmic nerves converging on the optic canal and superior orbital fissure. The middle fossa triangles are formed by the trigeminal divisions diverging as they pass from the gasserian ganglion to reach their foramina. Refer to figures 10.4

Table 10.1. Cavernous Sinus and Middle Fossa Triangles

Cavernous sinus	The Clinoidal Triangle
	The Oculomotor Triangle
	The Supratrochlear Triangle
	Infratrochlear Triangle (Parkinson's Triangle)
Middle fossa	Anteromedial Middle Fossa Triangle
	Anterolateral (Mullan's) Middle Fossa Triangle
	Posterolateral Middle Fossa Triangle (Glasscock's Triangle)
	Posteromedial Middle Fossa Triangle (Kawase's Triangle)
Paraclinoid Triangles	Inferolateral Paraclival Triangle
	Inferomedial Paraclival Triangle

10.2.4.1. Cavernous Sinus Triangles

10.2.4.1.1. The Clinoidal Triangle

This triangle is situated between the optic and oculomotor cranial nerves. This triangle is exposed by removing the anterior clinoid process. The optic strut is in its anterior part, the clinoid segment of the internal carotid artery is in the midportion, and the thin roof of the cavernous sinus is in the posterior part of this triangle.

10.2.4.1.2. The Oculomotor Triangle

This triangle is formed by the triangular patch of dura through which the oculomotor nerve enters the cavernous sinus at its roof. Two margins of this triangle are formed by the anterior and posterior petroclinoidal dural folds, extending from the anterior and posterior clinoid processes respectively to the petrous apex. The third side is formed by the interclinoidal dural fold that extends from the anterior to the posterior clinoid process.

10.2.4.1.3. The Supratrochlear Triangle

This triangle is situated between the lower surface of the oculomotor nerve and the upper surface of the trochlear nerve. A line joining the points of entrance of these nerves into the dura forms the third margin.

10.2.4.1.4. The Infratrochlear Triangle (Parkinson's Triangle)

This triangle is located between the lower margin of the trochlear nerve and the upper margin of the ophthalmic nerve. The third border is formed by a line connecting the point of entry of the trochlear nerve into the dura to the site where the trigeminal nerve enters Meckel's cave. The posterior bend of the internal carotid artery and the origin of the meningohypophyseal trunk from the posterior bend are located in this triangle.

10.2.4.2. Middle Fossa Triangles

10.2.4.2.1. Anteromedial Middle Fossa Triangle

This triangle is situated between the lower margin of the ophthalmic and the upper margin of the maxillary nerves. The third border is formed by a line connecting the point where the ophthalmic nerve passes through the superior orbital fissure and the maxillary nerve passes through the foramen rotundum (Fig. 10.4a+b). Removing bone in this space between the ophthalmic or maxillary nerve opens into the sphenoid sinus.

10.2.4.2.2. Anterolateral Middle Fossa Triangle

This triangle is located between the lower surface of the maxillary nerve, the upper surface of the mandibular nerve, and a line connecting between foramen ovale and foramen rotundum. Opening the bone in the medial wall of this triangle exposes the lateral wing of the sphenoid sinus.

10.2.4.2.3. Posterolateral Middle Fossa Triangle (Glasscock's Triangle)

This triangle is formed on the anteromedial side by the lateral surface of the mandibular nerve distal to the point at which the greater petrosal nerve crosses below the lateral surface of the trigeminal nerve. On its posterolateral side, it is formed by the anterior margin of the greater superficial petrosal nerve (GSPN). This triangle opens laterally to encompass the floor of the middle cranial fossa between these two structures. The middle meningeal artery passes through the foramen spinosum in this triangle. Opening the floor of the middle fossa in this triangle exposes the infratemporal fossa.

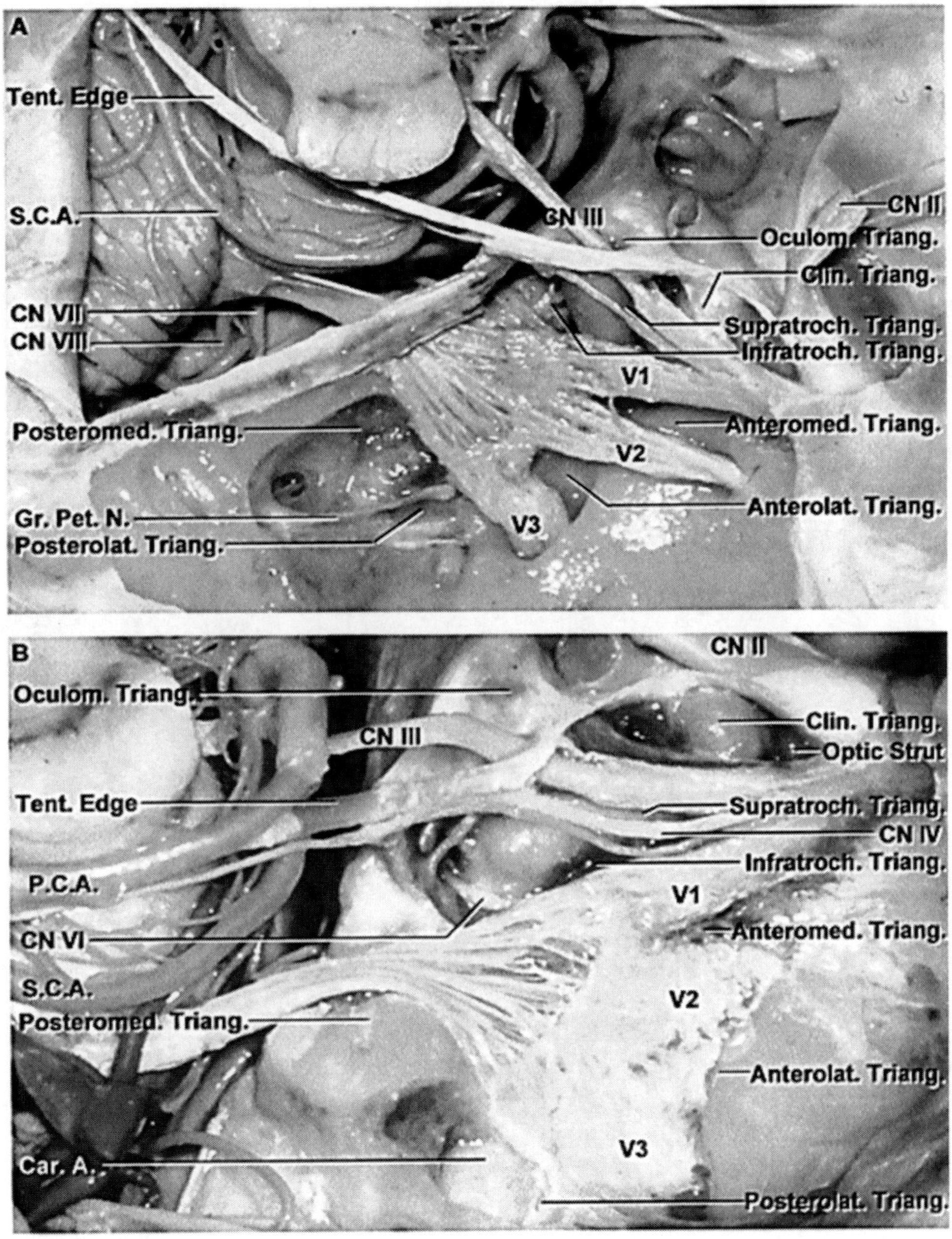

Figure 10.4. Triangles in the region of the cavernous sinus and middle fossa formed by the convergence and divergence of the cranial nerves. A+B, middle fossa and cavernous sinus triangles. C, paraclinoid triangles. A., artery; Anterolat., anterolateral; Anteromed., anteromedial; Bas., basilar; Car., carotid; Cav., cavernous; Clin., clinoid; CN, cranial nerve; Dors., dorsal; Fiss., fissure; Gr., greater; Inf., inferior; Infratroch., infratrochlear; Men., meningeal; Men. Hyp., meningohypophyseal; N., nerve; Oculom., oculomotor; Opticocar., opticocarotid; Orb., orbital; P.C.A., posterior cerebral artery; Pet., petrosal; Post., posterior; Posterolat., posterolateral; Posteromed., posteromedial; Prom., prominence; Pterygopal., pterygopalatine; Rec., recess; S.C.A., superior cerebellar artery; Seg., segment; Sup., superior; Supratroch., supratrochlear; Tent., tentorial; Tr., tract, trunk; Triang., triangle. Taken with permission from the Rhoton Collection.

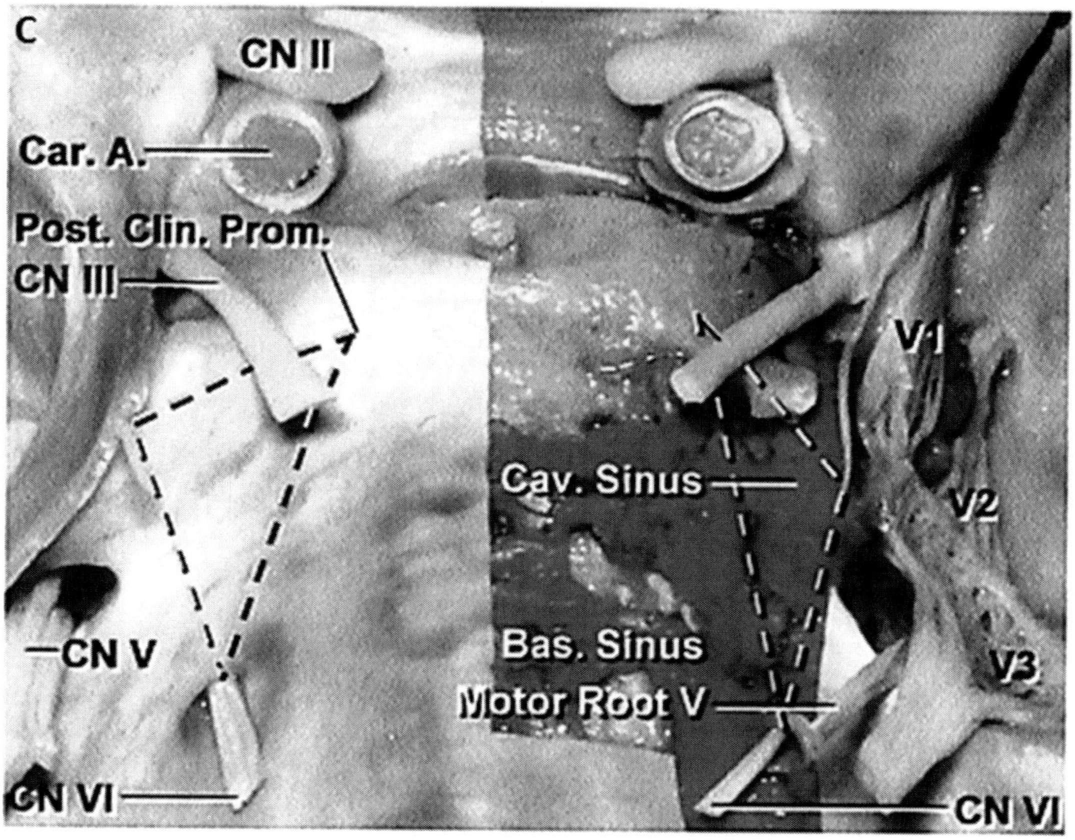

10.2.4.2.4. Posteromedial Middle Fossa Triangle (Kawase's Triangle)

This triangle is located between GSPN and the lateral edge of the trigeminal nerve behind the point where the greater petrosal nerve passes below its lateral surface and a line along the connecting hiatus fallopii to the dural ostium of Meckel's cave. The petrous C3-segment of the internal carotid artery crosses the anterior margin of this triangle. The cochlea is located below the floor of the middle fossa in the lateral apex of the triangle. Removing the bone in the lateral part of the Kawase's triangle exposes the cochlea and the anterior wall of the internal auditory canal. Removing the bone in the medial part of the Kawase's triangle exposes the side of the clivus and the inferior petrosal sinus.

10.2.4.3. Paraclinoid Triangles

10.2.4.3.1. Inferolateral Paraclival Triangle

This triangle is located on the posterior surface of the clivus and temporal bone (Figure 10.4c). The medial margin is formed by a line connecting the dural entry sites of the trochlear and abducens nerves; the upper margin extends from the dural entrance of the trochlear nerve to the point at which the first petrosal vein lateral to Meckel's cave joins the superior petrosal sinus; and the lower margin is formed by a line connecting the point at which the abducens nerve enters the dura to the site at which the first petrosal vein, lateral to the trigeminal nerve, joins the superior petrosal sinus. The porus through which the trigeminal root enters Meckel's cave is situated in the center of this triangle.

10.2.4.3.2. Inferomedial Paraclival Triangle

This triangle is formed above by a line extending from the posterior clinoid process to the dural entrance of the trochlear nerve; laterally by a line connecting the dural entrances of the trochlear and abducens nerves; and medially by a line extending from the dural entrance of the abducens nerve to the posterior clinoid process. The abducens nerve enters the cavernous sinus at the lower edge of this triangle. This triangle extends along the posterior sinus wall. Removing the medial part of the inferomedial triangle behind the internal carotid artery exposes the lateral edge of the dorsum sellae and CN-VI passing below Gruber's ligament.

10.3. The Jugular Foramen

10.3.1. Introduction

The jugular foramen is difficult to understand and to access surgically. It is difficult to conceptualize because it varies in size and shape in different crania, from side to side in the same cranium, and from its intracranial to extracranial end in the same foramen, and because of its complex irregular shape, its curved course, its formation by two bones, and the numerous nerves and venous channels that pass through it (refer to figures 10.5-10.6). The jugular foramen was discussed to some extent in chapter 3, as part of describing the cranial nerves anatomy (please refer to chapter 3).

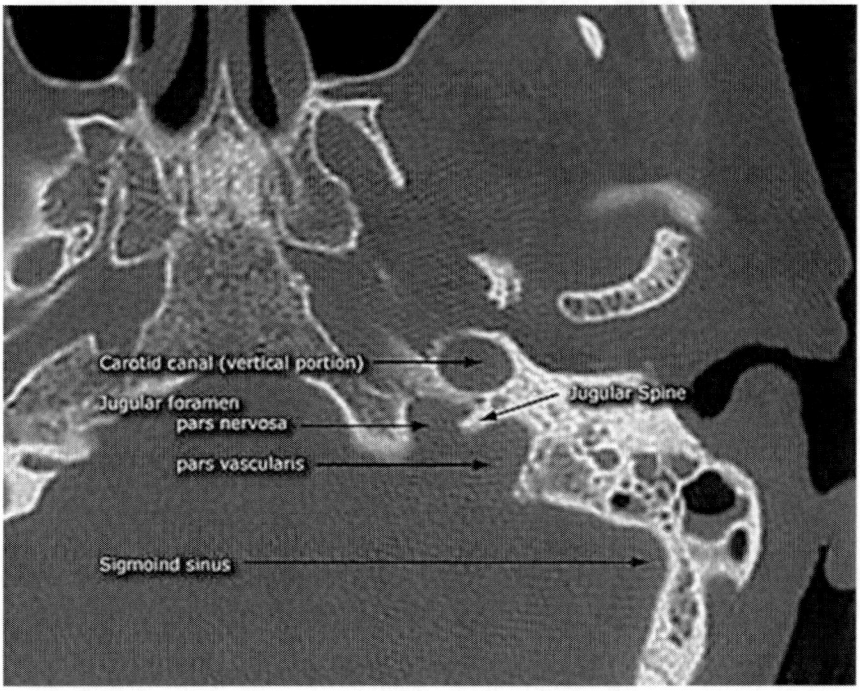

Figure 10.5. The Jugular foreman anatomy, annotated Computed tomography in bone window. Taken with permission from www.radiopaedia.org.

The jugular foramen is divided into three compartments: two venous and a neural or intrajugular compartment. The venous compartments consist of a larger posterolateral venous channel, the sigmoid part, which receives the flow of the sigmoid sinus, and a smaller anteromedial venous channel, the petrosal part, which receives the drainage of the inferior petrosal sinus. The petrosal part forms a characteristic venous confluens by also receiving tributaries from the hypoglossal canal, petroclival fissure, and vertebral venous plexus. The petrosal part empties into the sigmoid part through an opening in the medial wall of the jugular bulb between the glossopharyngeal nerve anteriorly and the vagus and accessory nerves posteriorly. The intrajugular or neural part, through which the glossopharyngeal, vagus, and accessory nerves course, is located between the sigmoid and petrosal parts at the site of the intrajugular processes of the temporal and occipital bones, which are joined by a fibrous or osseous bridge. The glossopharyngeal, vagus, and accessory nerves penetrate the dura on the medial margin of the intrajugular process of the temporal bone to reach the medial wall of the internal jugular vein.

10.3.2. Osseous Relationships

The jugular foramen is located between the temporal and occipital bones. One cannot see directly through the foramen from above because it is directed forward under the temporal bone. The sigmoid groove descends along the mastoid and crosses the occipitomastoid suture where it turns forward on the upper surface of the jugular process of the occipital bone and enters the foramen by passing under the posterior part of the petrous temporal bone. As shown in figure 10.6a, the foramen has a larger lateral sigmoid part through which the sigmoid sinus empties and a smaller anteromedial petrosal part through which the inferior petrosal sinus empties. The two parts are separated by the intrajugular processes of the occipital and temporal bones. The glossopharyngeal, vagus, and accessory nerves pass through the intrajugular portion of the foramen located between the sigmoid and petrosal parts. The foramen is asymmetric from side to side with the right side often being larger as shown. The cochlear aqueduct opens just above the anterior edge of the petrosal part. The vestibular aqueduct opens into the endolymphatic sac, which sits on the back of the temporal bone superolateral to the sigmoid part of the jugular foramen.

The entrance into the carotid canal is located directly in front of the medial half of the jugular foramen. The stylomastoid foramen is located lateral and the anterior half of the occipital condyle medial to the jugular foramen. The posterior condylar foramen is traversed by an emissary vein, which joins the sigmoid sinus. The hypoglossal canal passes above the middle third of the occipital condyle and opens laterally into the interval between the jugular foramen and carotid canal. The roof over the foramen formed by the jugular fossa of the temporal bone is shaped to accommodate the jugular bulb. The posterior margin of the foramen is formed by the jugular process of the occipital bone, which connects the basal (clival) part of the occipital bone to the squamosal part. The petroclival fissure intersects the anteromedial margin of the petrosal part of the foramen (refer to figure 10.6b-d).

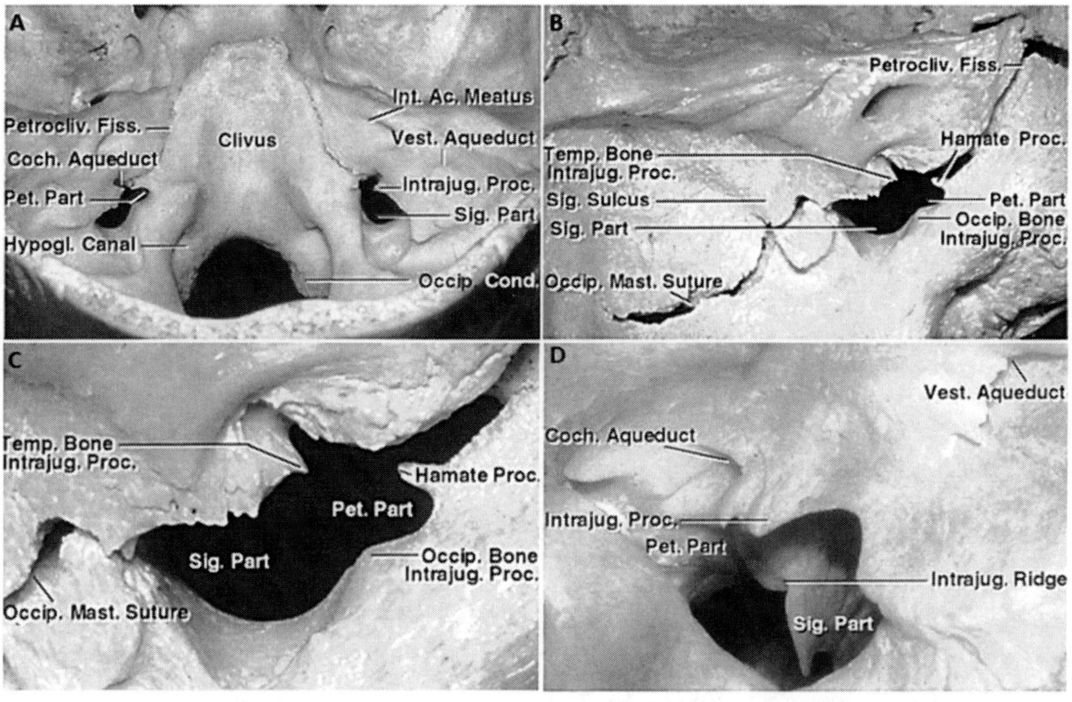

Figure 10.6. Osseous relationships. A, the view directed from posterior and superior shows the shape of the foramen, which is not seen on the direct superior view. B+C, another jugular foramen, Left side. B, the sutures have been forced open to show the relationship of the foramen to the petroclival and occipitomastoid sutures. The intrajugular process of the occipital bone is somewhat more prominent and projects forward toward the intrajugular process of the temporal bone. C, enlarged view. D, enlarged view. The cochlear aqueduct opens above the petrosal part of the foramen and the site where the glossopharyngeal nerve enters the intrajugular part of the foramen on the medial side of the intrajugular process. Ac., acoustic; Car., carotid; Coch., cochlear; Cond., condyle; Fiss., fissure; For., foramen; Hypogl., hypoglossal; Int., internal; Intrajug., Intrajugular; Jug., jugular; Mast., mastoid; Occip., occipital; Pet., petrous; Petrocliv., petroclival; Post., posterior; Proc., process; Sig., sigmoid; Squam., squamosal; Stylomast., stylomastoid; Temp., temporal; Vest., vestibular. Taken with permission from the Rhoton Collection.

A ridge, the intrajugular ridge, extends forward from the intrajugular process along the medial side of the jugular bulb. The glossopharyngeal nerve passes forward along the medial side of the intrajugular process and ridge. The vagus and accessory nerves enter the dura on the medial side of the process, but quickly descend and do not pass forward along the medial edge of the ridge as does the glossopharyngeal nerve (figure 10.6d). The jugular process of the occipital bone often has a small prominence on its surface that projects toward the intrajugular process of the temporal bone, and in some foramina, the intrajugular processes of the two bones are joined by an osseous bridge that converts the foramen into two osseous foramina. The cochlear aqueduct opens above the petrosal part of the foramen and the site where the glossopharyngeal nerve enters the intrajugular part of the foramen on the medial side of the intrajugular process. The vestibular aqueduct opens onto the posterior surface of the temporal bone superolateral to the jugular foramen.

10.3.3. Dural Architecture

The sigmoid sulcus makes a sharp turn just before emptying into the sigmoid portion of the jugular foramen. The inferior petrosal sinus extends along the petroclival fissure and enters the petrosal part of the foramen. The nerves enter the intrajugular part of the foramen located between the sigmoid and petrosal parts. The sigmoid sinus descends in the sigmoid sulcus and makes a sharp anterior turn to enter the jugular foramen. The jugular bulb extends upward under the petrous temporal bone toward the internal acoustic meatus. The endolymphatic sac is located above the lower portion of the sigmoid sinus on the back of the temporal bone and opens above through the vestibular aqueduct into the vestibule. Refer to figure 10.7a+b.

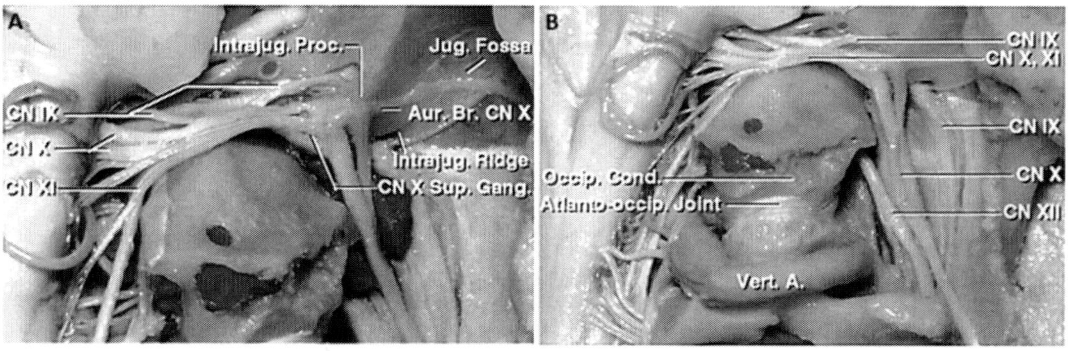

Figure 10.7. Posterior superior view of the jugular foramen. A, the dura covering the jugular foramen and the jugular bulb have been removed. The nerves penetrate the dura on the medial side of the intrajugular process of the temporal bone. The intrajugular ridge extends forward along the medial side of the jugular bulb. B, the hypoglossal nerve has been exposed on the lateral side of the occipital condyle. It exits the hypoglossal canal and joins the glossopharyngeal, vagus, and accessory nerves below the jugular foramen in the interval between the internal carotid artery and internal jugular vein. A., artery; Ac., acoustic; Aur., auricular; Br., branch; Car., carotid; CN, cranial nerve; Cond., condyle; Endolymph., endolymphatic; Gang., ganglion; Inf., inferior; Intrajug., intrajugular; Jug., jugular; Occip., occipital; Pet., petrosal, petrous; Petrocliv., petroclival; Proc., process; Sig., sigmoid; Sup., superior; Temp., temporal; Vert., vertebral; Vestib., vestibular. Taken with permission from the Rhoton Collection.

The glossopharyngeal nerve passes forward along the medial side of the intrajugular ridge, but the vagus and accessory nerves, although entering the dura on the medial side of the intrajugular process, almost immediately turn downward and do not course along the medial edge of the intrajugular ridge in the medial wall of the jugular bulb, as does the glossopharyngeal nerve. The auricular branch of the vagus nerve (Arnold's Nerve) arises from the vagus nerve, passes along the groove in the anterior wall of the jugular fossa, and penetrates the mastoid canaliculus in the lateral wall of the fossa. The intrajugular process of the temporal bone projects backward to join the intrajugular process of the occipital bone, thus forming an osseous bridge that divides the foramen into two parts. The vagus and accessory nerves pass lateral to the osseous bridge and the inferior petrosal sinus descends below the bridge to open into the internal jugular vein.

10.3.4. Stepwise Dissection of the Jugular Foramen

As shown in figure 10.8, the external acoustic meatus is located a little forward of the deep site of the jugular bulb. The internal carotid artery ascends to enter the carotid canal in front of the jugular foramen (figure 10.8a). Both the jugular foramen and carotid canal are situated behind the tympanic part of the temporal bone, which forms the posterior wall of the condylar fossa. The tensor and levator vela palatini muscles are attached to the eustachian tube in the area below the horizontal segment of the petrous carotid. The infratemporal fossa is located below the greater wing of the sphenoid. The mandibular nerve passes through the foramen ovale to enter the upper part of the infratemporal fossa. Branches of the ascending pharyngeal artery pass through the jugular foramen to supply the surrounding dura. The hypoglossal nerve passes forward across the external and internal carotid artery.

The glossopharyngeal nerve descends along the lateral side of the internal carotid artery (figure 10.8b). The accessory nerve passes backward across the lateral surface of the internal jugular vein. The hypoglossal nerve passes through the hypoglossal canal, which is located below and medial to the jugular foramen, and descends with the nerves exiting the jugular foramen. The occipital artery gives rise to a meningeal branch, which passes through the jugular foramen to supply the surrounding dura, and to the stylomastoid artery, which passes through the stylomastoid foramen with the facial nerve. The C1 transverse process and rectus capitis lateralis rest against the posterior surface of the internal jugular vein. The rectus capitis lateralis attaches to the jugular process of the occipital bone at the posterior margin of the jugular foramen. The vertebral artery, as it passes medially along the upper surface of the posterior arch of the atlas, is situated in the floor of the suboccipital triangle located between the superior and inferior oblique and rectus capitis posterior major.

The surface of the temporal and occipital bones surrounding the jugular foramen and carotid canal has an irregular surface that serves as the attachment of the upper end of the carotid sheath. The mastoid segment of the facial nerve and the stylomastoid foramen are situated lateral to the jugular bulb. The chorda tympani arises from the mastoid segment of the facial nerve and courses along the deep side of the tympanic membrane crossing the neck of the malleus. It exits the skull by passing through the petrotympanic and squamotympanic sutures and joins the lingual branch of the mandibular nerve distally. The carotid ridge separates the carotid canal and jugular foramen. The glossopharyngeal, vagus, accessory, and hypoglossal nerves exit the skull on the medial side of the internal carotid artery and jugular vein. The glossopharyngeal and hypoglossal nerves pass forward along the lateral surface of the internal carotid artery, and the accessory nerve descends posteriorly across the lateral surface of the internal jugular vein. The vagus nerve descends in the carotid sheath.

The tympanic segment of the facial nerve passes below the lateral semicircular canal and turns downward as the mastoid segment to exit the stylomastoid foramen (figure 10.8c). The stylomastoid foramen and the mastoid segment are located lateral to the jugular bulb. The semicircular canals are located above the jugular bulb. The chorda tympani crosses the inner surface of the tympanic membrane and neck of the malleus. The greater petrosal nerve courses along the floor of the middle fossa on the upper surface of the petrous carotid (figure 10.8d). The deep petrosal nerve arises from the sympathetic bundles on the internal carotid artery. The deep and greater petrosal nerves join to form the vidian nerve, which passes forward through the vidian canal to join the maxillary nerve and pterygopalatine ganglion in the pterygopalatine fossa. The cochlea is located above the lateral genu of the petrous carotid. The tympanic segment of the facial nerve passes posteriorly below the lateral semicircular canal.

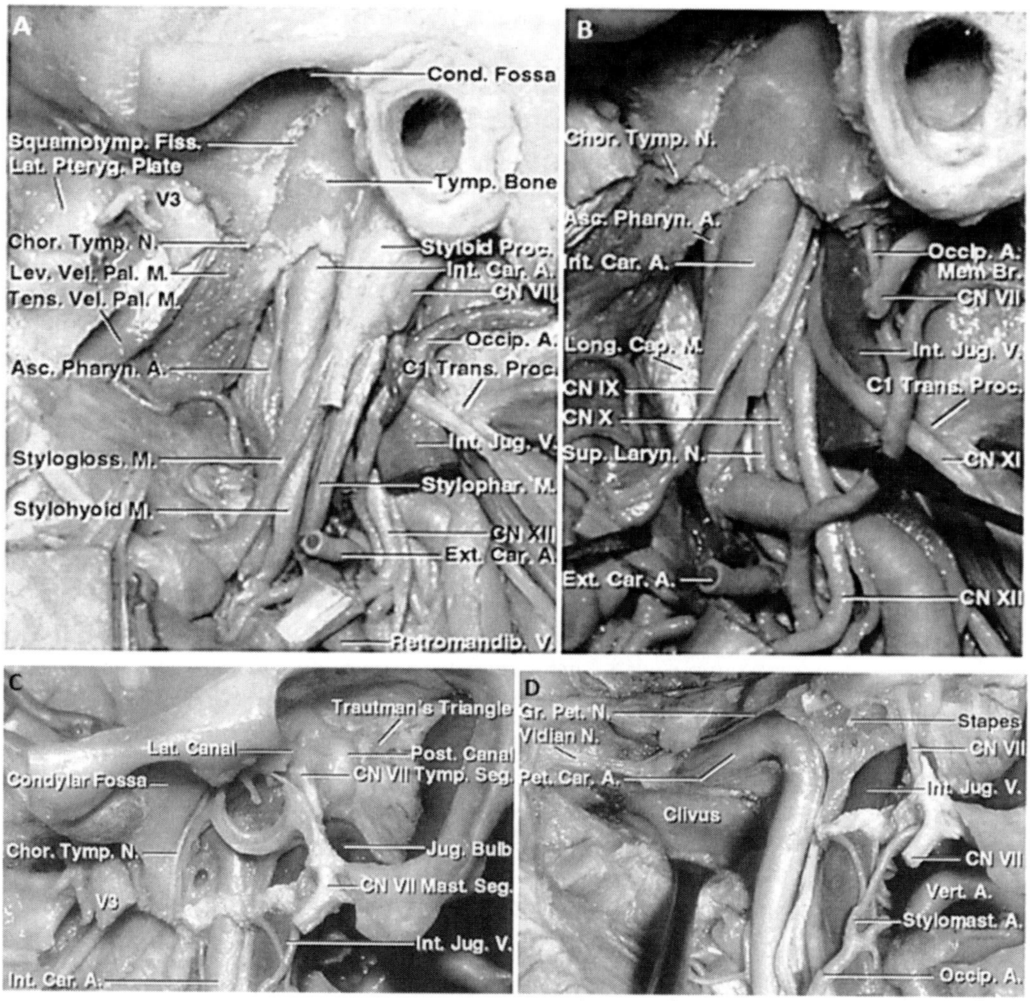

Figure 10.8. Stepwise dissection of the structures superficial to and surrounding the jugular foramen. A, the mandibular ramus and condyle, medial and lateral pterygoid muscles, and posterior belly of the digastric have been removed to expose the styloid process, which is located lateral to the jugular foramen. B, the styloid process has been removed to expose the glossopharyngeal, vagus, accessory, and hypoglossal nerves descending between the internal carotid artery and the internal jugular vein in the area immediately below the jugular foramen. C, lateral view of mastoid and tympanic cavity before removing the tympanic ring. D, the floor of the middle fossa and the tympanic sulcus has been removed to expose the jugular bulb and petrous carotid. A., artery; Asc., ascending; Aur., auricular; Br., branch; Cap., capitis; Car., carotid; Chor. Tymp., chorda tympani; CN, cranial nerve; Cond., condylar; Dors., dorsal; Eust., eustachian; Ext., external; Fiss., fissure; Gl., gland; Gr., greater; Inf., inferior; Int., internal; Jug., jugular; Laryn., laryngeal; Lat., lateral, lateralis; Lev., levator; Long., longus; M., muscle; Mast., mastoid; Men., meningeal; N., nerve; Obl., oblique; Occip., occipital; Pal., palatini; Pet., petrosal, petrous; Pharyn., pharyngeal; Post., posterior; Proc., process; Pteryg., pterygoid; Rec., rectus; Retromandib., retromandibular; Scap., scapulae; Seg., segment; Semicirc., semicircular; Sig., sigmoid; Squamotymp., squamotympanic; Sternocleidomast., sternocleidomastoid; Stylogloss., styloglossus; Stylomast., stylomastoid; Stylophar., stylopharyngeus; Submandib., submandibular; Sup., superior; Temp., temporal; Tens., tensor; TM., temporomandibular; Trans., transverse; Tymp., tympanic, tympany; V., vein; Vel., veli; Vent., ventral; Vert., vertebral. Taken with permission from the Rhoton Collection.

10.3.5. Jugular Foramen Syndromes

Different neoplastic and vascular processes can affect the jugular foramen region, both intracranially and extracranially. Some neoplastic processes follow anatomical pathways intracranially and within the petrous bone (like paragangliomas, glomus tumors etc). The jugular foramen syndromes are segregated according to the extent of the lesion spread, as presented by the different cranial nerves involved. Such a scheme is presented in table 10.2.

Table 2.11. Jugular foramen syndromes and clinical presentation

Foramen region	Cranial nerve	Clinical syndrome					
		Vernet	Collet Sicard	Villaret	Tapia	Schmidt	Jackson
Pars nervosa	IX	+	+	+			
Pars venosa	X	+	+	+	+	+	+
	XI	+	+	+	+/-	+	+
	XII		+	+	+		+
---	SNS*			+	+/-		

* Sympathetic trunk traveling on the internal carotid artery.

10.4. The Sphenoid Sinus

The sphenoid sinus and sellar region were discussed to some extent in the frame of the discussion on the diencephalon and pituitary gland. Refer to chapter 4 and related figures. Being such a unique structure in the skull base, gaining more and more popularity and access by neurosurgeons and ENT surgeons in recent years, we thought it deserves some more in-depth discussion. As shown in figure 10.9a, the upper part of the nasal cavity is separated from the orbits by the ethmoidal sinuses. The lower part of the nasal cavity is bounded laterally by the maxillary sinuses. The middle concha projects medially from the lateral nasal wall at the junction of the roof of the maxillary and ethmoidal sinuses. The posterior ethmoid air cells are located in front of the lateral part of the face of the sphenoid sinus. As shown in figure 10.9b, the posterior ethmoid air cells overlap the lateral margin of the sphenoid ostia.

Upon opening of the anterior wall of the sphenoid sinus, removing the sphenoid septa, the anterior sellar wall is exposed in the midline and the prominences over the optic canal and carotid arteries in the lateral walls of the sphenoid sinus (figure 10.9c). The medial part of the posterior wall of the left maxillary sinus can be removed to expose branches of the maxillary artery in the pterygopalatine fossa. The opticocarotid recesses extend laterally between the prominences over the carotid arteries and optic nerves. Removing the bone of the sinus wall (figure 10.9d) can expose the pituitary gland, intracavernous carotids, optic nerves, ophthalmic arteries, and cavernous sinuses. The inferolateral trunk passes above and lateral to the abducens nerve. The shortest distance between the paired carotid arteries is usually located just below the tuberculum sellae. The bony depression between the carotid prominence and the optic canal, the opticocarotid recess, extends into the medial end of the optic strut. The broad round prominence below the opticocarotid recess is produced by the structures passing through the superior orbital fissure.

As shown in figure 10.10a, the inferior hypophyseal arteries arise from the meningohypophyseal trunk, branch of the intracavernous carotid and pass to the capsule of the posterior lobe. Sympathetic nerves ascend on the carotid arteries. The abducens nerve passes through the cavernous sinus on the lateral side of the internal carotid artery and medial to the ophthalmic nerve. The anterior cerebral arteries are situated above and the pituitary gland is situated below the optic chiasm (figure 10.10b). The basilar apex is located behind the gland. The oculomotor nerve passes forward between the posterior cerebral and superior cerebellar arteries.

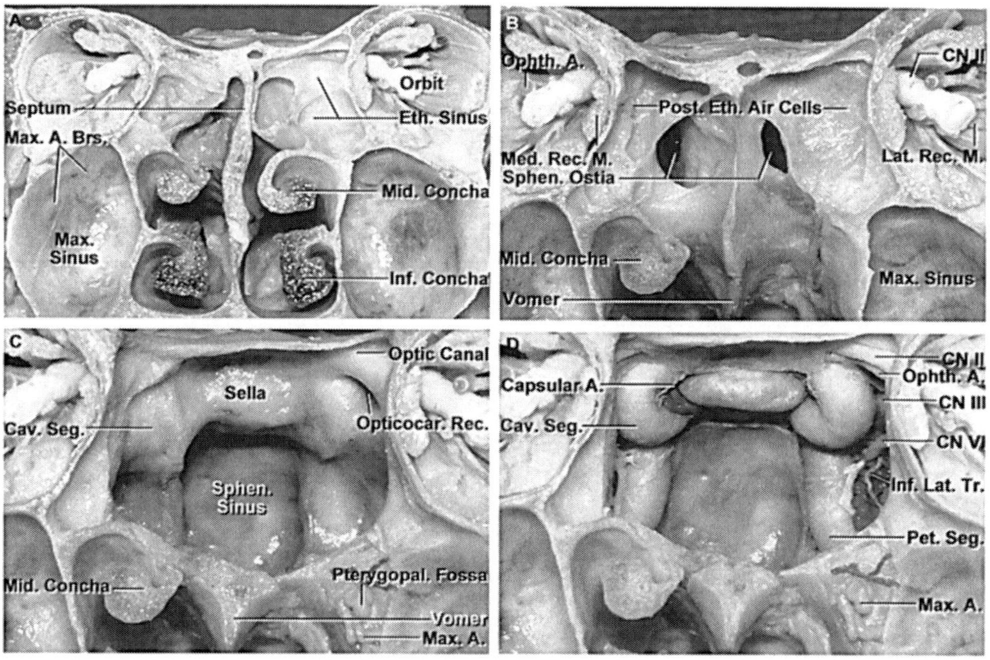

Figure 10.9. Anterior view of a coronal section in front of the sphenoid sinus, through the nasal cavity, orbits, and ethmoidal and maxillary sinuses. A, the upper part of the nasal cavity is separated from the orbits by the ethmoidal sinuses. The lower part of the nasal cavity is bounded laterally by the maxillary sinuses. The middle concha projects medially from the lateral nasal wall at the junction of the roof of the maxillary and ethmoidal sinuses. The posterior ethmoid air cells are located in front of the lateral part of the face of the sphenoid sinus. B, the middle and inferior nasal conchae on the left side and the nasal septum and the posterior ethmoidal sinuses on both sides have been removed to expose the posterior nasopharyngeal wall, the anterior aspect of the sphenoid body, and the sphenoid ostia. The posterior ethmoid air cells overlap the lateral margin of the sphenoid ostia. C, the anterior wall of the sphenoid sinus has been opened and the sphenoid septum has been removed to expose the anterior sellar wall in the midline and the prominences over the optic canal and carotid arteries in the lateral walls of this well-pneumatized sphenoid sinus. The medial part of the posterior wall of the left maxillary sinus has been removed to expose branches of the maxillary artery in the pterygopalatine fossa. D, the pituitary gland, intracavernous carotids, optic nerves, ophthalmic arteries, and cavernous sinuses have been exposed by removing the bone of the sinus wall. A., artery; Brs., branches; Cav., cavernous; CN., cranial nerve; Eth., ethmoid; Fiss., fissure; Inf., inferior; Lat., lateral; M., muscle; Max., maxillary; Med., medial; Mid., middle; Ophth., ophthalmic; Opticocar., opticocarotid; Orb., orbital; Pet., petrous; Pit., pituitary; Post., posterior; Pterygopal., pterygopalatine; Rec., recess, rectus; Seg., segment; Sphen., sphenoid; Sup., superior; Tr., trunk. Taken with permission from the Rhoton Collection.

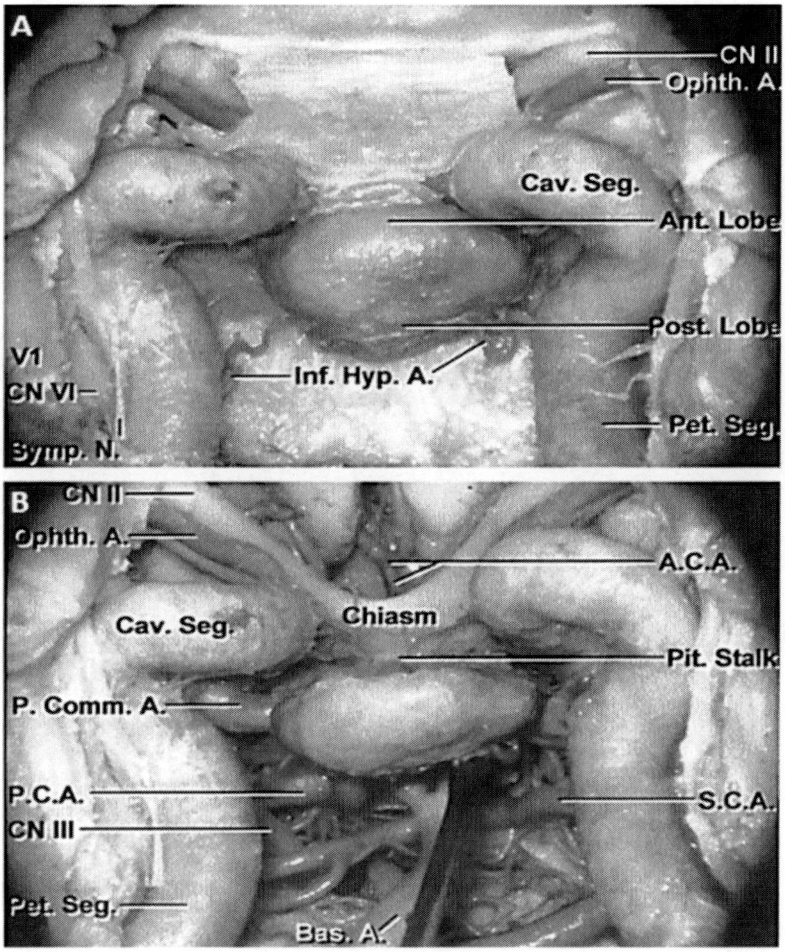

Figure 10.10. Stepwise dissection examining the relationship of the sphenoid sinus to the pituitary fossa, cavernous sinus, and sellar region. A, the venous space has been cleared to expose the intracavernous carotid and the anterior and posterior pituitary lobes. B, the dura has been removed to expose the intradural structures. A., artery; A.C.A., anterior cerebral artery; Ant., anterior; Bas., basilar; Car., carotid; Cav., cavernous; CN, cranial nerve; Comm., communicating; Eth., ethmoid; Hyp., hypophyseal; Inf., inferior; Intercav., intercavernous; N., nerve; Ophth., ophthalmic; Opticocar., opticocarotid; P.C.A., posterior cerebral artery; Pet., petrosal; Pit., pituitary; Post., posterior; Prom., prominence; Rec., recess; S.C.A., superior cerebellar artery; Seg., segment; Sphen., sphenoid; Symp., sympathetic; Tuberc., tuberculum. Taken with permission from the Rhoton Collection.

Chapter 11

The Visual System

11.1. Abstract

The different elements comprising the visual system have been discussed to some extent in their prospective locations. The visual motor system was discussed in the frame of the chapter on the brainstem and cranial nerves (chapter 3), the lateral geniculate nucleus (LGN) was discussed in the frame of the thalamus and diencephalon (chapter 4), and the optic radiation and visual cortex have been discussed in the frame of the description of cerebral hemispheral white matter and gray matter anatomy (chapter 7). The aim of this chapter is to provide an overview the visual system unified under function and not regional anatomy. The chapter begins with an overview of the structure of the eye, the retina, and retinal projections. Retro-chiasmal visual pathways lesions are described next, followed by a stepwise dissection through the optic system. The visual motor systems are described next, starting from the peripheral structures (extra-ocular, intraocular and eyelid muscles), followed by CNS visual structures and reflex eye movements. Key features in the clinical examination and manifestations of different lesions are presented.

11.2. Overview

The different elements comprising the visual system have been discussed to some extent in their prospective locations. The visual motor system was discussed in the frame of the chapter on the brainstem and cranial nerves (chapter 3), the lateral geniculate nucleus (LGN) was discussed in the frame of the thalamus and diencephalon (chapter 4), and the optic radiation and visual cortex have been discussed in the frame of the description of cerebral hemispheral white matter and gray matter anatomy (chapter 7). The aim of this chapter is to provide an overview the visual system unified under function and not regional anatomy. Like in other sensory systems, the visual system creates a somatotopic "map" of its sensory field, which is preserved at all levels of the visual system. Initial processing of the visual information begins as early as in the retina. The retina projects to several diencephalic structures, but mainly terminates in the thalamic relay nucleus (LGN), which in turn innervates a large cortical region (located at the occipital poles, termed as the visual cortex). From these primary and associated visual cortices, the information is sent to temporal and parietal lobes (association cortices). We will discuss the different stops and influences on this system.

11.3. Anatomy of the Eye

In brief, the cornea is a transparent protective coating for the optical structures of the eye. Its lateral margins are continuous with the conjunctiva. The conjunctiva is a specialized epithelium covering the "white" sclera. The cornea is not vascularized (unlike the conjunctiva and sclera). The eye can be subdivided into anterior and posterior chambers (refer to figure 11.1). The anterior chamber is fluid filled, located behind the cornea, bounded posteriorly by the iris and the opening of the pupil. The posterior chamber is bounded anteriorly by the iris and posteriorly by the lens and its encircling suspensory ligament (the zonule fibers of Zinn). The ciliary body, located around the rim of the posterior chamber, continuously produces the aqueous fluid. This fluid in turn, flows through the papillary opening into the anterior chamber. It is than drained by modified veins (the canals of Schlemm), which are located around the rim of the anterior chamber (in an angle where the iris meets the cornea, the so called limbus). The aqueous fluid here is in contact with the vitreous body (a gelatinous mass filling the main space of the eyeball between the lens and retina).

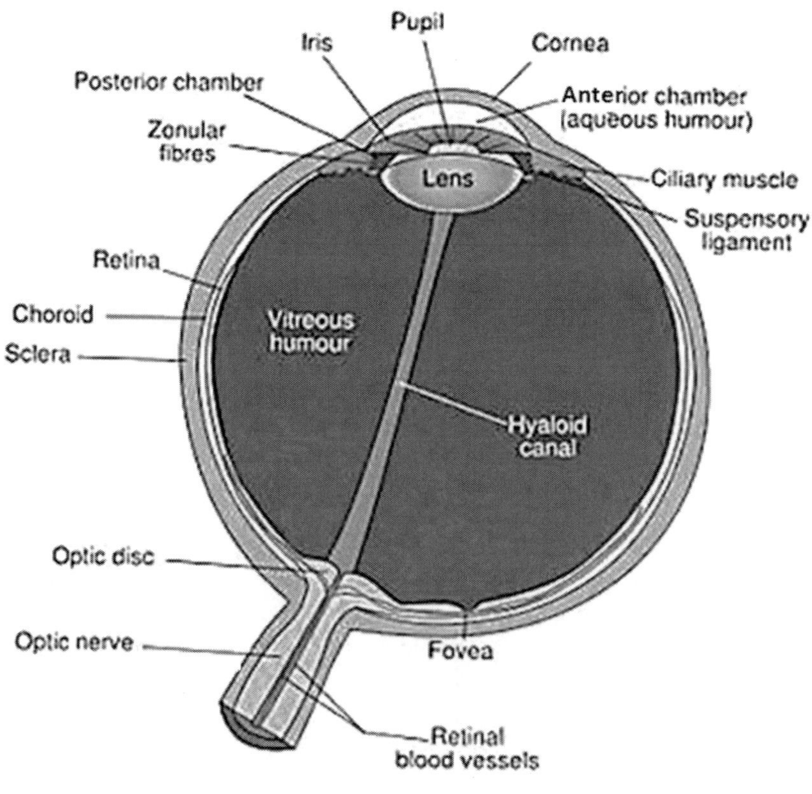

Figure 11.1. The human eye. Refer to text. Taken with permission from www.radiopaedia.org.

The iris is a pigmented structure, located directly anterior to the lens. Its stroma contains melanocytes, and muscle fibers. These muscle fibers belong to both the sphincter and dilator muscles. The sphincter muscle fibers are circumferentially organized whereas the dilator muscle fibers are radially arranged. The sphincter of the iris receives parasympathetic innervation from the Edinger-Westphal nucleus of the oculomotor nerve (CN-III, discussed later), via the ciliary ganglion. This results in the release of acetylcholine onto muscarinic receptors, resulting in a decrease in the diameter of the pupil (Miosis). The dilator muscle opposes the sphincter actions, and is innervation (sympathetics) arises in the intermediolateral cell column of upper thoracic levels spinal cord. Its postganglionic fibers originate in the superior cervical ganglion. These are adrenergic neurons, releasing norepinephrine which causes pupillary dilatation (mydriasis). Pupillary dilatation is a general a measure of the overall sympathetic tone. The iris, ciliary body, and choroid make up the vascular tunic of the eye (i.e., the uvea). The choroid is a highly vascularized, pigmented tissue layer lying between the retinal pigment epithelium and the sclera.

11.4. Neural Retina, Pigmented Epithelium

The inner surface of the posterior aspect of the eye is covered by the retina. This structure is in turn composed of the neural retina and the retinal pigment epithelium. The Retina cells are described in two layers: an inner layer and an outer layer. The inner layer refers to structures located towards the vitreous and center of the eyeball. The outer layer refers to structures located towards the pigment epithelium and choroid. The retinal pigment epithelium is a continuous sheet of pigment choroidal cells, bound by tight junctions, blocking the flow of plasma or ions across it.

The pigment epithelium has several functions: it supplies the neural retina with nutrition in the form of glucose and essential ions, it protects retinal photoreceptors from damaging levels of light and he has a role in maintaining the photoreceptor anatomy. The neural retina contains the photoreceptors and associated nerves, converting the light quanta impulses into an electrical signal (action and receptor potentials), processed by retinal nerves and sent by the ganglion cells via the optic nerve. The contact between the neural retina and the pigment epithelium layer is mechanically unstable.

11.4.1. Neural Retina Layers

The neural retina is composed of seven layers. Layers 2-7 are flanked by a pair of limiting membranes, consisting of glial cells processes joined by tight junctions. The outer limiting membrane is located between layers 1-2. The inner limiting membrane is between the neural layer and the vitreous. The photoreceptors outer segments interdigitate with the melanin filled processes of the pigment epithelium cells, which are mobile. These processes elongate into the pigment layer upon a bright light stimulus (the so called photopic conditions), and retract when the light is dim (i.e., in scotopic conditions).

The layers of the neural retina, presented from the outer layer inward are:

1) The photoreceptor cell layer composed of outer and inner segments.
2) The outer nuclear layer, which contains the photoreceptors cell nuclei.
3) The outer plexiform layer consisting of synaptic connections with second order retinal cells.
4) The inner nuclear layer which contains the cell bodies of secondary and tertiary order retinal cells.
5) The inner plexiform layer, representing another synaptic contact.
6) The ganglion layer, which contains the cell bodies of the ganglion cells.
7) The nerve fiber layer (i.e., optic fibers layer), converging at the optic disc.

The processing of the visual input in the retina, the functions of the outer and inner plexiform layers as does that of the horizontal, bipolar, amacrine and ganglion cells in visual processing, although fascinating, is not in the scope of this book.

11.5. Retinal Projections

Broadly classified, the retinal output can be segregated into geniculate and extra-geniculate pathways. The LGN anatomy and functions (i.e., the geniculate pathways) are discussed next. The extra-geniculate targets of retinal projections are a variety of locations in the diencephalon and midbrain. These include: The suprachiasmatic nucleus of the hypothalamus involved in the control of diurnal rhythms (hence the need for raw unconscious visual information), the accessory optic nucleus and the olivary pretectal nuclei subserving the pupillary light reflex, the superior colliculus involved in controlling eye movements, mediating visual reflexes, and the pulvinar nucleus of the thalamus, to which the superior colliculus projects, receiving input also from the pretectum and the visual cortex. The pulvinar in turn, sends the information to the visual association cortex.

11.5.1. Retino-geniculate Projections (The Geniculate Pathway)

The majority of retinal ganglion cells send their axons to the LGN nucleus of thalamus via CN-II (the optic nerve), optic chiasm and optic tract. Throughout its path, the visual information is conveyed in a way that a map of the visual space is maintained and the receptive fields lie in precise arrangement as they do on the retinal surface. This is termed as a retinotopic map. The visual fields consist of both a binocular and monocular zones. The binocular zone is the broad central region seen by both eyes. The right and left monocular zones are seen only by one eye. The visual fields are divided to hemi-fields (temporal and nasal fields), and to upper and lower quadrants. Only light passing through the pupil reaches the retina, than refracted by cornea and lens for image to be focused on the retina. Light from the inferior aspects of the visual field strikes the superior retina, while light from nasal visual field strikes the temporal retina. This results in an inverted (right to left and up to down) image to be perceived.

11.5.1.1. The Optic Nerve, Chiasm, Tract

The ganglion axons within the seventh nerve fiber layer of the neural retina are unmyelinated, but as they pass through the sclera they become ensheathed by myelin formed by oligodendrocytes. Thus, the myelin covering the optic nerve is central nervous system (CNS) in origin.

Thus, the optic nerve is considered part of the CNS and not the peripheral nervous system. This is also the reason why some CNS white matter diseases like multiple sclerosis affect only the optic nerve and no other cranial nerves. Since there are no photoreceptor cells in the optic disc part of the retina, it is a blind spot. In contrast, visual acuity is greatest at the fovea point of the retina, where a higher density of rods is found.

The optic nerve (CN-II) extends from the caudal aspect of the eyeball up to chiasm. CN-II is enclosed in dura and arachnoid layers, continuous with that of the brain. Thus, any increase in intracranial pressure is transmitted to the eyeball, resulting in papilledema. The optic chiasm is located rostrolaterally to the pituitary stalk. The optic chiasm allows for fibers from the nasal retina to cross (decussate) to the contralateral optic tract. Fibers from the temporal retina on the other hand remain on the same side (entering the ipsilateral optic tract). Von Wilbrand's knee is a microscopic exception. Some crossing fibers form a loop arching through caudal part of contralateral optic nerve. Its significance manifests in that lesions in this region can cause visual loss in both eyes. The optic tract, coursing over the crus cerebri, ending at the LGN is presented in the stepwise dissection subchapter. Refer to figures 11.2.

11.5.1.2. The Lateral Geniculate Nucleus

The LGN and metathalamus were discussed in detail in chapter 4. Briefly, the LGN is composed of six cellular layers, with myelinated fibers located between these layers. The layers are divided by morphology and origin of input. The LGN gives rise to the optic radiation. Layers 1-2 of the LGN contain large somata neurons, thus termed the magnocellular layers.

The magnocellular layers receive input from the retinal rods, having large receptive fields. Layers 3-6 of the LGN contain small somata neurons, thus termed the parvocellular layers. The parvocellular layers receive input from the retinal cones, having small receptive fields.

Fibers reaching LGN from the temporal retina remain uncrossed, terminating in layers #2, #3, and #5 of the ipsilateral LGN. Fibers reaching LGN from the nasal retina are crossed, terminating in layers #1, #4, and #6 of the contralateral LGN. The same point of the visual field is represented six times, in each layer of the LGN. The retinotopic map progresses from the midline to the periphery in visual space as the layers run from medial to lateral in LGN. Layers also run in a rostral to caudal direction, representing the inferior-superior axis. Representation of the blind spot in the LGN is as a blank column extending through all six LGN layers (refer to figure 11.2).

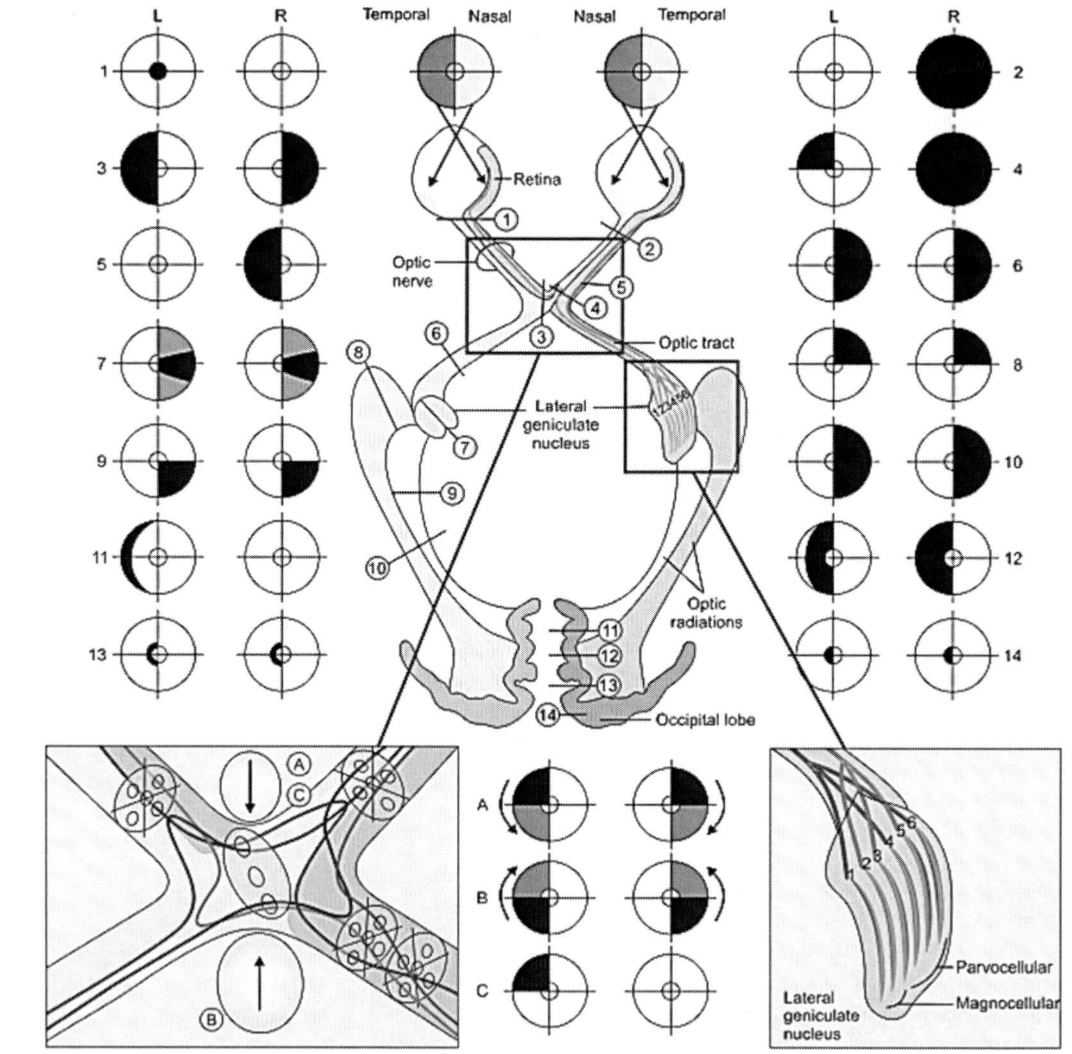

Figure 11.2. Visual pathway lesions and manifestations in visual fields. Modified from "Focused Neurosurgery", 2014.

11.5.2. The Optic Radiation

This white matter tract, discussed in chapter 7 in the frame of white matter hemispheral anatomy, extends from the LGN to ipsilateral primary visual cortex located on the banks of the occipital calcarine sulcus. It is also termed as the geniculostriate pathway. The optic radiation can be divided into two bundles, arising from the lower and upper quadrant of the contralateral visual hemi-fields. Fibers from the lower quadrant of the visual hemi-field originate from the dorsomedial portion of LGN, arching directly caudally to pass through the retrolenticular limb of the internal capsule. These fibers synapse on the superior bank of the occipital calcarine sulcus. Fibers from the upper quadrant of the visual hemi-field originate from the ventrolateral portion of LGN. These fibers do not pass directly to the visual cortex, rather arch rostrally, passing ventrally into the white matter of the temporal lobe, forming a broad "U-turn" termed as Meyer's or Archambault's loop. Only after forming this loop, the fibers pass caudally to synapse on the inferior banks of the occipital calcarine sulcus. Fibers arising from the retinal macula and fovea originate from central portion of LGN and pass to caudal portions of the occipital visual cortex.

11.5.3. The Primary Visual Cortex – Brodmann 17

This occipital cortex is a neocortex in its histology, having six cortical layers. Its layer-IV (the main receptive layer), contain an extra band of myelinated fibers termed as the stria of Gennari, indicative of a large geniculo-calcarine input. Its layer-VI is also prominent and is the source of cortical projection to the LGN. The superior bank of the primary visual cortex, as mentioned previously, receives input from the inferior contralateral hemi-fields. The inferior bank of the primary visual cortex receives input from the superior part of the hemi-fields. The central part of the visual field is represented in the cortical portion closest to the occipital pole. The central ten degrees of the visual field occupies over 50% of the visual cortex. The visual cortex is organized into cortical columns, extending perpendicularly from the pial surface to the white matter, discussed next.

11.5.3.1. Visual Cortical Columns

As mentioned, the visual cortex is organized into cortical columns, extending perpendicularly from the pial surface to the white matter. Here the central surround receptive field is transformed. The cells of layer-IV of the cortex, receiving the input from LGN, respond best to bars or edges of light rather than to spots or rings. These are thus termed simple cells. Progressing towards the white matter, into the deeper cortical layers, receptive field properties become even more complex (thus termed complex cells). Cells lying directly above or below one another in the primary visual cortex tend to respond to light stimuli in the same point in the visual space. This proves that the retinotopic map is preserved.

A superimposed architectural arrangement is the fact that the simple cells that respond to input from the right or left eye, form narrow parallel strips called ocular dominance columns. Stripes called orientation columns cross the cortex at right angles to the ocular dominance columns. These orientation columns contain cells that respond best to bars or edges of light with a particular orientation. A further discussion of cortical visual processing in not in the scope of this book.

11.5.3. Other Visual Cortical Areas

The visual information undergoes much more processing than that provided by the primary visual cortex. The visual world is broken down into elements (dots, stripes), for efficient processing. The reconstruction is in many aspects still unclear. Brodmann areas 18 and 19 (secondary and tertiary visual cortices respectively) continue the general pattern of organization seen in the primary motor cortex, receiving input from it and from the thalamic pulvinar nucleus.

Within the secondary visual cortex the magnocellular and parvocellular pathways diverge. Of note, up to this point these pathways are located in the same general region. The magnocellular stream proceeds to the V3 subregion of Brodmann 18, and to the medial temporal area (V5), to finally reach the posterior parietal area (7a). The information carried by this fiber bundle is largely originating from rod cells having large receptive fields. Thus, the information is used to determine where relevant visual stimuli are located, and to determine movement. The parvocellular stream reaches the V2 to V4 subregions of Brodmann 19. From there, the information continues to the inferior temporal cortex. The information carried by this bundle originates mainly from the retinal cones, coding mainly for form and color. This cortical subdivision is not in the scope of this book, and given here for completeness.

11.6. Retro-Chiasmal Visual Pathways Lesions

Lesions of the visual system posterior to the chiasm affect homonymous portions of the visual fields in both eyes. Optic tract lesions are caused by the same processes that affect the chiasm. Tract lesions produce relatively incongruous homonymous visual field defects and often produce a specific pattern of optic disc pallor. Optic tract lesions may also produce a relative affarent pupillary defect, because pupillomotor fibers travel in the optic tract before exiting at the brachium of the superior colliculus. Tract lesions are therefore characterized by contralateral incongruous homonymous visual field defects and a small RAPD and optic disc pallor in the eye contralateral to the lesion.

Axons in the optic tract synapse in the lateral geniculate nuclei. From there, superior retrogeniculate fibers travel directly through the parietal lobe to the occipital cortex and synapse superior to the calcarine fissure. Parietal lesions cause homonymous defects that are denser inferiorly. Inferior fibers take a more indirect route and sweep around the temporal horn of the ventricular system (Meyer's loop) and through the temporal lobe to neurons in the inferior occipital cortex. Lesions in the temporal lobe produce homonymous visual field defects that are denser in the superior quadrants.

From the chiasm posteriorly, corresponding axons move closer together as they converge on a single point in the occipital cortex; the more posterior the lesion, the more precise the homonymous defects approximate each other (i.e., greater congruity). Complete homonymous visual field defects are said to be non-localizing because they can be caused by lesions anywhere from the optic tract to the occipital lobe. A homonymous hemianopic visual field defect from a unilateral retrochiasmal lesion does not cause decreased visual acuity. However, bilateral retrochiasmal lesions (e.g., bilateral occipital infarcts) can profoundly affect vision in both eyes despite normal findings on ophthalmoscopy and normal pupillary responses. Refer to figure 11.2 for the different lesions effects on the visual fields.

11.7. Stepwise Dissection through the Optic System

Figures 11.3 - 11.9 present a stepwise dissection through the optic system. The aim of this subchapter is to recapitulate and emphasize the key gross anatomical points. As the optic nerve enters the optic canal and then the orbit, it remains within the central nervous system.

CN-II is therefore invested in the optic nerve sheath which is continuous with the dura (figure 11.3 - 11.4). The ophthalmic (CN-V1) and trochlear nerves (CN-IV) cross over the optic nerve in the apex of the orbit, while the abducens nerve (CN-VI) remains lateral (figure 11.4). Note the optic nerve sheath, which is present once the optic nerve enters the optic canal (figures 11.3 - 11.4). The optic nerve passes under the falciform ligament before entering the optic canal. The olfactory tract is superior to the optic nerve. In figure 11.4, the optic nerve is seen in the optic canal (optic nerve sheath has been opened).

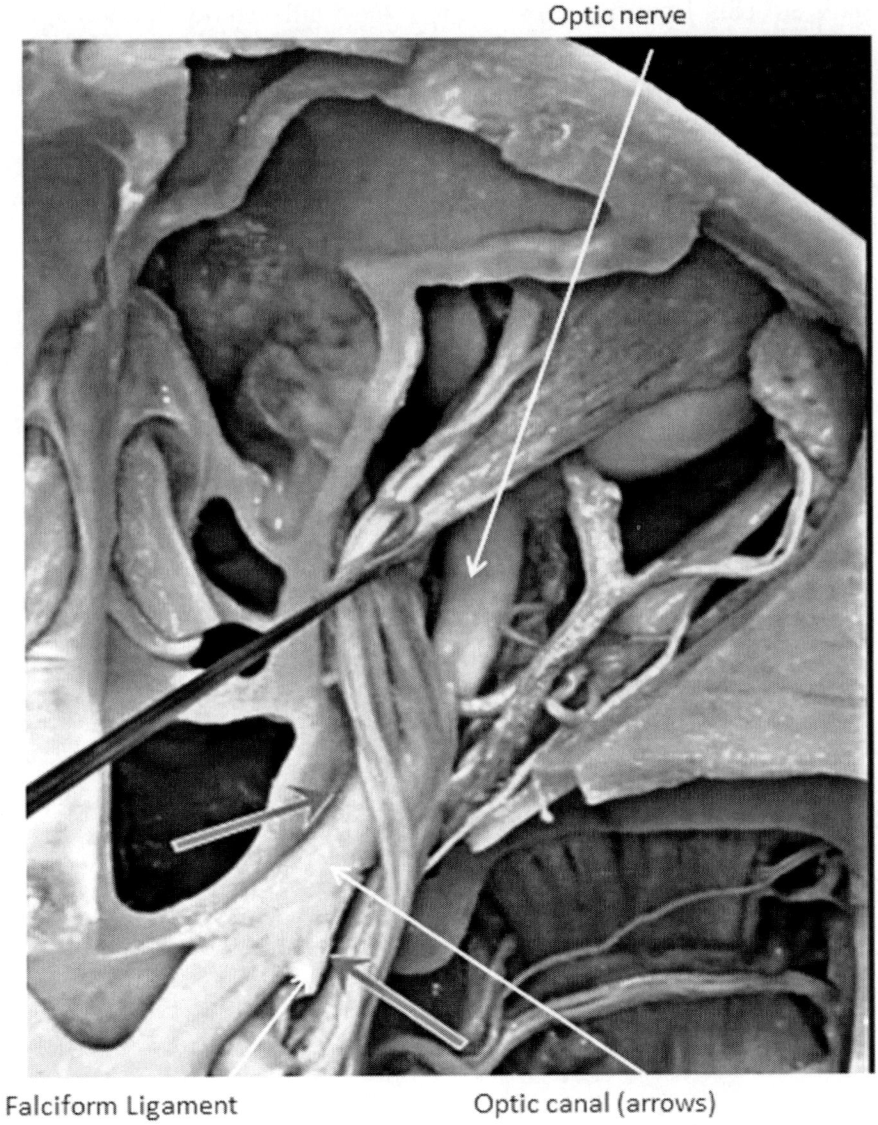

Figure 11.3. Axial view of the orbit and optic nerve. The roof of the orbit has been drilled and superior rectus muscles retracted. Taken with permission from the Rhoton Collection.

The anterior clinoid process contributes to the lateral wall of the optic canal and to the roof of the cavernous sinus. When drilling the anterior clinoid process to open the lateral part of the optic canal, the superiorly coursing trochlear and oculomotor nerves may be injured.

Within the posterior wall of the sphenoid sinus, the opticocarotid recess lies between the impression of the cavernous segment of the internal carotid artery and the impression of the optic nerve. In figure 11.5, the ophthalmic arteries are seen arising from the ophthalmic (supraclinoidal) segment of the internal carotid artery. They course inferior to the optic nerves as they enter the optic canal.

The optic nerve leads to the optic chiasm, which is intimately related to the anterior third ventricle (figure 11.6). The lamina terminalis blends with the posterior portion of the optic chiasm then projects superiorly with the supraoptic recess forming in the angle between. The pituitary stalk emerges from the hypothalamus and third ventricle posterior to the optic chiasm. The anterior communicating artery lies above the optic chiasm. The supraoptic recess lies between the lamina terminalis and the posterior projection of the optic chiasm in the third ventricle.

As shown in figures 11.7 - 11.8, the optic tract courses superior to the uncus and medial to the temporal horn before terminating in the lateral geniculate nucleus. The optic tract can be seen coursing medial to the amygdala, which marks the anterior portion of the uncus. The optic tract terminates in the lateral geniculate nucleus, which gives rise to the optic radiations in the roof and lateral wall of the temporal horn. Meyer's loop is comprised of the subset of the optic radiations that course anteriorly before looping back. Any approach to the temporal horn via the inferior limiting sulcus of the insula may damage these fibers and produce a superior quadrantanopia. Figure 11.9 presents the primary visual cortex, surrounding the calcarine sulcus.

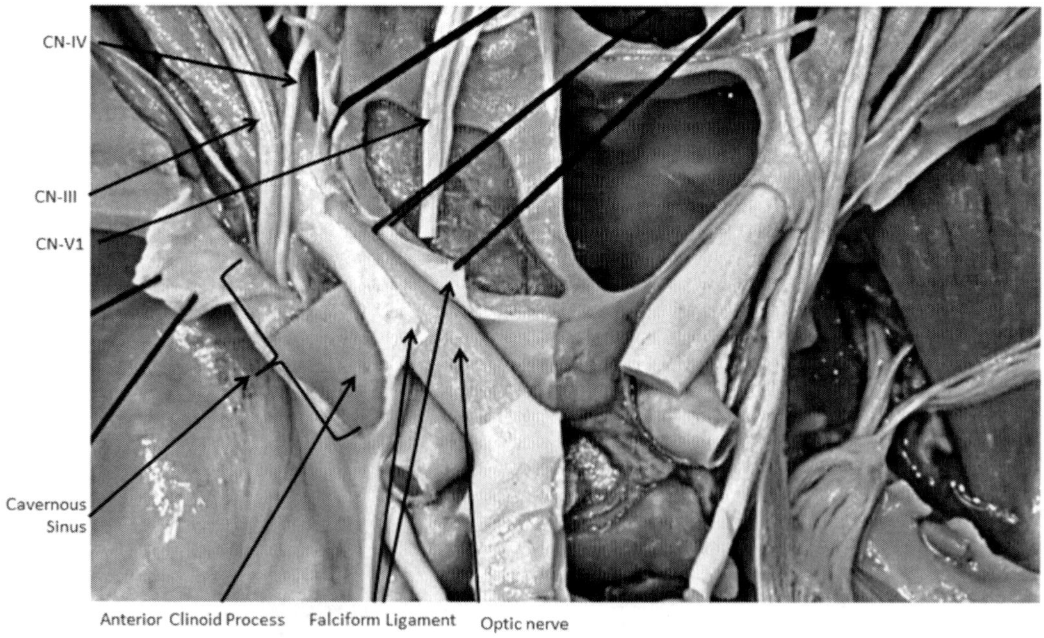

Figure 11.4. Optic nerve is seen in the optic canal (optic nerve sheath has been opened, orbital roof removed). Taken with permission from the Rhoton Collection.

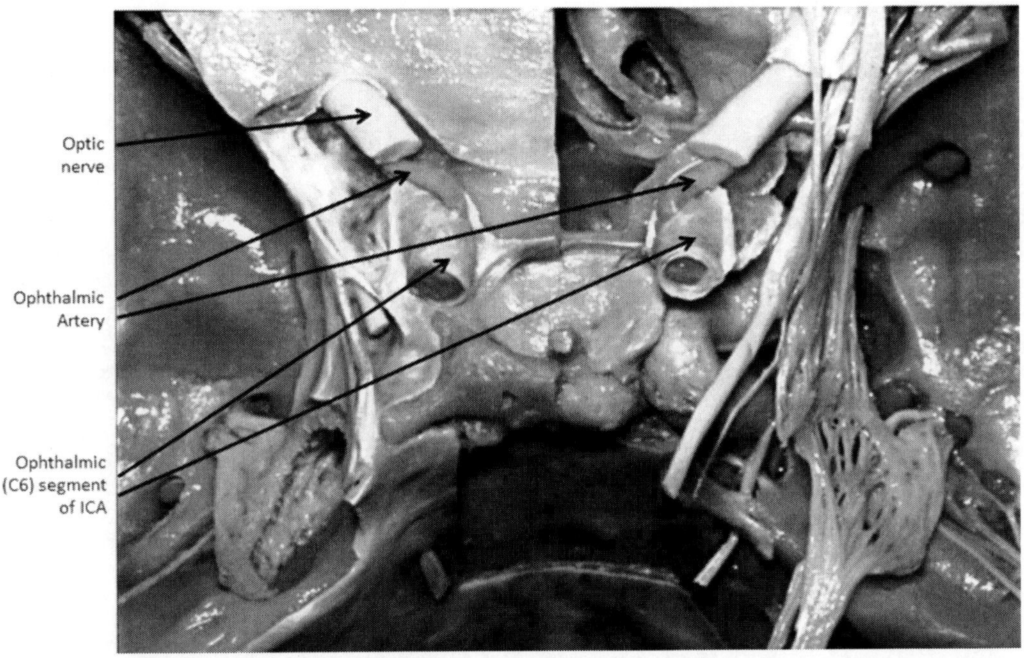

Figure 11.5. A Coronal – oblique view of the sellar region, showing the ophthalmic artery and optic nerves entering the optic canal. Taken with permission from the Rhoton Collection.

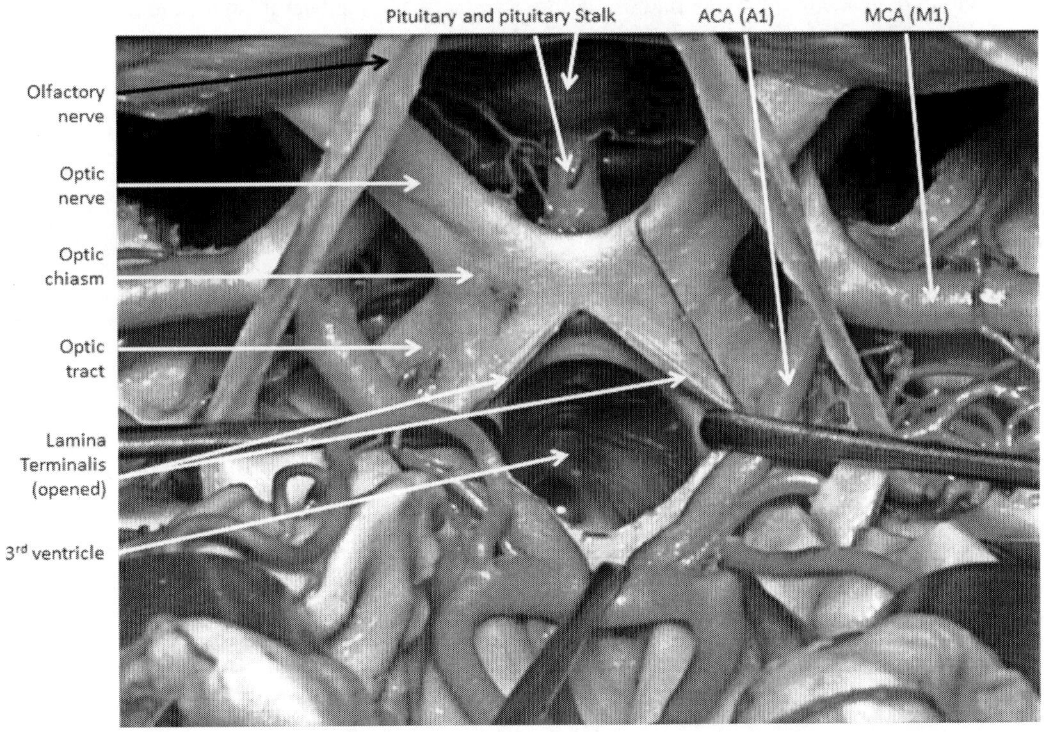

Figure 11.6. Superior axial view of the sellar region. The third ventricle as seen through the opened lamina terminalis. Taken with permission from the Rhoton Collection.

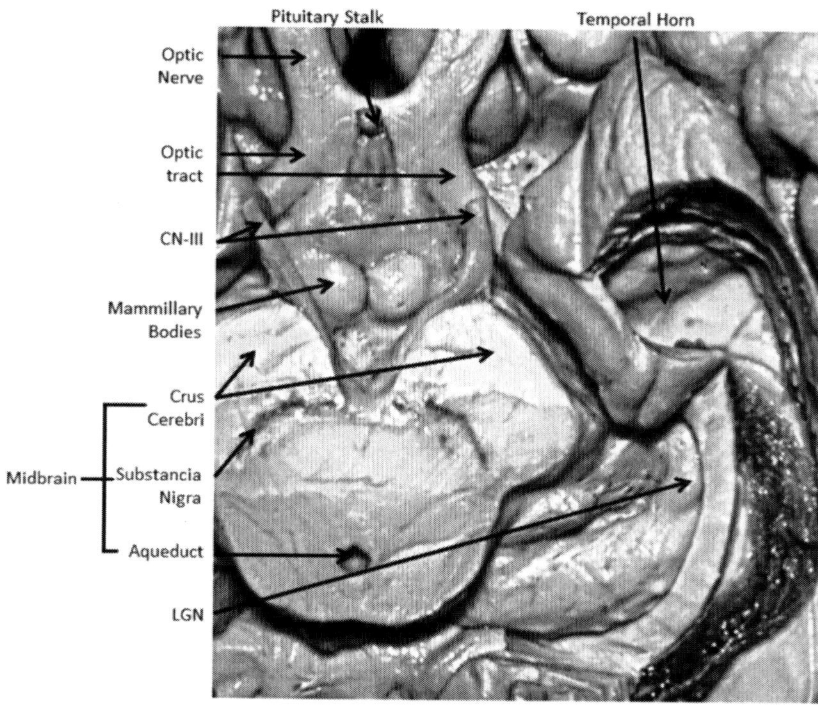

Figure 11.7. inferior brain shown, with brainstem cut at midbrain level. The optic tract courses superior to the uncus and medial to the temporal horn before terminating in the lateral geniculate nucleus. Taken with permission from the Rhoton Collection.

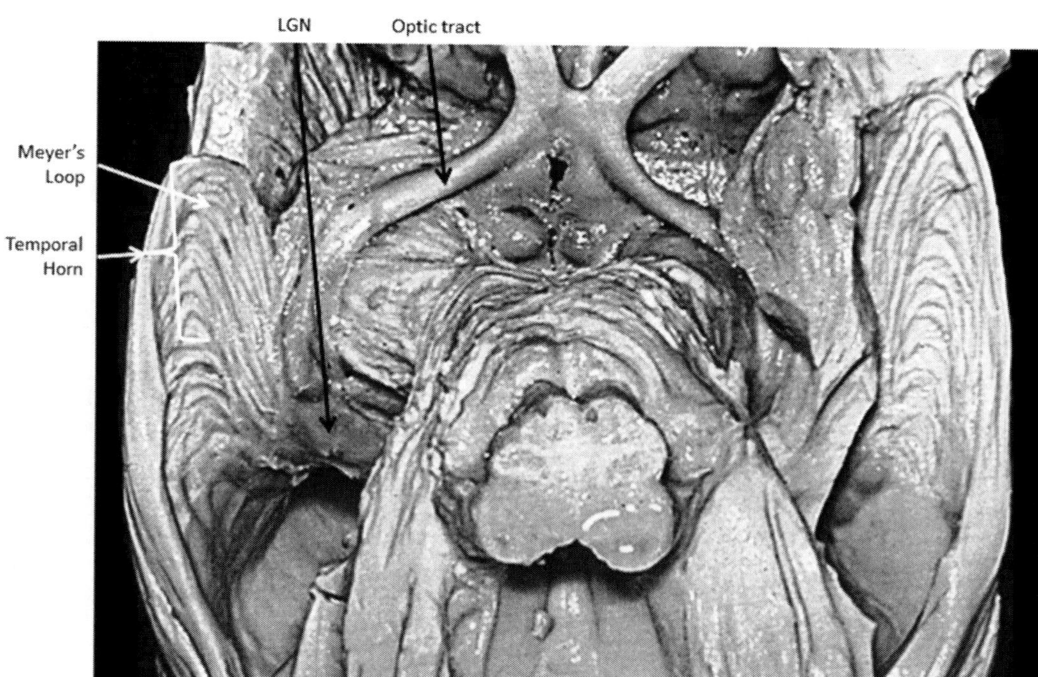

Figure 11.8. Superior view, white matter dissection, presenting the optic tract LGN and optic radiations. Taken with permission from the Rhoton Collection.

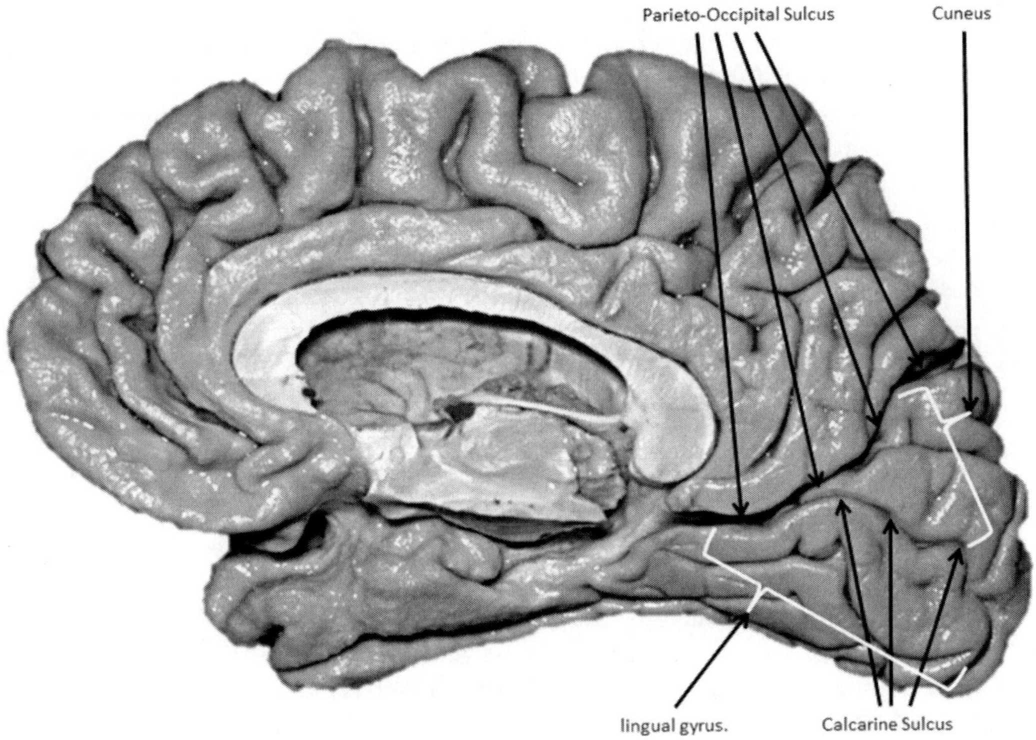

Figure 11.9. A midsagittal hemispherical view, presenting the occipital visual cortical areas and important anatomical landmarks. Taken with permission from the Rhoton Collection.

11.8. Visual Motor Systems

Each orbit contains seven extraocular muscles (including the levator palpebrae) driven by cranial nerves III, IV, VI. Both eyes move together to keep an object of regard imaged simultaneously on the fovea of each eye. These two retinal images are not identical because they view the object from slightly different angles. This disparity is processed by the brain to produce the perception of depth, or stereopsis. This "fusion" process can break down if there is a significant problem in the motor (efferent) visual system, with diplopia (double vision) usually being produced. For example, damage to cranial nerve VI (Abducens) causes a weakness of the lateral rectus muscle, and as a result the eye turns too far toward the nose. An object viewed with the fovea of the normal eye is also seen by the "crossed" eye but is imaged on the nasal retina and appears to be in the patient's temporal field. The patient has diplopia, with the object seen twice when both eyes are open: directly ahead with the fixing eye and in the temporal visual field of the crossed eye.

11.8.1. Peripheral Structures

11.8.1.1. Extraocular Muscles

The six extraocular muscles (all except the levator palpebrae) produce movements in the horizontal plane, around the vertical axis as well as torsional (rotational) movements. Two pairs of rectus muscles with each antagonistic pair arranged opposite one another:

1) The medial rectus muscle rotates the eye towards the nose (adduction).
2) The lateral rectus muscle rotates the eye towards the temple (abduction). It is innervated by CN-VI.
3) The superior rectus muscle rotates the eye upward (elevation).
4) The inferior rectus muscle rotates the eye downward (depression).
5) The superior oblique muscle action is modified, since its tendon passes through a loop of connective tissue (i.e., the trochlea found on the medial wall of the bony orbit). It performs intorsion, depression, and abduction. It is innervated by CN-IV.
6) The inferior oblique muscle actions are extorsion, elevation, and abduction.

The lateral rectus is innervated by CN-VI (abducens), the superior oblique is innervated by CN-IV (trochlear). All remaining 4 muscles are innervated by CN-III (oculomotor). Each muscle has an inner global layer (inserting onto the sclera), and an outer orbital layer (inserting into the connective tissue sheath, regulating the muscle pulling direction). Proprioceptive information from these muscles is carried by CN-V (trigeminal).

11.8.1.2. Intraocular Muscles

The Intraocular muscles encompass three intrinsic smooth muscles: the ciliary muscle, the sphincter and dilator pupillae. The ciliary muscle changes the curvature of the lens, to bring visual targets into focus on the retina. It is found in the ciliary body, connected to the lens by the suspensory ligament (which resembles the spikes of a bicycle wheel). Muscle constriction is produced by activation of cholinergic parasympathetic fibers from the ciliary ganglion. With age, since the lens is less elastic, the muscle contractions have less effect.

The sphincter and dilator pupillae control the size of the pupils in an antagonistic fashion, regulating the amount of light entering the eyes. The sphincter pupillae is a ring shaped muscle, lying along the pupillary margin, contracting in response to a cholinergic parasympathetic stimulus arriving from the ciliary ganglion. The resultant constriction of the pupil is termed miosis. The dilator pupillae muscle is radially arranged so that its action folds the iris and draws open the pupil. It is activated by adrenergic sympathetic postganglionic fibers arriving from the superior cervical ganglion.

11.8.1.3. The Eyelid Muscles

Three eyelid muscles belong to this group: the levator palpebrae, the orbicularis oculi, and the Müller tarsal muscles. Two of these muscles are striated muscles. The levator palpebrae muscle is a striated muscle supplied by CN-III. It originates and travels with the superior rectus muscle, but continues to reach the upper lid. The orbicularis oculi striated muscle is supplied by CN-VII, functions in closing the eye. It depresses the upper lid and elevates the lower lid. The Müller tarsal muscles are small smooth muscles at the edge of the bony orbit, supplied by postganglionic sympathetic fibers.

11.8.2. Central Nervous System Visual Structures

The detailed description of the different cranial nerves course and landmarks is given in chapter 3 with accompanying illustrations and dissection images.

11.8.2.1. The Oculomotor (CN-III) Complex

The oculomotor motor nucleus lies above the fibers of the medial longitudinal fasciculus (MLF), many of which synapse with it. The CN-III fibers pass around or through the red nucleus of the midbrain, exiting the midbrain at the interpeduncular fossa, passing along the wall of the cavernous sinus, to enter the orbit via the superior orbital fissure. The Edinger-Westphal nucleus gives rise to the cholinergic preganglionic parasympathetic fibers eventually controlling lens accommodation and pupillary constriction. These fibers travel with the ipsilateral CN-III, synapsing at the ciliary ganglion. Postganglionic fibers form the short ciliary nerve, supplying the ciliary muscle and pupillary constrictor. Refer to chapter 3.

The oculomotor nerve innervates all the extraocular muscles (including the levator palpebrae), except for the lateral rectus and superior oblique muscles. It also carries parasympathetic efferent fibers to the pupillary sphincter and ciliary muscle through the ciliary ganglion. Complete third cranial nerve palsy produces an eye that is turned down and out (because of remaining function of the superior oblique and lateral rectus muscles) and a dilated pupil with ptosis. Partial or incomplete paresis is more confusing. The pupillary fibers run superficially in the nerve and are preferentially affected by compression, such as from a posterior communicating artery aneurysm or brainstem herniation. Ischemic cranial mononeuropathy of the vasa nervosum of CN-III generally shows relative pupillary sparing, with the pupil being less affected than motility.

11.8.2.2. The Trochlear (CN-IV) Complex

This small midbrain nucleus, found in MLF of caudal midbrain. Its fibers cross the midline in the anterior medullary velum, exiting the dorsal surface of the midbrain at the base of the inferior colliculus. It next turns to the ventral surface, traveling in the wall of the cavernous sinus, to enter the orbit via the superior orbital fissure. The trochlear nerve innervates only the superior oblique muscle, but this muscle has a complex action. Because of its redirection at the trochlea and attachment to the globe, the superior oblique muscle intorts, depresses, and abducts the eye. When the globe is adducted, however, the angle of the muscle's insertion minimizes all actions except pure depression. The clinician looks at how well the right eye can move down in left gaze and how well the left eye moves down in right gaze. The vital role of the superior oblique muscle in ocular cyclotorsion explains why patients with trochlear palsy often describe diplopia with one image tilted.

11.8.2.3. The Abducens (CN-VI) Complex

The abducens nucleus is located in the depth of the facial colliculus, the elevation in the floor of the fourth ventricle at caudal pons level. Its fibers pass caudally-anteriorly to exit the pons at the pontomedullary junction, passing adjacent to the medial lemniscus. Within the subarachnoid space it ascends posteriorly to the clivus, passing under the petroclinoid ligament (in the so called Dorello's canal), to continue in the medial wall of the cavernous sinus, entering the orbit through the superior orbital fissure. Abducens intranuclear and internuclear nerves connections between the different motor nuclei (on both sides) allow transmitting signals to the medial rectus motor neurons on the contralateral side, via the MLF. This connection allows the lateral rectus in one eye, works in tandem with medial rectus muscle of the other eye.

In left abducens paresis, there may be no misalignment of right gaze because the left lateral rectus muscle is relaxed in this field of gaze. However, in left gaze, the left lateral rectus muscle cannot fully pull the left eye out, and an esotropia is evident. To avoid diplopia, the patient may assume a posture with the head turned to the left. Examination of the function of cranial nerve VI is performed by having the Patient look in far right and far left gaze.

11.8.2.4. Sympathetic Nerve Supply to the Orbit

Sympathetic innervation reaches the orbit from ipsilateral superior cervical ganglion. These adrenergic Postganglionic fibers enter the cranium on the walls of the internal carotid artery (through the carotid canal), running shortly with CN-VI, than join CN-III, and CN-V. Preganglionic sympathetic nerves are located at the T1-T3 spinal cord level, entering the sympathetic trunk, terminating in ipsilateral cervical (stellate) ganglion.

11.8.2.5. Horizontal and Vertical Gaze Centers

The Paramedian pontine reticular formation (PPRF) is the horizontal gaze center, projecting to extra-ocular motor nuclei. It occupies portions of the oral and caudal pontine reticular nuclei. Its cells show activity related to horizontal saccades. Its activity pattern is a product of signals sent from supranuclear structures, like the superior colliculus, and the frontal eye field. The PPRF is found adjacent and to some extent a part of the abducens nuclear complex. The "Where the eye is going" signal from PPRF is transformed into a "keep the eye in that position" signal by another brainstem structure (the nucleus prepositus hypoglossi).

The vertical gaze center is located in the rostral interstitial nucleus of MLF of midbrain, receiving supranuclear input from the superior colliculus and frontal eye field, as well as from omnipause cells. The tonic signal for the step in vertical gaze is provided by neurons of the interstitial nucleus of Cajal (the connections between these two nuclei is through posterior commissure).

11.8.2.6. Supranuclear Control of Vision

Directing saccadic movements is done by the cortical eye field (frontal lobe, Brodmann-8), the superior colliculus, and the supplemental eye field and the parietal eye field. The frontal eye field, located rostral to the primary motor cortex, receives input from the visual association cortices as well as from the basal ganglia, thalamic relays. The frontal eye field in turn, projects to the gaze centers. The superior colliculus, part of the optic tectum, is a layered structure found in the roof of the midbrain. Its superficial layer contains - visual sensory fibers projecting to LGN and to the pulvinar thalamic nucleus. Its intermediate layer has visual motor functions. It is a source of the crossed fibers running ventral to MLF, terminating in the gaze centers.

11.8.2.7. Smooth Pursuit Control

The control of smooth pursuit, or the ability to follow a moving target, is accomplished by the lateral parietal and mid-temporal cortices. These are sensitive to the speed and direction of targets across the retina. These in turn project to the flocculus and paraflocculus lobules of the cerebellum, which provides input to the brainstem vestibular nuclei. Premotor cortex neurons fire in a graded manner, not having the pulse and step form seen in saccades. The role of the cerebellum is in determining the rate of movement and predicting target trajectory.

11.8.3. Reflex Eye Movements

Compensatory reflexes keep the eyes on target despite body movements. The vestibule-ocular reflex compensates for acceleration sensed by the semicircular canals. The optokinetic reflex compensates for velocity and movement of the whole visual field (discussed next). The pupillary light reflex maintains the level of retinal illumination within the working range of the photo pigments in the photoreceptors. The blink reflex which provides protection of the eye.

11.8.3.1. Optokinetic Eye Movements

The optokinetic reflex compensates for continuous velocity movements and whole visual field movements (retinal slip). The eye automatically moves in a compensatory fashion to stabilize the image on the retina. These movements are usually slow, matching the retinal slip velocity. When the eyeball approaches the limit of its rotation, a quick saccade brings it back to its primary position and another slow following movement begins. Axons of retinal ganglion cells terminate in a series of small nuclei along the optic tract, termed as the accessory optic system. These include the nuclei of the optic tract, as well as the medial lateral and dorsal accessory nuclei. Each of these nuclei is sensitive to different movements. These nuclei in turn project to the pontine reticular formation (tegmentum), inferior olive, and vestibular nuclei.

11.8.3.2. The Pupillary Light Reflex

The pupil has also an ability to respond to the amount of ambient light. This ability evokes the action of the iris in both eyes. Thus, light directed into one eye results in pupillary constrictions in both eyes. The pupil changes its diameter to maintain luminance of the retina in the optimal range of the photo pigments. This reflex has a four neurons reflex arch. First, retinal ganglion cells having broad receptive fields, project through the optic nerve and tract to the midbrain (the decussation in the optic chiasm is responsible for the bilateral response). The olivary pretectal nucleus in turn, projects bilaterally to the Edinger-Westphal nuclei. The output of the Edinger-Westphal nuclei, the parasympathetic preganglionic fibers, terminates in the ciliary ganglion. The ciliary ganglion gives rise to the short postganglionic ciliary nerve to the sphincter and dilator pupillae.

11.8.3.3. Blinking and Other Lid Movements

The blink reflex is used to assess CN-V sensory and CN-VII motor functions (refer to chapter 3). The CN-V central processes terminate in the spinal CN-V nucleus. From there, via direct or indirect pathways, the reflex arch reaches the CN-VII-motor nucleus, producing lid closure. Eyelid blinks also occur at regular intervals, spreading the tear film over the cornea. The origin of this rhythmic blinking is still largely unknown.

Chapter 12

The Auditory System

12.1. Abstract

The different elements comprising the auditory system have been discussed to some extent in their prospective locations. The vestibulocochlear system was discussed in the chapter on the brainstem and cranial nerves (chapter 3), the medial geniculate nucleus (MGN) was discussed in the frame of the thalamus and diencephalon (chapter 4), and the auditory radiation and auditory cortex have been discussed in the frame of the description of cerebral hemispheral white matter and gray matter anatomy (chapter 7). The aim of this chapter is to provide an overview the auditory system unified under function and not regional anatomy. The cochlear system is presented with a short overview of the physiology of hearing. The central auditory pathways are reviewed next in different formats. Each processing center discussed shortly with its key unique features presented. Great thought was put into forming a cohesive view, stepwise discussion of this neuro-anatomically complex system, starting from the spiral ganglions to the auditory cortices. Finally, a short description of brainstem auditory evoked response measurements is given.

12.2. Introduction

The eighth cranial, or vestibulocochlear nerve consists of two distinct components: the cochlear and the vestibular nerves. The neurons of these primary afferent nerves are bipolar, with their dendrites synapsing on the inner and outer hair cells within the cochlea and on the type I and type II hair cells within the cristae and maculae of the vestibular end-organs. From an embryonic stand point, the neurosensory portions of the vestibulocochlear system are derived from ectoderm. With growth and development, these neurosensory epithelial structures become incorporated within the petrous portion of the temporal bone and are encased in the otic capsule. Concurrently, the middle ear space develops as an invagination from the first pharyngeal pouch and comes to lie lateral to the otic capsule. Meanwhile, the external ear develops from the overlying epithelium, and the fundus of its canal abuts the middle ear space at the tympanic membrane.

The vestibulocochlear labyrinth consists of a continuous complex of bony spaces encased in the otic capsule and within the petrous bone, called the bony labyrinth. It is filled with perilymph (similar to CSF), and suspended within it is an almost true, miniature replica of the bony spaces—the membranous labyrinth. The labyrinth is filled with endolymph. The different elements comprising the auditory system have been discussed to some extent in their prospective locations. The vestibulocochlear system was discussed in the frame of the chapter on brainstem and cranial nerves (chapter 3), the medial geniculate nucleus (MGN) was discussed in the frame of the thalamus and diencephalon (chapter 4), and the auditory radiation and auditory cortex have been discussed in the frame of the description of cerebral hemispheral white matter and gray matter anatomy (chapter 7). The aim of this chapter is to provide an overview the auditory system unified under function and not regional anatomy.

12.3. The Cochlear System

A transverse section through the cochlea (figure 12.1) shows that it is composed of three compartments: scala vestibuli, scala media, and scala tympani. The scala media, which contains endolymph, is separated from the scala vestibuli and tympani by Reissner's membrane and the basilar membrane, respectively. The scala vestibuli and scala tympani contain perilymph, and these two compartments communicate with each other at the cochlear apex through an opening at the tip of the basilar membrane called the helicotrema. At the base of the upper compartment, called the scala vestibuli, is the oval window, and at the base of the lower compartment, called the scala tympani, is the round window.

The basilar membrane has a complex structure resting on it that is best appreciated in cross section. The basilar membrane and the thin sloping membrane, called Reissner's membrane, form a tube that ends blindly and is sealed at the helicotrema. Extending along the entire basilar membrane and spiraling with the cochlea is the organ of Corti. It contains the structurally complex sensory epithelium innervated by the cochlear nerve. The basilar membrane is widest near the helicotrema and narrowest at the base. Maximal high-frequency vibration of the basilar membrane occurs at the base, and maximal low-frequency vibration occurs at the apex, thereby resulting in hair cell transduction of high frequencies at the base and low frequencies at the apex. The organ of Corti consists of a single row of inner hair cells and three rows of outer hair cells. The inner and outer hair cells slope toward each other to form a triangular canal between them called the tunnel of Corti. The tectorial membrane extends from a medial-to-lateral direction within the scala media and above the hair cells where the hair cell stereocilia are embedded.

12.3.1. The Physiology of Hearing

Air vibrations impinge on the tympanic membrane and cause it and the malleus to vibrate. This physical vibration is transmitted through the incus to the stapes and by way of its footplate to the fluids of the labyrinth. The fluid vibrations produce a stimulus along the basilar membrane that activates the organ of Corti. Impulses are transmitted through the cochlear nerve endings to the cochlear nuclei in the pontomedullary junction. The impulses then continue to the auditory areas of the cortex.

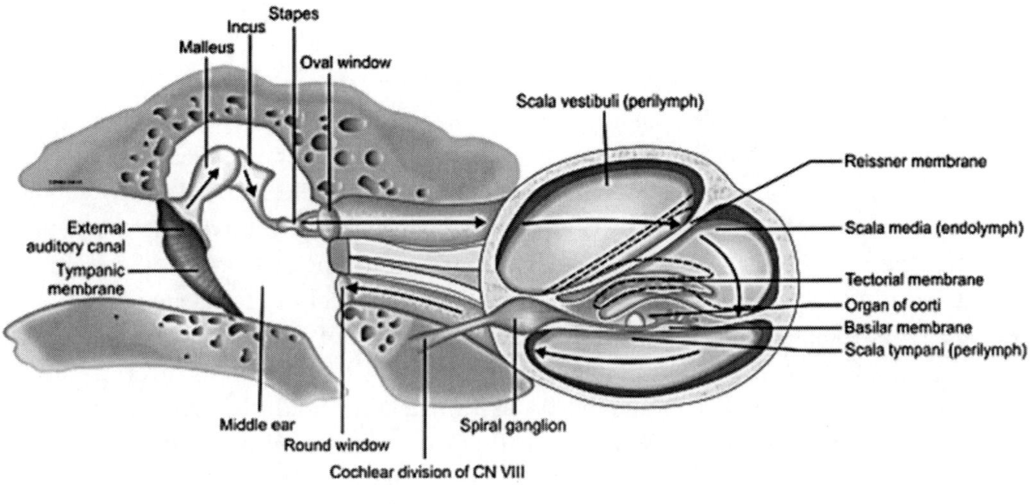

Figure 12.1. Sound waves contact the tympanic membrane, and the acoustic energy is transformed and transmitted to the inner ear through the ossicular chain in the middle ear. Displacement of the oval window by the stapes footplate results in instantaneous transmission of the pressure through perilymph in the scala vestibuli, Reissner's membrane, endolymph, basilar membrane, and perilymph in the scala tympani and in outward displacement of the round window membrane. Hair cell transduction occurs as the basilar membrane containing the organ of Corti moves relative to the tectorial membrane. Modified from "Focused Neurosurgery", 2014.

12.3.1.1. Transformer Mechanism of the Tympanum

Because the effective vibratory area of the tympanic membrane is about 17 times as large as the area of the footplate of the stapes and because the manubrium of the malleus is 1.3 times as long as the long process of the incus, the ratio of amplification from the tympanic membrane to the stapedial footplate is about 22 : 1. Because fluid is incompressible, the round window membrane acts as a compensating membrane to accommodate the vibrations of the stapes footplate. The intact tympanic membrane protects the round window from direct sound impingement; the tympanic membrane is connected to the oval window through the ossicular chain, thus making direct transmission by this route faster; and the round window membrane faces backward, at right angles to the plane of the tympanic membrane, and is recessed within the niche. These factors delay the impingement of sound onto the round window membrane, which produces the phase difference. As a consequence of these phenomena, a sizable perforation of the tympanic membrane results in a hearing loss of 30-35 dB by air conduction, whereas dislocation of the ossicular chain with an intact tympanic membrane produces an air conduction loss of about 55-60 dB.

12.3.1.2. Transmission in the Labyrinth

Cochlear signal transduction of high frequencies occurs near the basal portion, and transduction of low frequencies occurs near the apical regions of the basilar membrane and its organ of Corti.

12.3.2. Primary Afferent Innervation and Function

The spiral ganglion is made up to two types of bipolar sensory neurons. Type-I neurons, comprising about 90~95% of the cells in spiral ganglion, have radial branches. These synapse with only one to two inner hair cells. As many as 20 type-I cell fibers, converge on each inner hair cells, resulting in these type-I cochlear cell fibers responding to a narrow frequency range. Type-II neurons have widely distributed peripheral processes, traversing the tunnel of Corti, synapsing with Over 10 outer hair cells. Thus, type-II cochlear nerve fibers are more sensitive to low-intensity sounds than are type-I, but are less precisely frequency tuned.

Frequency is coded in the cochlear nerve by the position of the affarent fibers along the cochlear spiral ganglion. For loud sounds, each affarent fiber responds over a range of frequencies. As the intensity of the sound drops to near threshold, the frequency response range narrows. A tuning curve (threshold intensity vs. frequency) will show the characteristic frequency (namely that in which the fiber has the lowest threshold). Stimulus onset produces an initial high frequency discharge followed by a lower sustained level, relating to the stimulus intensity, and when the tone ends, the fiber activity drops back to the low spontaneous discharge activity. For low frequency fibers, the timing of each impulse is phase locked with the stimulus cycle, so that the fiber output preserves the timing information of the signal.

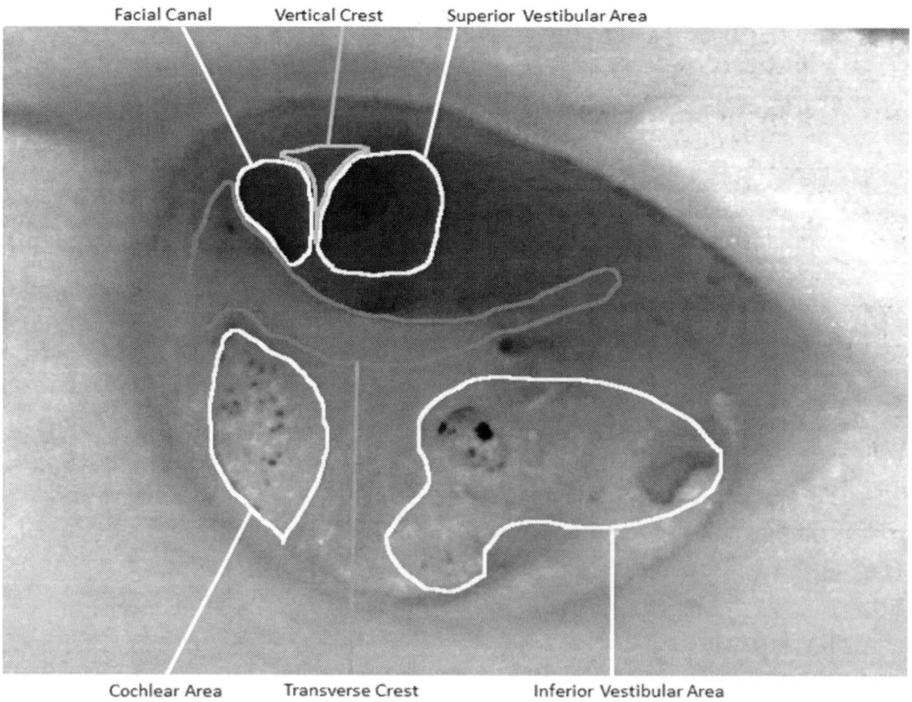

Figure 12.2. The internal acoustic meatus. The facial nerve enters the facial canal, which is at the superior and anterior quadrant of the internal auditory anal. The transverse crest separates the facial canal and superior vestibular area from the cochlear and inferior vestibular areas. The vertical crest separates the facial canal from the superior vestibular area. Taken with permission from the Rhoton Collection.

The hugh frequency range of the human ear cannot be coded in the response of a single nerve fiber. Intensity is coded both by the discharge rate of the cochlear nerve fibers and by recruitment of activity in additional affarent fibers as stimulus intensity increases. At higher stimulus intensities, additional cochlear nerve fibers with sequentially greater thresholds are recruited. The internal acoustic meatus and the spatial relationship shared by the facial and vestibulocochlear nerves, as well as the cochlea and vestibule are presented in figures 12.3-12.4. Refer to chapter 3 for further details.

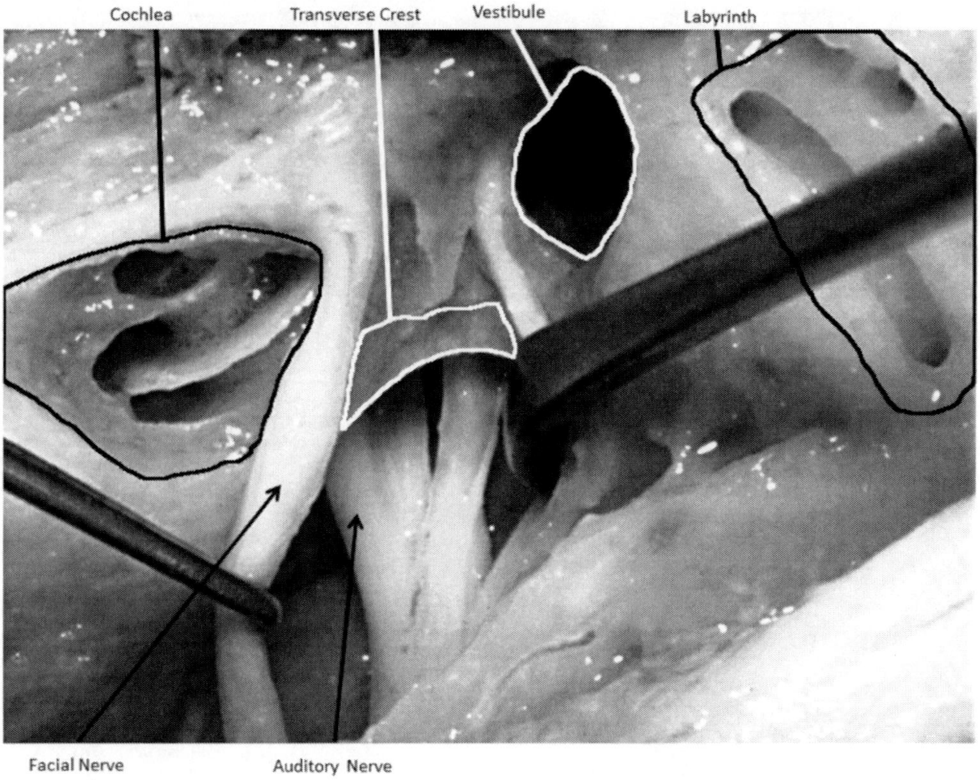

Figure 12.3. The fundus of the internal auditory canal has been drilled to expose the cochlea, vestibule and the labyrinth. The auditory nerve is seen coursing towards the cochlea inferior to the transverse crest and facial nerve. Taken with permission from the Rhoton Collection.

12.4. Central Auditory Pathways Overview

Throughout its path, the place-code of the cochlea is (as a rule) strictly maintained. This is referred to (in a corresponding manner to the other systems) as a tonotropic framework and a tonotopic frequency map. With this arrangement, the different white matter projections connect similar frequency regions of successive nuclei. Information processing is thus hierarchical with increasing complexity of feature extraction. Refer to chapter 3 for vestibulocochlear cranial nerve anatomy. Refer to figures 12.4-12.5 for a summary of the following. All fibers in the cochlear nerve synapse in the cochlear nuclei. As the information ascends to the cortex, it is distributed through multiple parallel pathways that finally converge in the inferior colliculus. Some of the stops in these pathways include the cochlear nuclei, the nuclei of the superior olive and trapezoid body, nuclei of the lateral lemniscus, the inferior colliculus, the medial geniculate nucleus (MGN) and the auditory cortex. The different fiber bundles conveying the information between these levels include the trapezoid body, the acoustic (medullary) stria, the lateral lemniscus, the brachium of the inferior colliculus (conveying the information from it to the MGN) and the sublenticular limb of internal capsule.

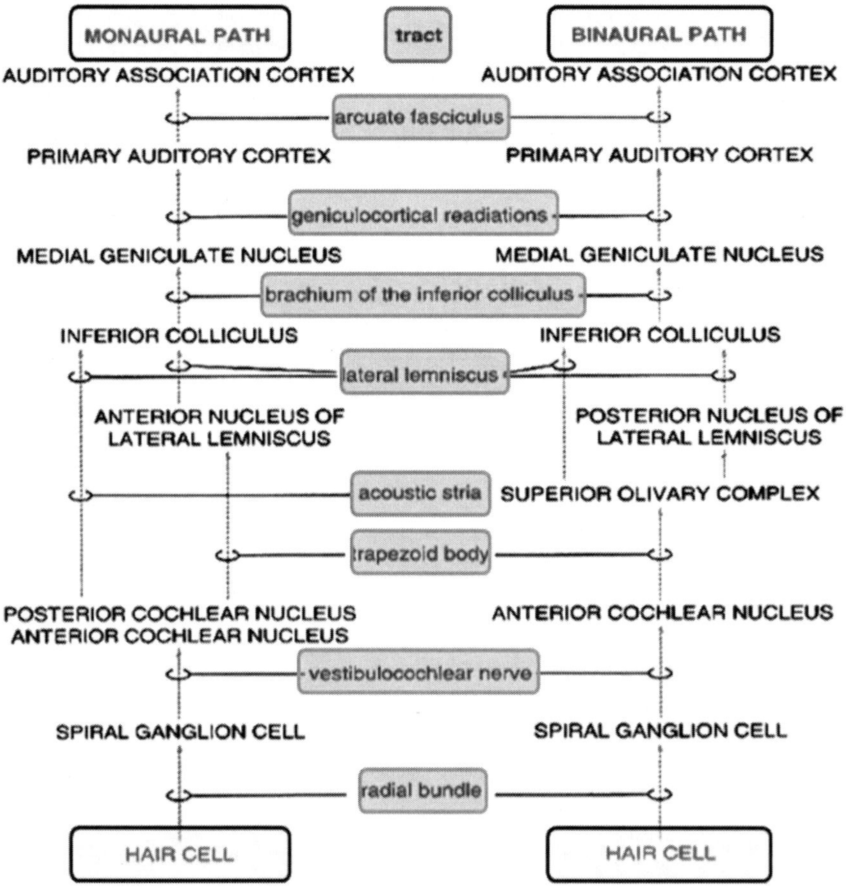

Figure 12.4. An overview of the central auditory pathways. Refer to text.

Although the auditory fibers decussate at several levels, the information is routed in one of two ways: a monaural or binaural pathway. Monaural information refers to acoustic information from a single ear, routed to the contralateral side. Binaural information refers to information about differences between sounds at both ears. This information is handled by central pathways that receive, compare, and transmit this input. These perform the computation needed to localize brief sounds. Unilateral damage to the cochlear nerve or nucleus results in monaural deafness. Unilateral damage at levels above the superior olivary complex, leaving intact binaural pathways, does not result in deafness. The auditory decussation, located at the trapezoid body, is functionally similar to the optic chiasm. It is termed as the functional acoustic chiasm.

The blood supply to the cochlea and auditory nuclei of the brainstem arise from the vertebrobasilar system, the internal auditory (or labyrinth) artery, usually branching off the anterior inferior cerebellar artery (AICA), and going to the inner ear. The superior olive and lateral lemniscus are supplied mainly by the short circumferential branches of the basilar artery. The inferior colliculus is supplied by branches coming off the superior cerebellar artery and quadrigeminal arteries. The MGN is supplied by the thalamogeniculate arteries, coming off the posterior cerebral artery. The primary auditory cortex is supplied by M2 segment branches of the middle cerebral artery (MCA).

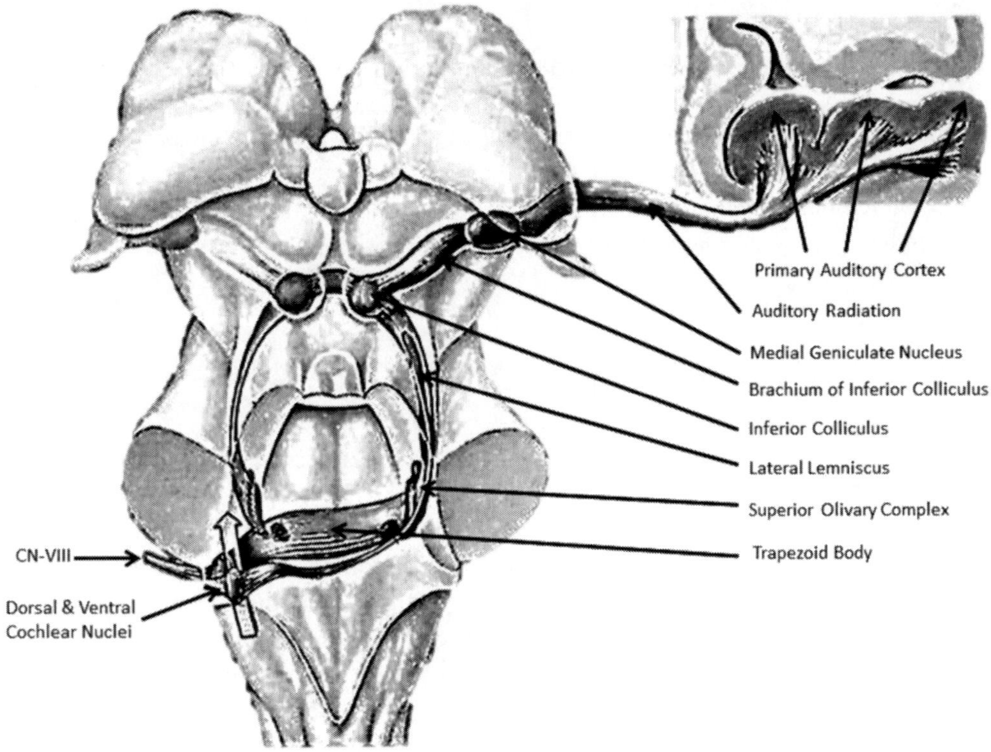

Figure 12.5. The auditory Pathways. Refer to text. Modified from Gray's anatomy (out of copyright and in the public domain).

12.5. Brainstem Auditory Nuclei and Pathways

12.5.1. Cochlear Nuclei

The dorsal and ventral cochlear nuclei are located lateral-posterior to the restiform body, partially on the surface of the brainstem at the pontomedullary junction level. The ventral cochlear nucleus extends more rostrally than the dorsal one, where it is covered by the cerebellar flocculus, and by the caudal fascicle of the middle cerebellar peduncle. Cochlear fibers enter the brainstem at the cerebellopontine angle, where they divide to ascending and descending bundles. The ascending fibers synapse in the anterior part of the ventral nucleus. The descending fibers synapse in the posterior part of ventral nucleus and dorsal nucleus.

Specific cell types give rise to parallel, but separate ascending pathways, that analyze and code different sound features, while preserving frequency information. These are divided to pathways conveying monaural information to the inferior colliculus, or to the superior olive for binaural processing. Most fibers from the ventral nucleus converge anterior to the restiform body to form the trapezoid body. Projections from the dorsal nucleus course posteriorly over the restiform body, as the posterior acoustic stria, decussating in the pontine tegmentum before joining the lateral lemniscus.

12.5.2. The Superior Olivary Complex

The superior olivary complex is located near the CN-VII motor nucleus. It serves as the first site where information from both ears converges. Myelinated fibers passing anterior to the superior olive intermingle with fibers of the lateral lemniscus, forming the trapezoid body. Its fibers end in the contralateral superior olive, or ascend in the contralateral lateral lemniscus.

12.5.3. Lateral Lemniscus and Nucleus

This lemniscus (white matter tract) is formed by second order nerve axons of the cochlear nuclei, third order neurons from superior olive, and fourth order neurons from adjacent nuclei of the lateral lemniscus. This heterogeneous collection prevents a simple correlation of nuclei or tracts with specific wave components. Two nuclear lemniscal groups are defined, the anterior and posterior groups. The anterior nuclei are larger, extending from the rostral limit of superior olive to the caudal edges of the inferior colliculus. These are an indirect monaural pathway. The posterior nuclei are located caudal to the inferior colliculus, receiving input mainly from the superior olivary complex. Its fibers decussate in the posterior tegmental commissure, terminating in the contralateral inferior colliculus.

12.5.4. The Inferior Colliculus

This part of the midbrain tectum serves as the location where all ascending auditory pathways terminate. It is composed of a central nucleus, a paracentral nuclear group and an external (or lateral) nuclear group. The central nucleus of the inferior colliculus is large, composed of parallel layers of disc-shaped dendritic fields. Affarent fibers arriving from the lateral lemniscus course parallel to these fields, forming a series of fibro-dendritic laminae. Each point along the cochlear spiral ganglion and nerve is represented in an isofrequency lamina (thus the tonotropic arrangement is maintained).

12.6. The Medial Geniculate Nucleus (MGN)

Grossly it is a small protuberance between LGN and the pulvinar nucleus of thalamus. The MGN is segregated into three divisions: anterior, medial and posterior. The anterior MGN division receives fibers from the central nucleus of the inferior colliculus. It projects to primary auditory cortex mainly. Fibers are tonotopically arranged in a way that low frequencies are located laterally while higher frequencies are located more medially. Its medial division, aka its magnocellular part, receives fibers from the external nucleus of the inferior colliculus, projecting to association areas of auditory cortex. Its posterior division receives fibers from the paracentral nuclei of the inferior colliculus, projecting to primary and secondary auditory cortices, still in a tonotopical manner. The auditory radiation connects the MGN with the auditory cortices.

12.7. Auditory and Related Association Cortices

The primary auditory cortex (marked as AI) is located at the transverse gyrus of Heschl (Brodmann 41, 42), at the inner depth of the superior temporal gyrus. It encompasses a granular cortex, with a well-developed layer-IV. It is reciprocally connected with the anterior division of MGN. The secondary auditory cortex is found adjacent to the granular cortex and planum temporale, referred to as Brodmann-42. It is reciprocally connected with the posterior division of MGB. The auditory association cortex, i.e., Brodmann-22, surrounds the primary auditory cortex in the superior temporal gyrus, connected to it by the arcuate fasciculus. It receives information from AI, as well as from the visual cortices and somatosensory information. It also functions as the speech receptive area (Wernicke's area), which may be as much as seven times larger on the left side than on the right. Higher association areas extend into the inferior parietal lobule. These are located at the angular gyrus (Brodmann–39), the supramarginal gyrus (Brodmann-40) etc.

12.8. Brainstem Auditory Evoked Response (BAER's) Measures

Brainstem Auditory Evoked Response (BAER's) measurements are possibly the most powerful clinical audiologic test available in differentiating between cochlear and retrocochlear lesions. BAER's is typically evoked with a short-duration pulse delivered to the ear at a predetermined intensity. At high-intensity levels, the acoustic stimulus evokes as many as seven amplitude peaks: Three of these peaks (waves I, III, and V) are the major peaks and are generally accepted as corresponding to firing of the first-order neurons of CN-VIII (wave I), the superior olivary complex (wave III), and the inferior colliculus (wave V). These three major waves are present at ~2-msec intervals (in normal-hearing children and adults). Only wave V is identifiable at threshold levels. Refer to table 12.1 for the BAER's wave localization and to figure 12.6 for a BAER's study sample.

Table 5.1. BAER's waves

Wave	Localization
I	Cochlear nerve
II	Cochlear nuclei (Pons)
III	Superior olivary complex (Pons)
IV	Lateral lemniscus
V	Inferior colliculus
VI	Medial geniculate (Thalamus)
VII	Auditory Radiation

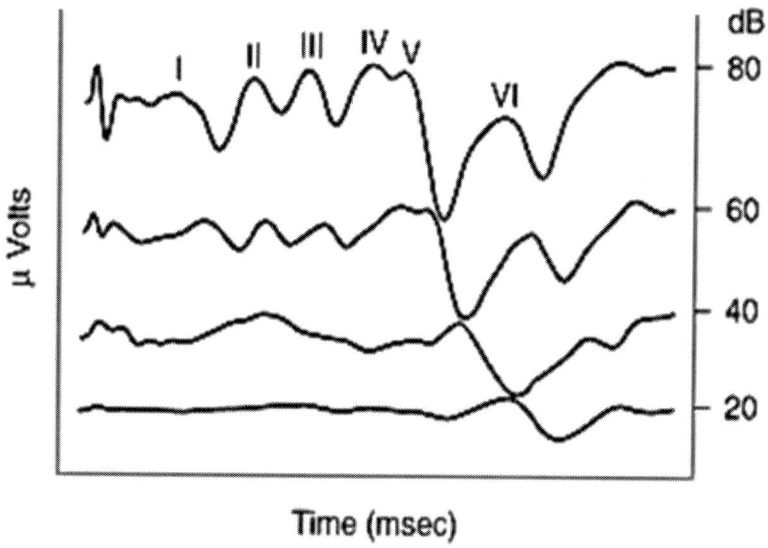

Figure 12.6. Wave latency results for auditory brainstem evoked responses are given as a function of decreasing stimulus level. The time window is 10 msec.

References

Abrahams PH, Marks SC Jr, Hutchings R. McMinn's Colour Atlas of Human Anatomy, 5th edition. *Churchill Livingstone,* 2002.

Aids to the Examination of the Peripheral Nervous System, 4th Edition. W B Saunders, 2000.

Albert L. Rhoton. The Rhoton Collection. *Neurosurgery,* Vol. 47, No. 3, Rhoton.inerurodb.org. 2000.

Alberts B, Johnson A, Lewis J, Raff M, Roberts K, Walter P. Molecular Biology of the Cell, 4th edition. *Garland Science Publishing,* 2002.

Andrew Kaye. Essential neurosurgery. *Blackwell Publishing Ltd*, 2005.

Atlas of Neuroanatomy and Neurophysiology Selections from the Netter Collection of Medical Illustrations. *Icon Custom Communications*, 2002.

Atlas of Neuroanatomy NTUMC 2008. Department of Anatomy and Cell Biology, National Taiwan University College of Medicine, 2008.

Atwood, H.L. and Lnenicka, G.A. Structure and function of synapses. Emerging correlations. *Trends in Neurosciences,* 248−250. 1986.

Barr, M.L. and Kiernan, J.A. The Human Nervous System, 5th edition. J.B. *Lippincott Company,* 1988.

Basar K, Sesia T, Groenewegen H, Steinbusch HW, Visser-Vandewalle V, Temel Y. Nucleus accumbens and impulsivity. *Prog. Neurobiol*. 92; 533–57. 2010.

Berkovitz BKB, Kirsh C, Moxham BJ, Alusi G, Cheeseman T. Interactive Head and Neck. *Primal Pictures,* 2002.

Boron W, Boulpaep E. Medical Physiology. *W B Saunders,* 2002.

Brodal, P. The Central nervous System. *Oxford University Press*, 1992.

Brown, A.G. Nerve Cells and Nervous Systems. An Introduction to Neuroscience. *Springer-Verlag,* 1991.

Brown, A.G. Organization in the spinal cord. The anatomy and physiology of identified neurons. *Springer-Verlag*, 1981.

Carlson, Neil R. Physiology of Behavior. 11th edition. *Pearson,* 2013.

Carol Turkington. The encyclopedia of the brain and brain disorders, 2nd edition. *Fact on file inc.,* 2002.

Carpenter, M.B. Core text of Neuroanatomy 3rd edition. *The Williams & Wilkins Company,* 1985.

Carpenter, R.H.S. Neurophysiology 3rd edition. *Arnold,* 1996.

Conn, P. M. (Ed). Neuroscience in Medicine. *J.B. Lippincott*, 1995.

Crockard Hayward Hoff. Neurosurgery, The scientific basis of clinical practice. *Wiley-Blackwell*. 3rd edition, 2000.

Crossman AR, Neary D. Neuroanatomy, 2nd edition. *Churchill Livingstone,* 2000.

Crossman AR, Neary D. Neuroanatomy: An Illustrated Colour Text, 5th edition. *Churchill Livingstone,* 2014.

Davies, A.M. and Lumsden, A. Ontogeny of the somatosensory system: Origins and early development of primary sensory neurons. *Annual Reviews in Neuroscience* 61–73, 1990.

De Groot, J. J. and Chusid, J.G. Correlative Neuroanatomy. *Appleton & Lange*, 1988.

Dean, P., Redgrave, P. and Westby, G.V.M. Event or emergency? Two systems in the mammalian superior colliculus. *Trends in Neurosciences* 137–147, 1989.

Duane E. Haines. Neuroanatomy an atlas of structures, sections and systems. 6th edition. *Lippincott Williams & Wilkins,* 2004.

Duane E. Haines. Neuroanatomy an atlas of structures, sections and systems. 8th edition. *Lippincott Williams & Wilkins,* 2011.

Eccles, J.C. and Schade, J.P. Organization of the Spinal Cord. Progress in Brain Research Volume 11. *Elsevier Publishing Company*, 1964.

Elliott L. Mancall, David G. Brock. Gray's Clinical Neuroanatomy: The Anatomic Basis for Clinical Neuroscience, 1st edition. *Elsevier,* 2011.

Fitzgerald MJT, Folan-Curran J. Clinical Neuroanatomy and Related Science, 4th edition. *Churchill Livingstone,* 2001.

Fitzgerald, M.J.T. Neuroanatomy Basic and Clinical, 3rd edition. *W.B. Saunders Company* Ltd, 1996.

Foote, S.L. and Morrison, J.H. Extrathalamic modulation of cortical function. *Annual Reviews of Neuroscience* 67–95, 1987.

George R. Leichnetz. Digital Neuroanatomy. *John Wiley & Sons, Inc.,* 2006.

Hal Blumenfeld. Neuroanatomy Through Clinical Cases, 1st edition. *Sinauer Associates,* 2002.

Hans J.ten Donkelaar, Martin Lammens, Akira Hori. Clinical Neuroembryology, Development and Developmental Disorders of the Human Central Nervous System. *Springer,* 2006.

HR Winn. Youmans Neurological Surgery, 6th edition. *Elsevier,* 2011.

James D. Fix. High yield neuroanatomy. *Lippincott Williams & Wilkins*, 2008.

John E. Hall. Guyton and Hall Textbook of Medical Physiology, 12th edition. *Sounders Elsevier,* 2010.

Jones, E.G. The Thalamus. *Plenum Press,* 1985.

Kahle, W. Nervous System and Sensory Organs 4th edition. *Georg Thieme Verlag*, 1993.

Kandel, E.R., Schwartz, J.H. & Jessell, T.H. (Eds.). Principles of Neural Science 3rd Edition. *Elsevier,* 1991.

Kenneth W. Lindsay and Ian Bone. Neurology and neurosurgery illustrated, 3rd edition. *Churchill livingstone,* 1997.

Kenneth W. Lindsay, Ian Bone and Geraint Fuller. Neurology and neurosurgery illustrated, 5th edition. *Churchill livingstone*, 2010.

Kerr JB. Atlas of Functional Histology. *Mosby,* 1999.

Kierszenbaum AL. Histology and Cell Biology: An Introduction to Pathology. St Louis: *Mosby,* 2002.

Kuffler, S.W., Nicholls, J.G. and Martin, R.WM. From Neuron to Brain 2nd edition. *Sinauer Associates Inc.,* 1984.

Kwang Ho Cho, Jose Francisco Rodríguez-Vázquez, Ji Hyun Kim, Hiroshi Abe, Gen Murakami, Baik Hwan Cho. Early fetal development of the human cerebellum. *Surg Radiol Anat:* 33(6);523-30, 2011.

Larsen, W.J. Human Embryology. *Churchill Livingstone Ltd.,* 1993.

Lasjaunias P, Berenstein A, ter Brugge K. Surgical Neuroangiography. Clinical Vascular Anatomy and Variations, 2nd edition. *Springer,* 2001.

Lennart Heimer. The Human Brain and Spinal Cord: Functional Neuroanatomy and Dissection Guide. *Springer,* 1983.

Lifemap discovery. Embryonic development & stem cell compendium. http://discovery.lifemapsc.com.

Lumley JSP. Surface Anatomy: The Anatomical Basis of Clinical Examination, 3rd edition. *Churchill Livingstone,* 2002.

M.G. Yasargil. Microneurosurgery in 4 Volumes. Georg Thieme Verlag Stuttgart, Thieme Stratton Inc., 1988.

Martin, John H. Neuroanatomy: text and atlas, 3rd edition. *McGraw-Hill,* 2003.

Melville P. Roberts, Joseph Hanaway, D. Kent Morest. Atlas of the Human Brain in Section. *Lea & Febiger,* 1987.

Meredith, G. E., C. M. Pennartz, and H. J. Groenewegen. The Cellular Framework for Chemical Signalling in the Nucleus Accumbens. *Progress in Brain Research* 99: 3–24, 2011.

Michael Salcman, Roberto C. Heros, Edward R. Laws, Volker K. H. Sonntag. Kempe's operative neurosurgery. *Springer,* 2003.

Micheal J. Aminoff, David A. Greenberg, Roger P. Simon. Clinical Neurology. *McGraw-Hill's inc.,* 2005.

Miguel Marín-Padilla. The Human Brain - Prenatal Development and Structure. *Springer,* 2011.

Moore KL, Persaud TVN. Before We Are Born: Essentials of Embryology and Birth Defects, 6th edition. *W B Saunders,* 2003.

Moruzzi, G. and Magoun, H.W. Brain stem reticular formation and activation of the EEG. *Electroencephalogram and Clinical Neurophysiology*. 455–473, 1949.

MS. Greenberg. Handbook of Neurosurgery, 7th edition. *Thieme,* 2010.

Neuroangio. www.neuroangio.org.

Nolte, John. A Study Guide to Accompany the Human Brain, 3rd edition. *Mosby,* 1993.

Norman L. Strominger, Robert J. Demarest, Lois B. Laemle. Noback's Human Nervous System, Structure and Function, 7th Edition. Humana press. *Springer Science and Business Media*. 2012.

Pollard TD, Earnshaw WC. Cell Biology. *W B Saunders,* 2002.

R. Joseph. Basal Ganglia, Striatum, Thalamus: Caudate, Putamen, Globus Pallidus, Limbic Striatum, Brainstem, Parkinson's Disease, Alzheimer's Disease, Psychosis, ...& Disorders of Movement. Neuroscience, Neuropsychiatry, Neuropsychology, 3rd & 4th editions. *Cosmology Science Publishers* (Cambridge), 2011.

R. Joseph. Brainstem and Cerebellum: Medulla, Pons, Midbrain, Reticular Formation, Arousal, Vision, Hearing, Norepinephrine, Serotonin, Dopamine, Sleeping, Dreaming,

REM, Cranial Nerves, Motor Control. Neuroscience, Neuropsychiatry, Neuropsychology, 3rd & 4th editions. *Cosmology Science Publishers* (Cambridge), 2011.

R. Nieuwenhuys J. Voogd C. van Huijzen. The Human Central Nervous System, 4th edition. *Springer,* 2007.

Radiology assistant. http://www.radiologyassistant.nl.

Radiopaedia. www.radiopaedia.org.

RD. Adams, M Victor. Principles of Neurology. *McGraw Hill,* 2008.

Rexed, B. The cytoarchitectonic organization of the spinal cord in the cat. *Journal of Comparative Neurology* 96, 415–495, 1952.

Ricardo Ramina, Paulo Henrique Pires de Aguiar, Marcos Tatagiba. Samii's Essentials in Neurosurgery, 2nd edition. *Springer-Verlag,* 2014.

Rohkamm. Color Atlas of Neurology. *Thieme,* 2004.

S Rengachary, R Ellenbogen. Principles of Neurosurgery, 2nd edition. *Mosby,* 2004.

Salmon M. Anatomic Studies: Book 1 Arteries of the Muscles of the Extremities and the Trunk, Book 2 Arterial Anastomotic Pathways of the Extremities. Ed. by Taylor G, Razaboni RM. St Louis: *Quality Medical Publishing Inc.*, 1994.

Saper, C.B. Function of the locus coeruleus. *Trends in Neurosciences* 343–344, 1987.

Scarabino, Salvolini, Di Salle, Rabischong, Duvernoy. Atlas of morphology and functional anatomy of the brain. *Gruppo Editoriale,* 2003

Schwienbacher I, Fendt M, Richardson R, Schnitzler HU. Temporary inactivation of the nucleus accumbens disrupts acquisition and expression of fear-potentiated startle in rats. *Brain Res*. 1027 (1–2): 87–93, 2004.

Seminars in Neurosurgery, volume 14, number 3. *Thieme Medical Publishers,* 2003.

Setti S. Rengachary and Robert H. Wilkins. Neurourgical operative atlas, *AANS publications committee,* 2000.

Shirayama, Yukihiko, and Shigeyuki Chaki. Neurochemistry of the Nucleus Accumbens and Its Relevance to Depression and Antidepressant Action in Rodents. Current Neuropharmocology 4.4 (2006): 277–91. *Bentham Science Publishers Ltd.,* 2011.

Snell, R.S. Clinical Neuoranatomy for Medical Students 7th edition. *Lippincott Williams & Wilkins,* 2009.

Sobotta. Atlas of Human Anatomy, 14th edition. *Fischer Gustav Verlag GmbH & Co,* 2006.

Stanley Monkhouse. Cranial nerves Functional Anatomy. *Cambridge University Press.* 2006.

Stephen Goldberg. Clinical Neuroanatomy Made Ridiculously Simple, 5th edition. *MedMaster inc.,* 2014.

Susan Standring. Gray's Anatomy, the anatomical basis of clinical practice, 39th edition. *Elsevier,* 2008.

Sydor A, Brown RY, Molecular Neuropharmacology: A Foundation for Clinical Neuroscience, 2nd edition. *McGraw-Hill,* 2009.

Tank, Patrick W. Grant's Dissector, 14th edition. Lippincott Williams & Wilkins, 2009.

UNSW Embryology. https://embryology.med.unsw.edu.au/embryology.

Walter J. Hendelman. Atlas of functional neuroanatomy, 2nd edition. *CRC Press Taylor & Francis Group,* 2006.

Wilkinson, J.L. Neuroanatomy for Medical Students 2nd edition. *Butterworth-Heinemann Ltd,* 1992.

Youmans JR. Neurological surgery. *W.B. Saunders Co.* 2004.
Zubieta JK, Stohler CS. Neurobiological mechanisms of placebo responses". *Ann. N. Y. Acad. Sci.* 1156: 198–210. 2009.

Index

S

T

U

V

W

Z